Foundations of Epidemiology

Foundations
of Epidemiology

THIRD EDITION

Revised by

David E. Lilienfeld
M.D., M.S. Eng., M.P.H., F.A.C.E.
Senior Epidemiologist, EMMES Corp.

Paul D. Stolley
M.D., M.P.H., F.A.C.E., F.A.C.P.
Professor and Chairman,
    Department of Epidemiology
    and Preventive Medicine
University of Maryland School of Medicine

Original edition by Abraham M. Lilienfeld,
M.D., M.P.H., D.Sc. (Hon.), F.A.C.E.

New York   Oxford   **Oxford University Press**   1994

Oxford University Press

Oxford   New York   Toronto
Delhi   Bombay   Calcutta   Madras   Karachi
Kuala Lumpur   Singapore   Hong Kong   Tokyo
Nairobi   Dar es Salaam   Cape Town
Melbourne   Auckland   Madrid

and associated companies in
Berlin   Ibadan

Library of Congress Cataloging-in-Publication Data
Lilienfeld, David E.
Foundations of epidemiology.—3rd ed.
revised by David E. Lilienfeld, Paul D. Stolley.
p. cm.
Rev. ed. of: Foundations of epidemiology
Abraham M. Lilienfeld and David E. Lilienfeld. 2nd ed. 1980.
Includes bibliographical references and index.
ISBN 0-19-505035-5
ISBN 0-19-505036-3 (pbk.)
1. Epidemiology.
I. Stolley, Paul D.
II. Lilienfeld, David E. Foundations of epidemiology.
III. Title.   [DNLM:
1. Epidemiologic Methods.
2. Epidemiology.
WA 950 L728f   1994]
RA651.L54   1994   614.4—dc20
DNLM/DLC for Library of Congress   93-5963

9 8 7 6 5 4 3 2 1

Printed in the United States of America
on acid-free paper

To Jo Ann and the luck of the Castel Felice (P.D.S.)

To Karen and Sam (D.E.L.)

PREFACE

The purpose of this book is to present the concepts and methods of epidemiology as they are applied to a variety of health problems. The broad scope of epidemiology is liberally illustrated with studies of specific diseases. Emphasis is placed on the integration of biological and statistical elements in the sequence of epidemiologic reasoning that derives inferences about the etiology of disease from population data. The epidemiologist's role in integrating knowledge obtained from a variety of scientific disciplines is described.

A knowledge of biostatistics is indispensable in the conduct of epidemiologic studies and the analysis of their results. This information is found in many textbooks of biostatistics. To provide the minimal background necessary for understanding the epidemiologic methods that are discussed, however, the statistical appendix has been expanded to cover correlation, regression, life tables and survivorship analysis, comparison of two sample means, and the kappa statistic.

This book has been designed as a text for introductory courses in epidemiology wherever they are offered. Thus, it can be used in schools of medicine, public health, allied health sciences, dentistry, nursing, and veterinary medicine, as well as in environmental health sciences and other programs offered by colleges of arts and sciences. To facilitate such use, a new chapter on the use of epidemiologic information in clinical settings has been added to this edition. This chapter includes a discussion of how health care providers should critically read reports in the medical literature.

The text has been divided into four parts. In Part I ("Introduction to Epidemiology"), Chapters 1 to 3 review the historical background and conceptual basis for epidemiology. Chapters 4 to 7 make up Part II ("Demographic Studies"); they discuss mortality and morbidity, and their application to epidemiologic problems. The next four chapters, 8 to 11, constitute Part III ("Epidemiologic Studies"); both experimental and observational epidemiologic studies are considered. The last section, Part IV ("Using Epidemiologic Information"), consists of Chapters 12 and 13. The ways in which the types of data obtained from the various demographic and epidemiologic studies are integrated into a conceptual whole and focused on the derivation of biologic inferences are described in Chapter 12, and the use of epidemiologic information in health care settings is discussed in the last chapter.

Several changes have been made in this edition. Many chapters have been extensively revised to include findings from recent epidemiologic studies. New examples illustrating a greater variety of epidemiologic problems, including such public health challenges as AIDS, have been included. In the discussion of morbidity and mortality, descriptions of surveillance and kappa as a measure of inter- and intra-observer variability have been added. The sequence of material on epidemiologic studies has also been changed: experimental studies are discussed before observational studies, cohort investigations before case-control studies. These revisions will assist students in their understanding of the epidemiologic study and should facilitate their assimilation of the material.

To enhance the teaching value of the book, answers to the study problems for the chapters have been added at the end of the text. The problem sets also have been revised to reflect current epidemiologic challenges. The problems give students an opportunity to apply the methods and reasoning process that constitute epidemiology. Some of them invite broad consideration of various epidemiologic issues and viewpoints.

Some Comments on Terminology. We have made some changes in the terms used in the previous edition to describe the different types of demographic and epidemiologic studies and their resultant measures. The changes are intended to reflect current terminology and to minimize confusion, and they are consistent with the second edition of the *Dictionary of Epidemiology* edited by John Last. It may be helpful to list some synonyms of commonly used terms here:

1. *Case-control studies,* in addition to being called ''retrospective'' studies, are also referred to as ''case-referrent'' studies.
2. *Cohort studies* are also termed ''prospective studies'' as well as ''longitudinal'' studies. What we call ''non-concurrent cohort'' studies are also referred to as ''historical cohort,'' ''retrospective cohort,'' ''retrospective longitudinal,'' and ''historical retrospective'' studies.
3. *Relative risk* is also termed ''risk ratio.''
4. *Attributable fraction,* as the term is used in this book, is synonymous with ''attributable risk'' and ''population attributable risk.''

This book was written for both students and practitioners of epidemiology. It seeks to present the reasoning used by epidemiologists in the context of both recent epidemiologic activity and classical epidemiologic investigations. It is through understanding these studies, and the concepts and methods on which they are based, that we can prepare to deal with the public health and medical challenges of the future.

February, 1994   D.E.L.
Baltimore, Md.   P.D.S.

ACKNOWLEDGMENTS

Dr. Tamar Lasky, co-author of Chapter 13, was of invaluable assistance in the preparation of this edition and her care and hard work are gratefully acknowledged. Her astute comments and suggestions have greatly improved the book. We thank Drs. Jack Mandel, Curt Meinert, Roger Sherwin, David Vlahov, J. Michael Sprafka, and Sankey Williams for their reviews of selected chapters and suggestions. Drs. Ellen Fisher, L. Ronald French, James Godbold, and Michael Osterholm also gave us some very helpful comments, and for that we thank them. Mr. Edward Parmalee assisted us with some of the questions for the book and Mrs. Hildred Griffeth typed the manuscript with her usual tact, efficiency, and good humor (sometimes sorely taxed). We greatly valued the advice and help we received from Jeffrey House of the Oxford University Press.

CONTENTS

I

INTRODUCTION TO EPIDEMIOLOGY

The first three chapters provide an introduction to the epidemiologic view of disease. The many facets of epidemiologic inquiry are explored in Chapter 1. The ways in which epidemiologic data may be used by clinicians, other health care providers, public health officers, or epidemiologists are also discussed. The essence of the epidemiologic approach to disease, which is focused on the occurrence of disease in *populations,* is described in the context of a food-borne outbreak.

Chapter 2 gives a brief account of the history of epidemiology, attempting to show how epidemiology evolved into its present form. The major figures in the development of epidemiology are mentioned. Many of the more notable historical examples of the uses of epidemiology, such as John Snow and the Broad Street Pump, are presented.

Chapter 3 deals with general epidemiologic principles in the study of diseases. One such principle, the triad of "time, place and persons," permits the epidemiologic description of a disease. Another triad, "agent, host, and environment," provides insight into the relationship between the agent or cause of a disease, the host in whom the disease develops, and the environment that facilitates the interaction of the agent and the host. The incubation period (also known as a latent period when studying chronic diseases) is used to determine the probable time of exposure to the agent for both infectious and noninfectious diseases. The epidemiologic importance of subclinical cases of disease is highlighted by the concept of a disease spectrum. Health care providers see only those cases that manifest clinical symptoms and require treatment, but epidemiologists are concerned with all cases of disease as they develop in the population. The chapter concludes with a discussion of herd immunity, the epidemiologic basis for the vaccination policies of several nations.

1

1

LAYING THE FOUNDATIONS: THE EPIDEMIOLOGIC APPROACH TO DISEASE

Epidemiology is concerned with the patterns of disease occurrence in human populations and the factors that influence these patterns. Epidemiologists are primarily interested in the occurrence of disease as categorized by **time, place, and persons.** They try to determine whether there has been an increase or decrease of the disease over the years, whether one geographical area has a higher frequency of the disease than another, and whether the characteristics of persons with a particular disease or condition distinguish them from those without it.

The personal characteristics that concern epidemiologists are:

1. Demographic characteristics such as age, gender, race, and ethnic group.
2. Biological characteristics such as blood levels of antibodies, chemicals, and enzymes; cellular constituents of the blood; and measurements of physiological function of different organ systems.
3. Social and economic factors such as socioeconomic status, educational background, occupation, and nativity.
4. Personal habits such as tobacco and drug use, diet, and physical exercise.
5. Genetic characteristics such as blood groups.

Much of this is encompassed by Hirsch's definition of historical and geographical pathology as a "science which ... will give, firstly, a picture of the occurrence, the distribution and the types of the diseases of mankind, in distinct epochs of time and at various points of the earth's surface; and secondly, will render an account of the relations of these diseases to the external conditions surrounding the individual and determining his manner of life" (Hirsch, 1883;

3

Frost, 1941). This statement has commonly served as a base for defining epidemiology as the "study of the distribution of a disease or a physiological condition in human populations and of the factors that influence this distribution" (Lilienfeld, 1978). A more inclusive description was given by Wade Hampton Frost, one of the architects of modern epidemiology, who noted that "epidemiology is essentially an inductive science, concerned not merely with describing the distribution of disease, but equally or more with fitting it into a consistent philosophy" (Frost, 1941). Thus epidemiology can be regarded as a sequence of reasoning concerned with biological inferences derived from observations of disease occurrence and related phenomena in human population groups. To this we can add that epidemiology is an integrative, eclectic discipline deriving concepts and methods from other disciplines, such as statistics, sociology, and biology, for the study of disease in a population.

GENERAL PURPOSES OF EPIDEMIOLOGIC INQUIRIES

The information obtained from an epidemiologic investigation can be utilized in several ways:

1. To elucidate the etiology of a specific disease or group of diseases by combining epidemiologic data with information from other disciplines such as genetics, biochemistry, and microbiology.
2. To evaluate the consistency of epidemiologic data with etiological hypotheses developed either clinically (at the bedside) or experimentally (in the laboratory).
3. To provide the basis for developing and evaluating preventive procedures and public health practices.

Examples of each of these three general purposes will be presented.

Etiological Studies of Disease

A simple example of the use of epidemiologic data to determine etiological factors would be the investigation of an outbreak of food poisoning to determine which food was contaminated with the microorganism or chemical responsible for the epidemic. Another example would be the study of a disease that occurs with higher frequency among workers in occupations exposing them to particular chemicals, as illustrated in the study of aniline, ortho-toluidine, and bladder cancer by Ward et al. (1991). Although the carcinogenicity of aniline-based dyes to the human bladder has been known for the past four decades, that for aniline and a related chemical, ortho-toluidine, is not yet established. At a western New York State plant in which aniline and ortho-toluidine were used to produce an antioxidant for tire production, the union had reported a cluster of bladder cancer cases among its members. During the subsequent investigation, lists were obtained of all employees in the plant since 1946. These workers were divided into three groups: those with definite exposure to these two chemicals (persons who worked in the department in which the chemicals were used), those with possible exposure to the chemicals (janitorial, maintenance, and shipping personnel), and those with no exposure (all other workers). Cases of bladder cancer among these employees were identified by the company and the union, with confirmation by review of medical records. Additional cases were ascertained from the New York State Cancer Registry. The observed numbers of cases were then compared with those that would be expected based on the bladder cancer incidence rates for New York State. A significantly larger number of bladder cancer cases (seven) was found to have occurred among the 708 persons definitely exposed to ortho-toluidine and aniline than would be expected (approximately one); for the 288 possibly exposed workers, there was also an excess number of cases, though less than for the definitely exposed group. The 753 persons not exposed had no significant excess in the number of bladder cancer cases. Further, this relationship between bladder cancer and exposure to aniline and ortho-toluidine showed a dose-response effect, i.e., the longer an employee was exposed to these two compounds, the greater was his or her chance of developing bladder cancer. The investigators concluded that a causal relationship existed between exposure to aniline and ortho-toluidine compounds and bladder cancer.

Only occasionally do investigators find that the increased exposure of individuals to certain agents results in a decreased frequency of disease. A classical example of this kind of relationship is that between the presence of fluorides in the water supply and dental caries. The investigation of this relationship is worth recounting as it illustrates in concise form how a sequence of studies can be conducted to develop a preventive measure for a disease.

By the late 1930s, it had been recognized that mottled enamel of teeth was due to the use of a water supply with a high fluoride concentration (Dean, 1938; Dean and Elvove, 1936; Dean et al., 1939). Earlier, a practicing dentist had formed a clinical impression that persons with mottled teeth had less caries than usual (Black and McKay, 1916; McKay, 1925; McKay and Black, 1916). This led the Public Health Service to conduct surveys of children 12–14 years old in thirteen cities in four states where the fluoride concentration in the water supply varied considerably (Dean et al., 1942). The results indicated that dental caries decreased with increasing content of fluoride in the water, thus suggesting that the addition of fluorides to the water supply should decrease the frequency of dental caries (Figure 1–1). This could best be demonstrated by comparative exper-

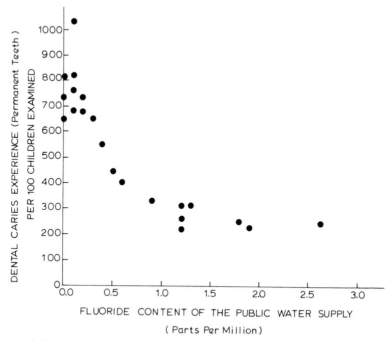

Figure 1–1. Relationship between the number of dental caries in permanent teeth and fluoride content in the public water supply. *Source:* Dean, Arnold, and Elvove (1942).

iment, where fluorides were added to the water supply of one community and the water supply remained untouched in a comparable community where the fluoride concentration was naturally low. The dental caries experience of school children in these communities could then be determined by periodic examinations over a number of years and compared. Several such studies were initiated, including one comparing Kingston and Newburgh, New York (Table 1–1) (Ast and Schlesinger, 1956). In the town with fluorides in the water supply, the index of dental caries (DMF) was found to be lower than in the one without fluorides. In this instance, a clinical impression led to both an epidemiologic survey and a comparative experiment, both of which demonstrated the relationship between a population characteristic, fluoride consumption, and a disease, dental caries.

Consistency with Etiological Hypotheses

The investigator attempts to determine whether an etiological hypothesis developed clinically, experimentally, or from other epidemiologic studies is consistent with the epidemiologic characteristics of the disease in a human population group(s). Many studies of the relationship between oral contraceptive use and various forms of cardiovascular disease illustrate this approach. Over a period of

Table 1-1. DMF* Teeth per 100 Children, Ages 6–16, Based on Clinical and Roentgenographic Examinations—Newburgh† and Kingston, New York, 1954–1955

	NUMBER OF CHILDREN WITH PERMANENT TEETH		NUMBER OF DMF TEETH		DMF TEETH PER 100 CHILDREN WITH PERMANENT TEETH§		
							PERCENT DIFFERENCE
AGE‡	NEWBURGH	KINGSTON	NEWBURGH	KINGSTON	NEWBURGH	KINGSTON	(N−K)/K
6–9‖	708	913	672	2,134	98.4	233.7	−57.9
10–12	521	640	1,711	4,471	328.1	698.6	−53.0
13–14	263	441	1,579	5,161	610.1	1,170.3	−47.9
15–16	109	119	1,063	1,962	975.2	1,648.7	−40.9

*DMF includes permanent teeth decayed, missing (lost subsequent to eruption), or filled.
†Sodium fluoride was added to Newburgh's water supply beginning May 2, 1945.
‡Age at last birthday at time of examination.
§Adjusted to age distribution of children examined in Kingston who had permanent teeth in the 1954–1955 examination.
‖Newburgh children of this age group were exposed to fluoridated water from the time of birth.
Source: Ast and Schlesinger (1956).

years, epidemiologic studies had shown a relationship between oral contraceptive use and both venous thromboembolism and thrombotic stroke (Collaborative Group for the Study of Stroke in Young Women, 1973; Vessey and Mann, 1978). Soon after these studies started to appear, the first of a series of case reports associated oral contraceptive use with myocardial infarction (Boyce et al., 1963). This stimulated several investigators to conduct epidemiologic studies of this issue (Mann et al., 1976a; Mann et al., 1976b). The statistically significant results of a study by Mann, Inman, and Thorogood (1976b) of women aged 40–44 who died from myocardial infarction are presented in Table 1-2.

Basis for Preventive and Public Health Services

Perhaps the simplest example of this objective is the epidemiologic evaluation of vaccines in controlled trials in human populations, such as the national study that was done to establish the effectiveness of the Salk vaccine in the prevention of poliomyelitis (Francis et al., 1955). In addition to controlled trials and the other types of epidemiologic studies already mentioned, information on the population distribution of a disease in itself provides the basis for developing certain aspects of community disease control programs. Knowledge of specific etiological factors is not essential for this purpose. For example, epidemiologic data on those persons with a higher frequency of a disease or a higher risk of developing one are useful

Table 1–2. Oral Contraceptive Practice Among Women Aged 40–44 Years Who Died from Myocardial Infarction (MI), and Controls

ORAL CONTRACEPTIVE PRACTICE	PATIENTS WITH MYOCARDIAL INFARCTION		CONTROLS	
	NO.	PERCENT	NO.	PERCENT
Never used	78	73.6	86	84.3
Current users (used during month before death or during same calendar period for controls)	18	17.0 ⎫ 28 (26.4%)	7	6.9 ⎫ 16 (15.7%)
Ex-users (used only more than one month before death or during same calendar period for controls)	10	9.4 ⎭	9	8.8 ⎭
Total	106	100.0	102	100.0
Not known	2		8	
Comparison between users and women not currently using oral contraceptives	$\chi^2 = 4.35$; $P < 0.05$			

Source: Mann et al. (1976b).

to the physician or public health administrator in indicating those segments of the population where health care activities should be focused.

The familial aggregation of diabetes mellitus illustrates this point. In a study of diabetic patients admitted to the Mayo Clinic, Steinberg and Wilder (1952) obtained a history of the presence or absence of diabetes among their parents and siblings (Table 1–3). Whether one hypothesizes a genetic etiological mechanism or environmental factors common to family members as an explanation for the observed familial aggregation, the higher-than-usual frequency of the disease in certain families suggests to the physician that the examination of parents and siblings of known diabetic patients will provide for the early detection of diabetes in a high-risk group of the population.

CONTENT OF EPIDEMIOLOGIC ACTIVITIES

Epidemiologists engage in three broad areas of study, each involving different methods: experimental epidemiology, natural experiments, and observational epidemiology.

Table 1–3. Frequency of Diabetes Among Siblings and Parents of Diabetic Patients Admitted to the Mayo Clinic

DIABETES STATUS OF PARENTS	NUMBER FAMILIES	SIBLINGS		
			DIABETES	
		TOTAL	NUMBER	PERCENT
Both diabetic	22	100	16	16.0
One diabetic	370	1,620	185	11.4
Neither diabetic	1,589	6,664	311	4.7
Total families	1,981	8,384	512	6.1

Source: Steinberg and Wilder (1952). Reprinted by permission of The University of Chicago Press, Copyright © 1952. The American Society of Human Genetics, Waverly Press, Inc.

Experimental Epidemiology

In planned experiments, the investigator controls the population groups being studied by deciding which groups are exposed to a possible etiological factor or preventive measure. The Newburgh-Kingston dental caries study, for instance, was a planned, controlled experiment. An important feature of many experiments is that the investigator can randomly allocate subjects to experimental and control groups. This method is discussed in greater detail in Chapters 8 and 9.

Natural Experiments

Occasionally, the investigator is fortunate enough to observe the occurrence of a disease under natural conditions so closely approximating a planned, controlled experiment that it is categorized as a "natural experiment." Any inferences about etiological factors derived from such situations are considerably stronger than if they had been derived solely from an observational study. The studies in England by Doll, Hill, and Peto of the relationship between tobacco use and lung cancer illustrate this approach (Doll and Hill, 1950; Doll and Peto, 1976; Doll et al., 1980; Report of the Royal College of Physicians, 1971). In 1951, these investigators ascertained the smoking habits of British male physicians, aged thirty-five and over, and followed them to determine their mortality from different causes, in particular lung cancer. Initially, this study indicated that physicians who smoked cigarettes had a mortality rate from lung cancer that was about ten times that of nonsmoking physicians (Doll and Hill, 1950). Questionnaires were sent to these physicians again to determine their cigarette smoking habits in 1956,

1966, and 1971 (Doll and Peto, 1976; Report of the Royal College of Physicians, 1971). The findings of these surveys in terms of the ratio of number of cigarettes smoked by the male physicians to the numbers smoked by all British men in the same age group is shown in Figure 1–2. There was about a 50 percent decline in cigarette smoking among these male physicians. During this same period of time, the investigators continued to obtain information on the mortality experience of the physicians, comparing it with the mortality among all British men (Doll and Peto, 1976; Report of the Royal College of Physicians, 1971). Figure 1–3 presents the trend of the physicians' mortality experience from lung cancer and from all other cancer as a percentage of national mortality. There was an approximately 40 percent decline in mortality from lung cancer with essentially no decline in other cancer deaths.

Observational Epidemiology

This refers to the observation and analysis of the occurrence of disease in human population groups and to the inferences that can be derived about etiological factors that influence this occurrence. Appropriate methods for selecting specific groups in the population and for analyzing information obtained from them have been developed. Much of what the epidemiologist does falls into this category and, therefore, several of the later chapters as well as the Appendix deal with it. The studies of aniline- and ortho-toluidine-exposed employees, dental caries, and familial aggregation of diabetes already cited are examples of observational investigations.

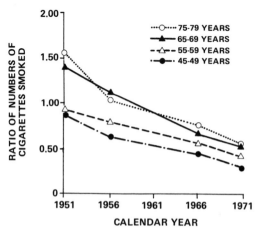

Figure 1–2. Trend in ratio of numbers of cigarettes smoked by male physicians of same ages, by age groups, 1951–1971. *Source:* Doll and Peto (1976).

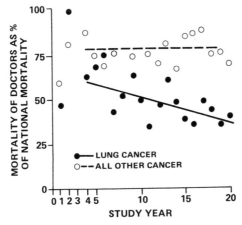

Figure 1–3. Trend in mortality of male doctors as percentage of national mortality of same ages for lung cancer and all other cancer, 1951–1971. *Source:* Doll and Peto (1976).

Development and Evaluation of Study Methods

As the scope of epidemiology has been broadened to include new and/or different types of diseases, epidemiologists have had to develop new methods of study. In some cases these methods have been adapted from other disciplines, such as sociology, statistics, biology, and demography. However, the appropriateness of such new methods for particular epidemiologic situations is not always apparent. Thus, they need to be evaluated for different epidemiologic circumstances to determine their utility.

One often hears the statement that there are "two epidemiologies," one for infectious diseases and the other for noninfectious diseases. This is a misconception. In general, the methods used and the inferences derived are the same for both disease groups; this will be illustrated throughout our discussions. The reader should note that epidemiology is essentially a *comparative* discipline. It is mainly concerned with studying diseases and related phenomena at different time periods, in different places, and among different types of people (i.e., "time, place, and persons") and then comparing them. This approach is used for all categories of disease, infectious and noninfectious alike (Lilienfeld, 1973).

THE SEQUENCE OF EPIDEMIOLOGIC REASONING

Epidemiology was defined at the beginning of this chapter in terms of a reasoning process. The observational study, one of the major tools of epidemiology, affords an excellent view of the reasoning process by which one achieves the objective of elucidating etiological factors of a disease. Basically, the epidemiologist uses a two-stage sequence of reasoning:

1. The determination of a statistical association between a characteristic and a disease.
2. The derivation of biological inferences from such a pattern of statistical associations.

The methods used to determine the statistical associations fall into one of two broadly defined categories: (a) associations based on group characteristics, and (b) associations based on individual characteristics. Although there is a certain degree of overlap between these two categories, their distinction has proved to be extremely useful.

In studying *group* characteristics, the epidemiologist concentrates on the comparison of the mortality and/or morbidity experience from a given disease in different population groups in the hope that any observed differences can be related to differences in the local environment, in personal living habits, or even in the genetic composition of these groups. In these **demographic studies,** information on the characteristics of the individual members of the population groups is not usually obtained. Generally, existing mortality and morbidity statistics are utilized. For example, let us assume that Community A has a higher mortality rate from cancer of the liver than Community B. Furthermore, Community A is engaged primarily in mining, while Community B is engaged in agriculture. Comparison would suggest that mining may be of etiological importance in liver cancer. Usually, the results of such studies provide *clues* to etiological hypotheses and serve as a basis for more detailed investigations. Such an observed relationship, generally termed an ''ecological correlation,'' may suffer from an **''ecological fallacy'';** that is, the two communities differ in many other factors, and one or more of those may be the underlying reason for the differences in their observed mortality or morbidity experience (Goodman, 1953; Robinson, 1950; Selvin, 1958; Piantadosi et al., 1988). The various types of studies of group characteristics will be discussed in Chapters 4–7.

After an association has been established in a study of group characteristics, or when a lead has been developed from either clinical studies of patients, experimental work, or other sources, the investigator attempts to determine whether this association is also present among *individuals*. Answers will be sought to such questions as:

1. Do persons with the disease have the characteristic more frequently than those without the disease?

2. Do persons with the characteristic develop the disease more frequently than those who do not have the characteristic?

Such associations are established in epidemiologic studies, i.e., by cohort or case-control studies, which will be discussed in Chapters 10 and 11.

These two general methods of determining statistical associations—those between groups and those among individuals—must be distinguished since a relationship derived from a study of individuals is less likely to result from an ecological fallacy and is, therefore, more likely to be biologically significant than one derived from a study of group characteristics. Conversely, an association derived from studies of groups has a greater likelihood of being the result of a third common factor (Piantadosi et al., 1988).

AN EXAMPLE OF THE EPIDEMIOLOGIC APPROACH

The essentials of the epidemiologic approach in determining the specific etiological agent of a disease are perhaps best demonstrated by the investigation of the origin of a food poisoning outbreak. This usually includes ascertaining whether a statistical association is found between the consumption of a specific food at some event and the specific form of the disease. This is accomplished by computing food-specific attack rates, defined as follows:

$$\text{Food-specific attack rate} = \frac{\begin{array}{c}\text{Number of persons who ate}\\ \text{a specific food and became ill}\end{array}}{\begin{array}{c}\text{Number of persons who ate}\\ \text{the specific food}\end{array}},$$

and comparing them with attack rates for those who had not eaten the specific food. The report of a salmonellosis outbreak caused by *Salmonella typhimurium* DT4 illustrates this approach (Ortega-Benito and Landridge, 1992).

During late July, 1989, the guests and staff of a private club experienced a striking increase in gastrointestinal symptoms. Most of the people affected had eaten at the club between Saturday, July 22, and Monday, July 24. Those who had consumed hot foods did not appear to develop any illness. During that weekend, the club had also supplied sandwiches for tea break to members of a cricket team. Symptoms of gastrointestinal illness among team members began to increase on July 23, although regional public health officials were not notified until August 1, 1989. The limited nature of the exposure of the cricket team members suggested that the sandwiches (specifically, eggs or mayonnaise) may have contained the etiologic agent.

Two groups were selected for study: 129 club staff members who ate their meals at the club and 105 persons involved with the cricket team (team members, umpires, scorers, and guests). Each of these persons was given a self-administered questionnaire; 177 (110 club staff and 67 cricket group) completed questionnaires were returned. Since not all the members of the two groups completed questionnaires, one must assume that those who did so are a representative *sample* of all the members.

A case was defined as anyone who had diarrhea or vomiting or had *Salmonella typhimurium* isolated from his stools between July 20 and July 26, 1989. From the club staff group, 33 persons met the case definition, as did 35 cricket group members. A crude attack rate was computed:

$$\text{Crude attack rate} = \frac{\text{Number of persons ill with the disease}}{\text{Number of persons eating at the club}}.$$

The crude attack rate among club staff was 30 percent (33/110) and among the cricket team group, 5 percent (35/67). Meal-specific attack rates were computed for the club staff (Table 1–4). They showed a definite statistical association between salmonellosis and sandwiches. Additional analyses of the attack rates for consumption of specific sandwiches by the cricket group and on specific days for club staff were also calculated (Tables 1–5 and 1–6). Among the cricketers, statistical associations between illness and egg mayonnaise, tuna mayonnaise, and tuna and cucumber sandwiches were found. Among club staff, statistical associations between illness and egg mayonnaise sandwiches were found regardless of which day they were consumed; an association could also be discerned between illness and tuna and cucumber sandwiches consumed on July 24. The investigators concluded that only sandwiches containing mayonnaise were associated with the illness.

Laboratory investigations were undertaken to identify the specific form of salmonellosis. Salmonella was identified in 36 of 68 stool specimens examined. *Salmonella typhimurium* was the only type isolated. This information allowed the investigators to trace the source of the outbreak. Eggs, a component of mayonnaise, are often found to be contaminated in investigations of food-borne salmonellosis outbreaks. The eggs used in the mayonnaise had been provided by one supplier. Investigation of that supplier's environment did not reveal a source of the salmonella. However, that supplier had also used three supplementary sources for the eggs, which the investigators also examined. Two flocks in two farms were found to be infected with salmonella; one with *Salmonella enteritidis* and the other with *Salmonella typhimurium* DT4 in 2,580 infected birds. These

Table 1–4. Attack Rates by Meal and for Sandwiches among 110 Club Staff

| | EATEN | | | | NOT EATEN | | | | DIFFERENCE IN ATTACK RATES |
| | ILL | NOT ILL | TOTAL | ATTACK RATE (%) | ILL | NOT ILL | TOTAL | ATTACK RATE (%) | (4)–(8)=(9). |
MEAL	(1)	(2)	(3)	(4)	(5)	(6)	(7)	(8)	
Breakfast	9	20	29	31	24	45	69	35	–4
Lunch	18	42	60	30	15	23	38	39	–9
Dinner	11	19	30	37	22	46	68	32	5
Sandwiches	25	24	49	51	8	41	49	16	35*

*The only difference that was statistically significant (p=0.006) was for sandwiches.

Source: Adapted from Ortega-Benito and Landridge (1992).

Table 1–5. Attack Rates for Specific Sandwiches among 110 Club Staff on July 24, 1989[+]

| SANDWICH | EATEN | | | | NOT EATEN | | | | DIFFERENCE IN ATTACK RATES |
	ILL (1)	NOT ILL (2)	TOTAL (3)	ATTACK RATE (%) (4)	ILL (5)	NOT ILL (6)	TOTAL (7)	ATTACK RATE (%) (8)	(4)–(8)=(9)
Egg Mayonnaise	4	1	5	80	18	47	65	28	52*
Tuna Mayonnaise	2	1	3	67	21	47	68	31	36
Egg and Tomato	0	1	1	0	24	47	71	34	−34
Tuna and Cucumber	5	1	6	88	16	47	63	25	53*
Cheese and Tomato	1	0	1	100	23	48	71	32	68
Cheese and Pickle	0	1	1	0	24	47	71	34	−34
Lettuce and Tomato	0	1	1	0	23	47	70	33	−33
Turkey Salad	0	0	0	0	24	48	72	33	−33
Ham Salad	2	0	2	100	21	48	69	30	70
Roast Beef	2	0	2	100	23	48	71	32	68
Liver Sausage	0	1	1	0	24	47	71	34	−34

[+]For July 23 and July 25, similar results were found, except for the absence of an association between illness and tuna and cucumber.
*The only differences that were statistically significant were for egg mayonnaise (p=0.03), and tuna and cucumber (p=0.008).
Source: Adapted from Ortega-Benito and Landridge (1992).

Table 1–6. Attack Rates for Specific Sandwiches among 55 Cricketers

SANDWICH	EATEN				NOT EATEN				DIFFERENCE IN ATTACK RATES (4)−(8)=(9)
	ILL (1)	NOT ILL (2)	TOTAL (3)	ATTACK RATE (%) (4)	ILL (5)	NOT ILL (6)	TOTAL (7)	ATTACK RATE (%) (8)	
Egg Mayonnaise	14	3	17	82	7	18	25	28	54*
Tuna Mayonnaise	7	2	9	78	13	18	31	42	36
Egg and Tomato	3	0	3	100	18	21	41	44	56
Tuna and Cucumber	12	3	15	80	9	16	25	36	44*
Cheese and Tomato	6	6	12	50	16	15	31	52	−2
Cheese and Pickle	5	6	11	45	18	14	32	56	−11
Lettuce and Tomato	2	0	2	100	23	21	44	52	48
Turkey Salad	0	0	0	0	26	21	47	55	−55
Ham Salad	11	5	16	69	11	16	27	41	28
Roast Beef	2	0	2	100	22	20	42	52	48
Liver Sausage	1	0	1	100	25	21	46	54	46

*The only differences that were statistically significant were for egg mayonnaise (p=0.0017), and tuna and cucumber (p=0.017).

Source: Adapted from Ortega-Benito and Landridge (1992).

17

flocks were slaughtered. In summary, the findings were:

1. Chickens at two farms were infected with salmonella.
2. These eggs had not been pasteurized before use.
3. The eggs supplied by one of these farms were used by the club staff to make mayonnaise for sandwiches during the third weekend in July, 1989.
4. The contaminated mayonnaise was consumed by club staff and the cricket group.

The pattern of statistical associations and the laboratory findings showing that a flock which had provided some of the eggs was infected with the same type of *Salmonella typhimurium* that had been found among the ill club staff and cricketers clearly implicated the infected eggs as the cause of this epidemic.

SUMMARY

Epidemiology is a comparative science in which the occurrence of disease in population groups is related to the presence or absence of factors in those groups. Epidemiologists place these associations into a biological framework to provide insights into the causes of disease. Epidemiologic activities include experimental studies, in which the investigators control the exposure of the individuals to a factor; observational studies, in which the investigators follow the health experiences of individuals exposed and not exposed to a factor (the control of the individuals' exposures was beyond the investigators' control); and the development and evaluation of new study methods.

Factors studied by the epidemiologist include demographic characteristics, biological characteristics, social and economic characteristics, personal habits, and genetic traits. The factors may be associated with either an increased risk of disease (suggestive of a causal relationship) or a decreased risk (suggestive of a protective relationship). Such associations are best discerned in studies of individuals in a population. The finding of an association between a disease and group characteristics in a study of population (rather than individual) characteristics can lead to an ''ecological fallacy.'' The determination of a statistical relationship between a characteristic and a disease is only the first step in epidemiologic reasoning. The second step is deriving a biological inference from the patterns of statistical associations.

Epidemiologists use two approaches to discern a statistical relationship between a characteristic and a disease. In one approach, the demographic study, the relationship between group characteristics and disease is examined. In the other approach, the epidemiologic study, the relationship between individual characteristics and disease is examined. An example of the latter can be found in the investigation of a food-borne outbreak. The source of an outbreak may be found by comparing the attack rates among persons who consumed a given food with those for persons who did not consume that food. The food item with the greatest disparity in attack rates among those who consumed it and those who did not consume it was the source of the outbreak.

STUDY PROBLEMS

1. What is the epidemiologic significance of the expression "time, place, persons"?
2. What is an "ecological fallacy"? Why is it important to the epidemiologist?
3. Why should epidemiologists be interested in population-based statistics such as mortality rates? Why should they be cautious in the use of such rates?
4. What are the major steps in an investigation of a food-borne outbreak?
5. An outbreak of food poisoning occurred at a Coast Guard training station a few hours after the communal breakfast meal. The symptoms were mainly nausea, vomiting and diarrhea. An investigation revealed the findings listed in the table below.

| TYPE OF FOOD | CONSUMED FOOD | | | DID NOT CONSUME FOOD | | |
	NUMBER OF INDIVIDUALS	NUMBER ILL	ATTACK RATE (%)	NUMBER OF INDIVIDUALS	NUMBER ILL	ATTACK RATE (%)
Tomato juice	204	47		263	21	
Cantaloupe	290	53		177	15	
Chipped beef with sauce	147	60		320	8	
Potatoes	161	44		306	24	
Eggs	169	39		298	29	
Pastry	204	34		263	34	
Toast	238	46		229	22	
Milk	301	50		166	18	

(a) Calculate the attack rates for each food for those who consumed and those who did not consume each food item.
(b) Which food do you think is the likely cause of this "common source" epidemic? Explain your choice.

(c) What additional investigations could be done to determine the source of the likely microorganism?

(d) How can such food poisoning epidemics be prevented in the future?

REFERENCES

Ast, D. B., and Schlesinger, E. R. 1956. "The conclusion of a ten-year study of water fluoridation." *Am. J. Pub. Health* 46:265–271.

Black, G. V., and McKay, F. S. 1916. "Mottled teeth: an endemic developmental imperfection of the teeth, heretofore unknown in the literature of dentistry." *Dent. Cosmos.* 58:129–156.

Boyce, J., Fawcett, J. W., and Neal, E.W.P. 1963. "Coronary thrombosis and conovid." *Lancet* 1:111.

Collaborative Group for the Study of Stroke in Young Women. 1973. "Oral contraception and increased risk of cerebral ischemia or thrombosis." *New Eng. J. Med.* 288:871–878.

Dean, H. T. 1938. "Endemic fluorosis and its relation to dental caries." *Pub. Health. Rep.* 54:1443–1452.

Dean, H. T., and Elvove, E. 1936. "Some epidemiological aspects of chronic endemic dental fluorosis." *Am. J. Pub. Health* 26:567–575.

Dean, H. T., Jay, P., Arnold, F. A. Jr., McClure, F. J., and Elvove, E. 1939. "Domestic water and dental caries, including certain epidemiological aspects of oral *L. acidophilus.*" *Pub. Health Rep.* 54:862–888.

Dean, H. T., Arnold, F. A. Jr., and Elvove, E. 1942. "Domestic water and dental caries. V. Additional studies of the relation of fluoride domestic waters to dental caries experience in 4,425 white children, aged 12 to 14 years, of 13 cities in 4 states." *Pub. Health Rep.* 57:1155–1179.

Doll, R., and Hill, A. B. 1950. "Smoking and carcinoma of the lung: Preliminary report." *Br. Med. J.* 2:739–748.

Doll, R., and Peto, R. 1976. "Mortality in relation to smoking: 20 year's observations on male British doctors." *Br. Med. J.* 2:1525–1536.

Doll, R., Gray, R., Hafner, B., and Peto, R. 1980. "Mortality in relation to smoking: 22 years' observations on female British doctors." *Br. Med. J.* 1:967–971.

Francis, T. Jr., Korns, R. F., Voight, R. B., Boisen, M., Hemphill, F. M., Napier, J. A., and Tolchinsky, E. 1955. "An evaluation of the 1954 poliomyelitis vaccine trials: summary report." *Am. J. Pub. Health* 45:1–63.

Frost, W. H., 1941. "Epidemiology." In *Papers of Wade Hampton Frost, M.D.,* K.E. Maxcy, ed., New York: The Commonwealth Fund, pp. 493–542.

Goodman, L. A. 1953. "Ecological regressions and behavior of individuals." *Am. Soc. Rev.* 18:663–664.

Hirsch, A. 1883. *Handbook of Geographical and Historical Pathology, Vol. I.* London: New Sydenham Society.

Lilienfeld, A. M. 1973. "Epidemiology of infectious and non-infectious disease: some comparisons." *Am. J. Epidemiol.* 97:135–147.

Lilienfeld, D. E. 1978. "Definitions of epidemiology." *Am. J. Epidemiol.* 107:87–90.

Mann, J. I., Doll, R., Thorogood, M., Vessey, M. P., and Waters, W. E. 1976a. "Risk factors for myocardial infarction in young women." *Br. J. Prev. Soc. Med.* 30:97–100.

Mann, J. I., Inman, W. H., and Thorogood, M. 1976b. "Oral contraceptive use in older women and fatal myocardial infarction." *Br. Med. J.* 2:445–447.

McKay, F. S., and Black, G. V. 1916. "An investigation of mottled teeth." *Dent. Cosmos.* 58:477–484.

McKay, F. S. 1925. "Mottled enamel: A fundamental problem in dentistry." *Dent. Cosmos.* 67:847–860.

Ortega-Benito, J. M. and Landridge, P. 1992. "Outbreak of food poisoning due to Salmonella typhimurium DT4 in mayonnaise." *Public Health* 106:203–208.

Piantadosi, S., Byar, D. P., and Green, S. B. 1988. "The ecological fallacy." *Am. J. Epidemiol.* 127:893–904.

Report of the Royal College of Physicians. 1971. *Smoking and Health Now.* London: Pitman Medical and Scientific Publishing Co.

Robinson, W.S. 1950. "Ecological correlations and the behavior of individuals." *Am. Soc. Rev.* 15:351–357.

Selvin, H. C. 1958. "Durkeim's suicide and problems of empirical research." *Am. J. Soc.* 63:607–619.

Steinberg, A. G., and Wilder, R. M. 1952. "A study of the genetics of diabetes mellitus." *Am. J. Human Genet.* 4:113–135.

Vessey, M. P., and Mann, J. I., 1978. "Female sex hormones and thrombosis. Epidemiological aspects." *Br. Med. J.* 34:157–162.

Ward, E., Carpenter, A., Markowitz, S., Roberts, D., Halperin, W. 1991. "Excess number of bladder cancers in workers exposed to ortho-toluidine and aniline." *J. Nat. Cancer Inst.* 83:501–506.

2

AN OVERVIEW OF THE HISTORY
OF EPIDEMIOLOGY

The development of epidemiology has spanned many centuries. As an eclectic discipline, epidemiology has borrowed from sociology, demography, and statistics, as well as other fields of study. Hence, the reader should not be surprised to learn that its history is interwoven with that of other scientific disciplines. It was not until the nineteenth century that the fabric of epidemiology was woven into a distinct discipline with its own philosophy, concepts, and methods.

This chapter first describes the social and medical environment within which epidemiology developed. The emergence of epidemiology in the 1800s as an area of medical inquiry is then discussed. Stimulated by the observation of patterns of disease in the population, nineteenth-century epidemiologists devised methods to investigate the causes of these diseases and the means by which they could be prevented. The overwhelming of this demographic focus by the rise of bacteriology in the 1880s and 1890s is then examined. Epidemiologists turned their attention from the occurrence of disease in a population to the spread of bacteria by individual contact. The reemergence of epidemiology in the early and mid-twentieth century, associated with the entry of demographers and sociologists into the field, is then described.

THE SOCIAL AND MEDICAL ENVIRONMENT

Humankind has experienced disease for as long as records of human culture have existed. Along with these plagues and pestilence there have been attempts, crude at first, to understand and prevent such occurrences. The fourteenth century witnessed perhaps the most severe plague in recorded history in Europe and Asia: a worldwide pandemic of bubonic plague called the Great Plague. It is estimated that as many as one-third of the inhabitants of Europe died during this plague. Agriculture, economic relationships, and family life itself were altered by this horrific epidemic. Explanations put forth at the time to explain the occurrence of the plague included person-to-person spread of some mysterious disease-causing agent, deliberate poisoning by the Jews of Europe, divine retribution, and so on. However, the state of medical science did not provide much understanding of the causes of the Great Plague. When the Great London Fire of 1666 killed the rodent population that had served as a reservoir of the etiologic agent, *Yersinia pestis,* epidemics of the plague declined in London.

The underlying logic for modern epidemiologic investigations evolved from the scientific revolution of the 1600s, which indicated that the orderly behavior of the physical universe could be expressed in terms of mathematical relationships (Mason, 1962). During this period, Francis Bacon developed the basis of inductive logic and, with it, the concept of "inductive laws" (Copleston, 1963). Many seventeenth-century scientists reasoned that if mathematical relationships could be found to *describe, analyze,* and *understand* the physical universe, then similar relationships, known as *"laws of mortality,"* must exist in the biological world (Lilienfeld, 1979b; Merz, 1976). Laws of mortality were considered to be generalized statements about the relationships between disease (as manifested by mortality) and man. These laws formed the basis of the life table, which attempted to both quantitate and express them mathematically. From this philosophical base, the epidemiologic study evolved.

For specific aspects of disease, such as epidemics, attempts were made to formulate "laws of epidemics." In fact, the contagium vivum theory was regarded in a like manner. It was a generalization of the observed facts that several diseases (smallpox, measles, cholera) were thought to be caused by contagia viva.

Inspired by Bacon's writings, the Royal Society of London was founded in 1662. Its initial members included Robert Boyle, for formulator of Boyle's Law, William Petty, one of the founders of economics, and John Graunt, a tradesman who was a close friend of Petty and one of the Society's financial patrons. That same year, Graunt published his *Natural and Political Observations Mentioned in a Following Index and Made Upon the Bills of Mortality,* a pioneering work in a comparative study of mortality and morbidity in human populations (Lorrimer, 1959).

An intellectually curious man, Graunt collected the Bills of Mortality, which had been initiated in 1603 by the parish clerks, in London and in a parish town of Hampshire. After organizing the published Bills, he derived from them inferences about mortality and fertility in the human population, noting the usual excess of male births, the high infant mortality, and the seasonal variation in

Table 2–1. Life Table of Deaths in London
Adapted from Graunt's *Observations*

EXACT AGE	DEATHS	SURVIVORS
0	—	100
6	36	64
16	24	40
26	15	25
36	9	16
46	6	10
56	4	6
66	3	3
76	2	1
80	1	0

Source: Graunt (1662).

mortality. Graunt attempted to distinguish two broad causes of mortality, the acute and the "chronical diseases," and to discern urban-rural differences in mortality. From collected data, he constructed the first known life table, summarizing the mortality experience in terms of the number, percent, or probability of living or dying over a lifetime, a truly outstanding achievement (Table 2–1). Further, Graunt noted that one could attempt to formulate a law of mortality from such tables; he proposed that each country should prepare similar tables so that they could be compared to construct a general law of mortality (Lorrimer, 1959). Reviewing Graunt's work at the tercentenary of the publication of his *Observations,* D. V. Glass (1963) said:

> But, whatever the particular and varying emphases, demographers in general would agree that probably the most outstanding qualities of Graunt's work are first, the search for regularities and configurations in mortality and fertility; and secondly, the attention given—and usually shown explicitly—to the errors and ambiguities of the inadequate data used in that search. Graunt did not wait for better statistics; he did what he could with what was available to him. And by so doing, he also produced a much stronger case for supplying better data.

As mathematical principles developed during the late 1600s and early 1700s, Graunt's ideas were refined and extended. During this period, the idea of using comparative groups in studies also began to emerge. The control group was initially viewed as another group in which a law of mortality, formulated from a different ("experimental" or "study") group, could be tested. In light of this development, it is not surprising that the two noteworthy epidemiologic papers, each the first of its kind, appeared in the middle of the eighteenth century.

The first, a report of an experiment that was conducted in 1747 by James Lind (1753), who had developed certain hypotheses from epidemiologic observations regarding the etiology and treatment of scurvy. He decided to evaluate these hypotheses in the following way:

On the 20th of May, 1747, I took twelve patients in the scurvey, on board the SALISBURY at sea. Their cases were as similar as I could have them. They all in general had putrid gums, the spots and lassitude, with weakness of their knees. They lay together in one place, being a proper apartment for the sick in the fore-hold; and had one diet common to all, viz., water-gruel sweetened with sugar in the morning; fresh mutton broth often times for dinner; at other times puddings, boiled biscuit with sugar, etc.; and for supper, barley and raisins, rice and currents, sago and wine, or the like. Two of these were ordered each a quart of cyder a day. Two others took twenty-five gutts of elizir vitriol three times a day, upon an empty stomach; using a gargle strongly acidulated with it for their mouths. Two others took two spoonsful of vinegar three times a day, upon an empty stomach; having their gruels and their other food well acidulated with it, as also the gargle for their mouth. Two of the worst patients, with the tendons in the ham rigid (a symptom none of the rest had), were put under a course of sea water. Of this, they drank half a pint every day, and sometimes more or less as it operated by way of a gentle physic. Two others had each two oranges and one lemon given them every day. These they eat with greediness, at different times, upon an empty stomach. They continued but six days under this course, having consumed the quantity that could be spared. The two remaining patients took the bigness of a nutmeg three times a day, or an electuary recommended by a hospital-surgeon, made of garlic, mustard seed, rad raphan, balsam of Peru, and gum myrrh; using for common drink, barley-water well acidulated with tamarinds; by a decoction of which, with the addition of cremor tartar, they were gently purged three or four times during the course.

   The consequence was, that the most sudden and visible good effects were perceived from the use of the oranges and lemons; one of those who had taken them being at the end of six days fit for duty. The spots were not indeed at that time quite off his body, nor his gums sound; but without any other medicine, then a gargarism of elixir vitriol, he became quite healthy before we came into Plymouth, which was on the 16th of June. The other was the best recovered of any in his condition; and being now deemed pretty well, was appointed nurse to the rest of the sick.

From these results, Lind inferred that citric acid fruits cured the scurvy and that this would also provide a means of prevention. The British Navy eventually accepted his analysis, requiring the inclusion of limes or lime juice in the diet on ships from 1795; hence, the nicknaming of British seamen as ''limeys.''

   The other paper, an epidemiologic analysis, was published in 1760 by Daniel Bernoulli, a member of the noted European family of mathematicians. Having evaluated the available evidence, Bernoulli concluded that inoculation protected against smallpox and conferred life-long immunity. Using a life table, not unlike those of today, he determined that inoculation at birth would increase life expectancy.

EPIDEMIOLOGY EMERGES IN THE NINETEENTH CENTURY

The French Revolution at the end of the eighteenth century had a far-reaching influence on epidemiology. It stimulated an interest in public health and preventive medicine, thereby facilitating the development of the epidemiologic approach to disease. Furthermore, it permitted several individuals from the lower classes to assume positions of leadership in medicine. One such person was Pierre Charles-Alexandre Louis, one of the first modern epidemiologists. The characteristic that distinguished Louis's work was the comparison of groups of individuals.

Louis (1836) conducted several observational studies, the most famous of which demonstrated that bloodletting was not efficacious in the treatment of disease and, thus, helped reverse a trend toward its increasing use in medical practice. His approach to epidemiology is illustrated by a comment, in 1836, on the question of the inheritance of phthisis (tuberculosis) (Louis, 1837): "To determine the question satisfactorily, tables of mortality [life tables] would be necessary, comparing an equal number of persons born of phthisical parents with those in an opposite condition." Louis was not the first to use statistical methods in medicine, which he termed "la méthode numerique," but he pioneered in emphasizing their importance in medicine (Lilienfeld, 1979a; Lilienfeld, 1979b; Shyrock, 1947).

Louis was a well-known teacher with students from both England and the United States (Lilienfeld, 1979b). His influence was international and had an astounding impact on the growth of epidemiology that extends to the present (Lilienfeld, 1977a; Lilienfeld, 1977b; Lilienfeld, 1979b). Many of his students were from England and the United States. Lacking a vital statistics system to provide information on the health condition of the population, French epidemiology declined in the mid-1800s (Lilienfeld, 1980c), Louis's students, including William Farr and William Augustus Guy, assumed leadership in the field. They acted as "santiary physicians" involved in epidemiologic and other public health activities.

SANITARY PHYSICIANS—EPIDEMIOLOGY IN ACTION

Between 1835 and 1845, the center of epidemiologic activity moved from Paris to London (Lilienfeld, 1979b). For the following half century, Victorian epidemiology flourished. Physicians in London and elsewhere in England applied Louis's numerical method to the health problems of the day. Their activities were directed toward both disease prevention and treatment, including epidemiologic assessments of the efficacy of smallpox vaccination, specific medical practices, and the morbidity and mortality experiences of persons in various trades. Victorian epidemiology flourished, led by two institutions: the Registrar-General's Office and the London Epidemiological Society.

The Registrar-General's Office

In 1836, the Registrar-General's Office was legislated into existence by the English Parliament as a centralized registry for information on births, deaths, and marriages (Registrar-General, 1839; Szreter, 1991a). As Goldman (1991) noted, this action was a political one and it is not surprising that the first annual report of the Registrar-General (for 1837–1838) viewed the data collected and analyzed from the commercial perspective of life insurance companies. However, by the second such report, William Farr had assumed command of the office and had shifted the focus toward public health (Eyler, 1979). This orientation was to remain characteristic of the Registrar-General's Office and its successor agencies (e.g., the Office of Population Censuses and Surveys) up to the present.

Under Farr's direction, the Registrar-General's Office became a major force in the Victorian public health movement. It provided the statistical facts that were often necessary for initiatives to be developed in response to public health problems (Eyler, 1979; Wohl, 1983). An example of the Office's influence is illustrated by Farr's 1843 analysis of mortality in Liverpool (Szreter, 1991b). Farr found that barely half the native residents of this city lived to see their sixth birthday, while in England in general, the median age of death was 45 years. At the request of the municipal leaders of Liverpool, Parliament passed the landmark Liverpool Sanitary Act of 1846 (Frazer, 1947; Wohl, 1983). This act created a sanitary code for Liverpool, established a local public health authority to enforce it, and introduced the position of the "Medical Officer of Health," the physician who was charged with implementing the code and managing the authority. It served as a model for the organization of English local public health administration during the second half of the nineteenth century.

Farr also developed the concept of mortality surveillance, in which mortality data are regularly reviewed and analyzed to discern changes in the health of the public. These activities represent the first regular use of vital statistics and other demographic data for epidemiologic purposes, and they were a major reason for the vitality of Victorian epidemiology.

The London Epidemiological Society

Another institution of Victorian epidemiology was the London Epidemiological Society (LES) (Lilienfeld, 1979b). Among its founding members were Farr, William Augustus Guy (Dean of the King's College Medical School and a President of the Royal Statistical Society), Thomas Addison (describer of Addison's disease), and Richard Bright (who provided the first description of end-stage renal disease) (Lilienfeld and Lilienfeld, 1980a; 1980b; 1980c; Brockington, 1965). The influence of Louis was also apparent in this society when, at its inaugural, the President (Dr. Benjamin Babbington) remarked: "Statistics, too, have supplied us with a new and powerful means of testing medical truth, and we learn from the labours of the accurate Louis how appropriately they may be brought to bear upon the subject of epidemic disease" (Epidemiological Society, 1850).

The initial purpose of the London Epidemiological Society was to determine the etiology of cholera, but its activities quickly expanded. Its report on smallpox vaccination in 1853, for example, was the major reason for the passage of the Vaccination Act of 1853, mandating vaccination on a nationwide basis. One of the Society's founding members, John Snow (1936), conducted a series of classical studies of cholera. Snow, who was known for his administration of chloroform to Queen Victoria during childbirth, investigated the occurrence of cholera in London during 1848–1854 in addition to reviewing reports of epidemics occurring aboard ships and in Europe.

In London, several water companies were responsible for supplying water to different parts of the city. In 1849, Snow noted that the cholera rates were particularly high in those areas of London that were supplied by the Lambeth Company and the Southwark and Vauxhall Company, both of whom obtained their water from the Thames River at a point heavily polluted with sewage. Between 1849 and 1854 the Lambeth Company had its source of water relocated to a less contaminated part of the Thames. In 1854, when another epidemic of cholera occurred, an area consisting of two-thirds of London's resident population south of the Thames was being served by both companies. In this area, the two companies had their water mains laid out in an interpenetrating manner, so that houses on the same street were receiving their water from different sources. Snow ascertained the total number of houses supplied by each water company, calculated cholera death rates per 10,000 houses for the first seven weeks of the epidemic and compared them with those for the rest of London; the data were supplied to Snow by Farr (Table 2–2). His findings were indisputably clear; the mortality rates in the houses supplied by the Southwark and Vauxhall Company were between eight and nine times greater than those in homes supplied by the Lambeth Company. From these findings, integrated with his investigation of the Broad Street Pump cholera outbreak and his assssment of other characteristics of

Table 2–2. Deaths from Cholera per 10,000 Houses by Source of Water Supply,
London, 1854

WATER SUPPLY	NUMBER OF HOUSES	DEATHS FROM CHOLERA	DEATHS IN EACH 10,000 HOUSES
Southwark and Vauxhall Company	40,046	1,263	315
Lambeth Company	26,107	98	37
Rest of London	256,423	1,422	59

Source: Snow (1936).

cholera epidemics, Snow inferred the existence of a "cholera poison" transmitted by polluted water.

John Snow's achievement was based on his logical organization of observations, his recognition of a natural experiment, and his quantitative approach in analyzing the occurrence of a disease in a human population. The influence of his report was more widespread than has been realized. It led to legislation mandating that *all* of the water companies in London filter their water by 1857, only two years after the report's publication. (It was not until 1883 that Robert Koch identified the cholera vibrio).

A somewhat different approach to the epidemiologic study of disease is embodied in William Budd's studies of typhoid fever, which were published during the years 1857–1873 (Budd, 1931). Budd, an active member of the LES and a student of Louis, practiced medicine in his native village of North Tawton, a remote rural community in England. From his observations of the environmental conditions of the village, he argued against the miasmatic origin of typhoid fever.

> Much there was, as I can myself testify, offensive to the nose, but [typhoid] fever there was none. It could not be said that the atmospheric conditions necessary to [typhoid] fever was wanting, because while this village remained exempt, many neighbouring villages suffered severely from the pest. . . . Meanwhile privies, pig-styes, and dungheaps continued, year after year, to exhale ill odours, without any specific effect on the public health. . . . I ascertained by an inquiry conducted with the most scrupulous care that for fifteen years there had been no severe outbreak of this disorder, and that for nearly ten years there had been but a single case. For the development of this fever a more specific element was needed than either the swine, the dungheaps, or the privies were, in the common course of things, able to furnish.

From his epidemiologic observations of an outbreak of typhoid fever that occurred in North Tawton between July and November 1839, Budd inferred that it was a contagious disease. During this period, he saw more than eighty patients with typhoid fever. Noting instances of three or four successive cases occurring in the same household, he ascribed these to contagion. Considerably more important was his observation that three individuals who left the village during the epidemic for other villages spread the disease to some of their new contacts. He traced specific instances of person-to-person contact that resulted in the appearance of typhoid fever in villages previously free of the disease despite environmental conditions similar to North Tawton. Budd concluded that typhoid fever is a "contagious, or self-propagating fever," that the intestinal disturbance is its distinctive manifestation, and that "the contagious matter by which the fever is propagated is cast off, chiefly, in the discharges from the diseased intestine." It was not until 1880 that the typhoid fever bacillus was described.Other members of the LES were active in research on such issues as whether smallpox vaccination should be mandatory and whether occupation influenced health and if so, how. They also testified before Parliament and provided data for Parliamentary debates. The vitality in the field of epidemiology, however, diminished as the bacteriological revolution swept through medicine in the late nineteenth and early twentieth centuries.

THE BACTERIOLOGICAL REVOLUTION

The Bacteriological Revolution, in which the cause of various diseases was attributed to bacteria, marked a major change in the development of modern medicine (Shyrock, 1947). For the first time, there was a scientific understanding of the etiology of disease and thus a basis for public health efforts. However, the bacteriological revolution posed a major challenge for epidemiology. Once the cause of a disease was known, the major epidemiologic question was how the disease propagated itself in a population. In the late nineteenth and early twentieth centuries epidemiologists responded to this question by tracing the "point-contact spread" of infection; i.e., from which individuals did the cases of the disease become infected with the etiologic agents? In this manner, it might be possible to find out which individual brought the disease into the community so that contacts between this individual, those already infected, and uninfected persons in the community could be minimized (Eyler, 1986, 1989; Leavitt, 1992). Epidemiologic expertise could thus be brought to bear on disease control through knowledge of the etiologic agent. The focus on populations, an essential aspect of epidemiologic investigation into disease etiology that was characteristic of Victorian epidemiology, waned.

THE DEMOGRAPHIC FOCUS REESTABLISHED

The poulation focus in epidemiology regained strength during the first half of the twentieth century through the activities of demographer-sociologists and statis-

ticians. Some of this impetus came from professionals in the life insurance industry, which had an economic interest in determining which individuals were at
greatest risk of morbidity and mortality. Outside the life insurance industry, three
individuals, Edgar Sydenstricker, A. Bradford Hill, and Harold Dorn, were of
special importance. The epidemiologic activities of these individuals will be discussed briefly since they illustrate the role that population studies had in the
reemergence of epidemiology in the early 1900s and in the expansion of epidemiologic activities to include noninfectious diseases during 1930–1970.

Sydenstricker, an economist and sociologist by training, joined the United
States Public Health Service in 1915 (Wiehl, 1974). After some initial studies of
sickness insurance in Europe, Sydenstricker was assigned to work with Dr. Joseph
Goldberger in his studies of pellagra in South Carolina. Sydenstricker organized
a series of surveys to discern the diets, illnesses, housing, sanitary conditions, and
economic status of families living in cotton mill villages in South Carolina during
1916–1918. These extensive epidemiologic studies identified the etiology of pellagra and made it possible to develop interventions.

Toward the end of his pellagra studies, Sydenstricker was assigned to work
with a young Public Health Service physician, Wade Hampton Frost, on the 1918
influenza pandemic. Sydenstricker quickly determined that existing data on the
epidemiology of the disease were inadequate. He organized field studies to provide the necessary information. (During this collaboration, Frost was summoned
to the Johns Hopkins University School of Hygiene and Public Health to direct
the first epidemiology training program but Sydenstricker and Frost continued to
collaborate despite this move.) Based on the successful conduct of the influenza
studies, Sydenstricker was appointed to direct the Public Health Service's Office
of Statistical Investigations. In this role, he undertook a series of morbidity surveys in Hagerstown, Maryland, which established a model for other workers to
follow in determining public health priorities in a population.

A. Bradford Hill was an English statistician who, as a result of illness, was
unable to pursue his desire to become a physician (Doll, 1993). His early work
in the 1920s dealt with the analysis of vital statistics, particularly demographic
characteristics such as the difference in mortality among urban and rural residents
(e.g., Hill, 1925). Later he was instrumental in the development of the randomized
clinical trial and its widespread adoption as a means of assessing the efficacy of
a new treatment for a disease (Doll, 1993; Hill, 1990). He was also among the
leaders in discerning the role of cigarette smoking in the epidemic of lung cancer.
This work was completed with his colleague and student, Professor Richard Doll.

Harold Dorn was trained as a demographer and developed an interest in
urban-rural differences in mortality (Dorn, 1934). As a result, he became familiar
with the work of both Sydenstricker and Hill. Soon after he completed his doctoral
work in 1936, Dorn joined the United States Public Health Service. As part of
the Social Security Act of 1936, which created the Social Security system, the

Public Health Service had been given research funds with which it would undertake a national morbidity survey; one major concern was the morbidity related to cancer (Fox, 1987; Mountin et al., 1939). Dorn was appointed director of a national cancer survey to provide data on this issue. The result was the First National Cancer Survey in 1937, the predecessor of the current Surveillance, Epidemiology, and End Results (SEER) cancer surveillance system in the United States.

The National Cancer Institute was established in 1937 and Dorn was assigned to it. The First National Cancer Survey provided much information on the burden of cancer in the population, and Dorn sought to use it as the basis for an epidemiologic profile of cancer. To do so, he would need a biostatistics and epidemiology unit. World War II interrupted these efforts, and Dorn was not able to organize this group at the National Cancer Institute until the late 1940s (Ellenberg, 1993). The group that he recruited to the National Cancer Institute included Jerome Cornfield, Samuel Greenhouse, and Nathan Mantel. Many of the statistical and epidemiologic techniques now routinely used in epidemiologic work (e.g., the odds ratio estimate of the relative risk) were developed in Dorn's unit.

SUMMARY

The basis of epidemiologic inquiry evolved from the Scientific Revolution of the 1600s, which suggested an ordering of nature explicable in mathematical relationships. This concept was extended to biological phenomena and led to the development of the life table. However, until 1830, most epidemiologic activities were the result of isolated efforts by individuals such as John Graunt and James Lind. In the 1830s, the emergence of the Parisian school of medicine fostered the development of a quantitative comparative approach to investigations into the etiology of disease and the efficacy of medical practices. The major figure in this development was Pierre Charles-Alexandre Louis, who created the "numerical method" to undertake epidemiologic investigations. Louis's research and teaching attracted many foreign students, including several from England and the United States. It was Louis's English students who would assume leadership of epidemiology during the middle and late nineteenth century.

William Farr, the first director of the Registrar-General's Office, was one of Louis's English students. Under Farr's supervision, the Registrar-General's Office served as the national center for health statistics. It provided the statistical data that underlay many of the public health initiatives taken in Victorian England. In one instance, the data culled by Farr led to the development of the position of the Medical Officer of Health. Farr's activities were not restricted to the direction of the Registrar-General's Office; he was also a member of the London Epidemiological Society.

The London Epidemiological Society provided a forum for the discussion of epidemiologic activities by its members. The Society also investigated issues, such as vaccination, and issued reports of such work. One member of the Society, John Snow, investigated the relationship between consumption of water from one of the water companies in London and the development of cholera. His epidemiologic study suggested that such a relationship existed, and Snow inferred that a "cholera poison" was transmitted by the water. Another of the Society's members, William Budd, undertook an epidemiologic study of typhoid fever. Forty years before the discovery of the typhoid fever bacillus, he concluded that typhoid fever was propagated through "discharges from the diseased intestine."

The development of bacteriology in the late nineteenth century led epidemiologists to focus on the "point-contact spread" of the agents of disease, i.e., bacteria. With the agents of disease identified, however, the need for epidemiology lessened. It was not until demographers and sociologists, such as Edgar Sydenstricker, A. Bradford Hill, and Harold Dorn, began to undertake epidemiologic investigations in the early and middle twentieth century that epidemiology was reinvigorated. These individuals brought a population focus back into epidemiology. They also trained the next generation of leaders in epidemiology, many of whom are active in the field today.

REFERENCES

Bernoulli, D. 1760. "Mathematical and physical memoirs, taken from the registers of the Royal Academy of Sciences for the year 1760: An attempt at a new analysis of the mortality caused by smallpox and of the advantages of inoculation to prevent it." In *Smallpox Inoculation: An Eighteenth Century Mathematical Controversy. Translation and Critical Commentary* by L. Bradley, 1971. Nottingham, England: Univesity of Nottingham.

Brockington, C. F. 1965. *Public Health in the Nineteenth Century.* Edinburgh: E. & S. Livingstone.

Budd, W. 1931. *Typhoid Fever: Its Nature, Mode of Spreading and Prevention.* Original publication 1873. New York: American Public Health Association.

Copleston, F. 1963. *A History of Philosophy, Vol. 3, Pt. II.* Garden City, N.Y.: Image Books.

Doll, R. 1993. "Sir Austin Bradford Hill, 1897–1991." *Stat. Med.* 12:795–806.

Dorn, H. F. 1934. "The effect of rural-urban migration upon death-rates." *Population* 1: 95–114.

Ellenberg, J. 1993. "Remarks." Presented at: Conference on Current Topics in Biostatistics, National Institutes of Health, Bethesda, Md., January 25, 1993.

"Epidemiological Society." 1850. *Lancet* 2:641.

Eyler, J. M. 1979. *Victorian Social Medicine. The Ideas and Methods of William Farr.* Baltimore: Johns Hopkins University Press.

————. 1986. "The epidemiology of milk-borne scarlet fever: the case of Edwardian Brighton." *Am. J. Pub. Health* 76:573–584.

————. 1989. "Poverty, disease, and responsibility: Arthur Newsholme and the public health dilemmas of British liberalism." *Milbank Q.* 67(Suppl 1):109–126.

Fox, D. M. 1987. "Politics of the NIH extramural program, 1937–1950." *J. Hist. Med. Allied Sci.* 42:447–466.

Frazer, W. M. 1947. *Duncan of Liverpool.* London; Hamish Hamilton Medical Books.

Glass, D. V. 1963. "John Graunt and his natural and political observations." *Proc. Roy. Soc. (Biology)* 159:2–37.

Goldman, L. 1991. "Statistics and the science of society in early Victorian Britain: an intellectual context for the General Register Office." *Soc. Hist. Med.* 4:415–434.

Graunt, J. 1662. *Natural and Political Observations Mentioned in a Following Index, and Made Upon the Bills of Mortality.* London. Reprinted. Baltimore: The Johns Hopkins Press, 1939.

Hill, A. B. 1925. *Internal Migration and its Effects upon the Death-Rates: with Special Reference to the County of Essex.* Medical Research Council Special Report Series No. 95, London: HMSO.

————. 1990. "Memories of the British Streptomycin Trial in tuberculosis: the first randomized clinical trial." *Controlled Clinical Trials* 11:77–79.

Leavitt, J. W. 1992. " 'Typhoid Mary' strikes back: bacteriological theory and practice in early twentieth-century public health." *Isis* 83:608–629.

Lilienfeld, A. M., and Lilienfeld, D. E. 1979a. "A century of case-control studies: Progress?" *J. Chron. Dis.* 32:5–13.

————. 1980a. "The 1979 Heath Clark Lectures. 'The Epidemiologic Fabric.' I. Weaving the Threads." *Int. J. Epid.* 9:199–206.

————. 1980b. "The 1979 Heath Clark Lectures. 'The Epidemiologic Fabric.' II. The London Bridge—It Never Fell." *Int. J. Epid.* 9:299–304.

Lilienfeld, D. E. 1979b. "The greening of epidemiology: Sanitary physicians and the London Epidemiological Society (1830–1870)." *Bull. Hist. Med.* 52:503–528.

Lilienfeld, D. E., and Lilienfeld, A. M. 1977a. "Teaching preventive medicine in medical schools: An historical vignette." *Prev. Med.* 6:469–471.

————. 1977b. "Epidemiology: A retrospective study." *Amer. J. Epid.* 106:445–459.

————. 1980c. "The French influence on the development of epidemiology." In *Times, Places, Persons.* A. M. Lilienfeld, ed. Baltimore: The Johns Hopkins University Press.

Lind, J. 1753. *A Treatise on the Scurvy.* Edinburgh: Sands, Murray, and Cochran.

Lorrimer, F. 1959. "The development of demography." In *The Study of Population.* P. M. Hauser and O. D. Duncan, eds. Chicago: University of Chicago Press, pp. 124–179.

Louis, P.C.-A. 1836. *Researches on the Effects of Bloodletting in Some Inflammatory Diseases, and on the Influence of Tartarized Antimony and Vesication in Pneumonitis.* Translated by C. G. Putman with Preface and Appendix by James Jackson. Boston: Milliard, Gray and Co.

————. 1837. "Pathological researches on phthisis." *Amer. J. Med. Sci.* 19:445–449.

Mason, S. F. 1962. *A History of the Sciences.* New York: Collier Books.

Merz, J. T. 1976. *A History of European Scientific Thought in the Nineteenth Century, Vol. 2.* Glouceseter, Mass.: Peter Smith.

Mountin, J. W., Dorn, H. F., and Boone, B. R. 1939. "The incidence of cancer in Atlanta, Ga., and surrounding counties." *Pub. Health Rep.* 54:1255–1273.

Registrar-General. 1839. "First annual report of the Registrar-General on births, deaths, and marriages in England in 1837–8." *J. Stat. Soc. London* 2:269.

Shyrock, R. H. 1947. *The Development of Modern Medicine.* New York: Knopf.

Snow, J. 1936. "On the mode of communication of cholera." In *Snow on Cholera.* New York: The Commonwealth Fund, pp. 1–175.

Szreter, S. 1991a. "Introduction: the GRO and the historians." *Soc. Hist. Med.* 4:401–414.

———. 1991b. "The GRO and the public health movement in Britain, 1837–1914." *Soc. Hist. Med.* 4:435–463.

Wiehl, D. G. 1974. "Edgar Sydenstricker: a memoir." In *The Challenge of Facts.* R. V. Kasius, ed. New York: PRODIST.

Wohl, A. S. 1983. *Endangered Lives.* Cambridge, Mass.: Harvard University Press.

3

SELECTED EPIDEMIOLOGIC CONCEPTS
OF DISEASE

Many of the fundamental epidemiologic concepts have evolved from studies of infectious diseases, but they are equally applicable to noninfectious diseases and conditions. Only those that have proved to be of practical value will be considered in this chapter.

AGENT, HOST, AND ENVIRONMENT

Essentially, the epidemiologic patterns of infectious diseases depend upon factors that influence the probability of contact between an infectious agent and a susceptible person known as a host. The presence of the infectious material by which the disease may be transmitted varies with the duration and extent of its excretion from an infected person, the **environmental** conditions affecting survival of the **agent,** the route of entry into the **host,** and the existence of alternative reservoirs or hosts of the agent. The availability of susceptible hosts depends upon the extent of mobility and interpersonal contact within the population group and the degree and duration of immunity from previous infections with the same or related agents.

Relationships similar to those among infectious agents of disease, human hosts, and their environment also exist among noninfectious etiological agents, hosts, and environment. For example, whether or not a person develops a specific form of cancer may depend upon the extent of his exposure to the carcinogenic agent, the dose of the agent, and his susceptibility, which may be influenced by genetic and/or immunological factors. A classification of agent, host, and environmental factors is presented in Table 3–1 as a frame of reference in the search for determinants of disease occurrence in a population.

A specific scientific discipline is usually concerned with a particular category of the factors listed in Table 3–1. For instance, the geneticist concentrates on genetic factors; the microbiologist on infectious agents; the sociologist on human behavior, ethnic groups, and socioeconomic environments. The epidemiologist, however, attempts to integrate from diverse disciplines the data necessary to analyze a particular disease. The need for evaluating the *interaction* of these factors relative to **time, place,** and **persons** is the main reason for viewing this frame of reference as primarily an epidemiologic concept.

Table 3–1. A Classification of Agent, Host, and Environmental Factors That Determine the Occurrence of Diseases in Human Populations

I. *Agents of Disease—Etiological Factors*

		Examples
A.	Nutritive elements	
	excesses	Cholesterol
	deficiencies	Vitamins, proteins
B.	Chemical agents	
	poisons	Carbon monoxide, carbon tetrachloride, drugs
	allergens	Ragweed, poison ivy, medications
C.	Physical agents	Ionizing radiation, mechanical
D.	Infectious agents	
	metazoa	Hookworm, schistosomiasis, onchocerciasis
	protozoa	Amoebae, malaria
	bacteria	Rheumatic fever, lobar pneumonia, typhoid, tuberculosis, syphilis
	fungi	Histoplasmosis, athlete's foot
	rickettsia	Rocky mountain spotted fever, typhus, Lyme disease
	viruses	Measles, mumps, chickenpox, smallpox, poliomyelitis, rabies, yellow fever, HIV

II. *Host Factors* (Intrinsic Factors)—Influences Exposure, Susceptibility, or Response to Agents

		Examples
A.	Genetic	Sickle cell disease
B.	Age	Alzheimer's disease
C.	Sex	Rheumatoid arthritis
D.	Ethnic group	—
E.	Physiologic state	Fatigue, pregnancy, puberty, stress, nutritional state

(continued)

Table 3–1. A Classification of Agent, Host, and Environmental Factors That Determine the Occurrence of Diseases in Human Populations (continued)

F.	Prior immunologic experience	Hypersensitivity, protection
	active	Prior infection, immunization
	passive	Maternal antibodies, gamma globulin prophylaxis
G.	Intercurrent or preexisting disease	
H.	Human behavior	Personal hygiene, food handling, diet, interpersonal contact, occupation, recreation, utilization of health resources, tobacco use

III. *Environmental Factors* (Extrinsic Factors)—Influences Existence of the Agent, Exposure, or Susceptibility to Agent

		Examples
A.	Physical environment	Geology, climate
B.	Biologic environment	
	human populations	Density
	flora	Sources of food, influence on vertebrates and arthropods, as a source of agents
	fauna	Food sources, vertebrate hosts, arthropod vectors
C.	Socioeconomic environment	
	occupation	Exposure to chemical agents
	urbanization and economic development	Urban crowding, tensions and pressures, cooperative efforts in health and education
	disruption	Wars, floods

MODE OF TRANSMISSION

As is evident from Table 3–1, infectious diseases are usually classified by the etiological agent, such as a virus or a bacterium. This classification, based on the biological features of the agent, is satisfactory from many points of view, including that of potential preventive measures. However, it is also possible to classify diseases by their epidemiologic features. In many instances, this may be more advantageous for applying preventive measures than an etiological classification. Infectious diseases, for example, can be divided according to the way they are spread through human populations:

  1. *Common-vehicle epidemics.* The etiological agent is transmitted by water, food, air, or inoculation (Table 3–2). Common-vehicle epidemics can result from a single exposure of a population group to the agent, from repeated multiple exposures, or from continued exposure over a period

of time. They are usually characterized by explosiveness of onset and limitation or localization in time, place, and persons. This type of epidemic can be illustrated by a food poisoning outbreak, which is the result of a single source of exposure.

2. *Epidemics propagated by serial transfer from host to host.* The agent is spread through contact between infected and susceptible individuals by means of the respiratory, anal, oral, genital, or other route; by serial transfer of infected blood or sera; by dust; or by insects and arthropods (vectors) (Table 3–2). The course of such an epidemic is illustrated in Figure 3–1.

This simple classification of infectious diseases by mode of transmission provides a basis for considering possible measures to prevent epidemics in the community. But several types of infections, particularly from viral and parasitic agents, may have more complicated modes of transmission. An example is given in Figure 3–2.

Table 3–2. Classification of Human Infections by Selected Epidemiologic Features*

	Examples
I. *Dynamics of Spread through Human Populations:*	
A. Spread by a "common vehicle"	
ingestion with water, food or beverage	Salmonellosis
inhalation in air breathed	Legionnaire's disease
inoculation (intravenous, subcutaneous)	Hepatitis B
B. Propagation by serial transfer from host to host	
respiratory route of transfer	Measles
anal-oral route	Shigellosis Hepatitis B
genital route	Syphilis, AIDS
II. *Portal of Entry (and Portal of Exit) in Human Host:*	
Upper respiratory tract	Diphtheria
Lower respiratory tract	Tuberculosis
Gastrointestinal tract	Typhoid fever
Genitourinary tract	Gonorrhea
Conjunctiva	Trachoma
Percutaneous	Leptospirosis
Percutaneous (bite of arthropod)	Yellow fever
	(continued)

Table 3–2. Classification of Human Infections by Selected Epidemiologic Features*
(continued)

III. *Principal Reservoir of Infection:*	
Man	Hepatitis A
Other vertebrates (zoonoses)	Tularemia
Agent free-living (?)	Histoplasmosis
IV. *Cycles of Infectious Agent in Nature:*	
(arrows designate transfer to occasional host)	
Man-man	Influenza
Man-arthropod-man	Malaria
Vertebrate-vertebrate↘	Psittacosis
man	
Vertebrate-arthropod-	Viral encephalitis
vertebrate↘	
man	

V. *Complex Cycles*—seen especially in certain helminth infections. For example, in paragonimiasis the cycle is as follows:

Ovum——miracidium——cercaria——adult——ovum
(in snail)   (in crab,   (in man)
crayfish)

The agent is free-living in fresh water during a part of its existence as ovum, miracidium, and cercaria.

*Some diseases may be classified in more than one category in this classification; the most usual situation is given in the examples cited.

THE INCUBATION PERIOD

One important epidemiologic feature of a disease is the incubation period, first described by Fracastoro in 1546 (Fracastoro, 1930). This is the interval between the time of contact and/or entry of the agent and onset of illness. In infectious diseases, it is generally thought of as the time required for the multiplication of the microorganism within the host up to a threshold point where the pathogen population is large enough to produce symptoms in the host.

Each infectious disease has a characteristic incubation period, largely dependent upon the rate of growth of the organism in the host (Benenson, 1990). Other factors that play a role include the dosage of the infectious agent, its portal of entry, and the rate and degree of immune response by the host. An incubation period will vary among individuals; and, in a group of cases, its distribution will be asymmetrical, so that the part of the curve with longer incubation periods has a long "tail," that is, the curve is "skewed to the right" (Figure 3–3). Sartwell pointed out that this asymmetrical curve resembles a log-normal distribution. Indeed, when one graphs the frequency of incubation periods against the loga-

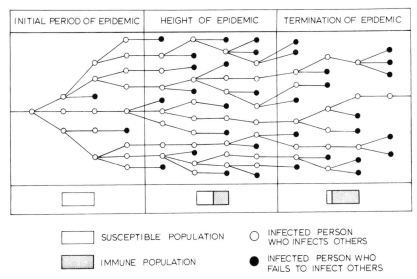

Figure 3–1. Course of a typical propogated epidemic in which the agent is transmitted by contact between individuals. *Source:* Burnet and White (1972).

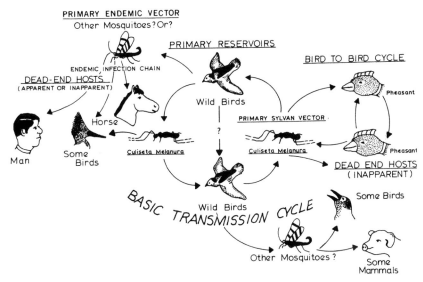

Figure 3–2. Summer infection chains for eastern equine encephalitis. *Source:* Hess and Holden (1958).

41

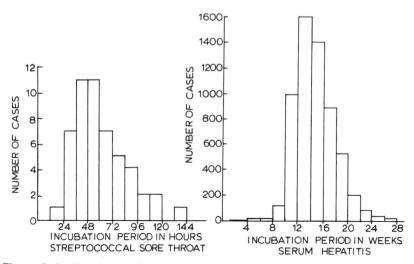

Figure 3–3. Distribution of incubation periods in an epidemic of food-borne strepto-coccal sore throat and a series of serum hepatitis following administration of icterogenic lots of yellow fever vaccine. *Source:* Sartwell (1950).

rithm of time, the skewness essentially disappears and the curve resembles a normal distribution; hence, the name "log-normal distribution" (Armenian and Khoury, 1981; Polednak, 1974; Sartwell, 1950, 1966).

In a graph of a common-vehicle epidemic from a single source, the curve resulting from plotting the times of onset of the disease also represents the distribution of incubation periods. Knowing the incubation period for a disease in a single-source common-vehicle epidemic enables one to estimate the time of exposure to the disease agent.

Only three factors are necessary to describe this type of epidemic:

1. Distribution of times and onset of illness, known as the **epidemic curve**.
2. The specific disease, which is characterized by its incubation period.
3. The time of exposure.

In practice, if only two of these factors are known, it is possible to deduce the third factor.

If one recognizes an infectious disease from its clinical characteristics, the incubation period is then also known. In a single-source common-vehicle epidemic, the epidemic curve represents the distribution of incubation periods and the median point on the curve represents the median incubation period (Figure 3–4). The median is preferred as a measure of central tendency because of the usual skewness of the distribution of the incubation periods. Using the median incubation period, one can estimate the time of exposure to the etiological agent

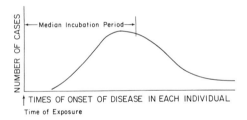

Figure 3–4. Distribution of times of onset of disease (the epidemic curve) and median incubation period in a single-source common-vehicle epidemic.

and investigate the events that occurred about that time to determine the cause of the epidemic. Likewise, if sufficient information is available to construct the epidemic curve and the time of exposure is known, one can determine the type of infectious disease if the incubation period of that disease is already known.

Although the prototype for this kind of reasoning is the previously described single-source food poisoning outbreak, it is also applicable to diseases caused by several possible etiological agents, one of which may be known (Armenian and Khoury, 1981). Cobb, Miller, and Wald (1959) attempted to apply this approach to leukemia, where exposure to radiation is recognized as one etiological factor for some forms of the disease. They analyzed the cases of leukemia that occurred after the 1945 atomic bomb explosion in Hiroshima, which can be regarded as a single exposure. Figure 3–5A compares the annual incidence of leukemia following explosion of the bomb among those who were located less than 1,000 meters (m) from the hypocenter (the location of the bomb in the air at the time of the explosion) with the incidence among those who were 2,000 m or more from the center, generally considered an unexposed group. The annual leukemia incidence rate proved to be higher in the first group, but interestingly, the peak incidence of leukemia occurred in 1951 or 1952, about six years after the radiation exposure. Admittedly, the data for the earlier years are probably incomplete, but, nonetheless, the shape of the curve resembles that of an epidemic curve observed in single-exposure common-vehicle epidemics. The incidence pattern for those who were between 1,000 to 1,999 m from the bomb site is similar although their rates are lower (Fig. 3–5B). Continued follow-up of these survivors still shows an excessive rate of leukemia in the exposed group.

Cobb, Miller and Wald also collated several reports of ankylosing spondylitis patients who developed leukemia following radiation treatment by either a single exposure or multiple exposures over a number of years. In the latter case, they determined the central point of the exposure period and adjusted for the size of the administered dose. Assuming the interval between the time of exposure and onset of leukemia to be the incubation period, they obtained the results presented in Figure 3–6. These results show that the curve peaks at about four years after

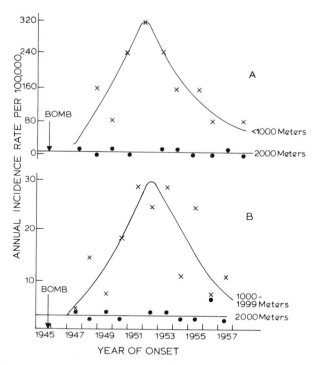

Figure 3–5. Annual incidence rate of leukemia following the atomic bomb explosion among survivors who were residents of Hiroshima City at the time of diagnosis. (A) Persons less than 1000 meters from hypocenter compared with persons 2000 or more meters from the hypocenter at time of explosion. (B) Persons 1000 to 1999 meters from hypocenter compared with persons 2000 or more meters from hypocenter at time of explosion. *Source:* Cobb, Miller, and Wald (1959).

exposure to radiation and that 90 percent of the cases have occurred within nine years of such exposure.

If one is willing to assume from these data that the incubation period of leukemia induced by unknown factors is similar to that of leukemia caused by radiation, it would suggest that the search for etiological factors of leukemia should focus on the ten-year period before the onset of the disease in adults. However, data obtained from future studies may change these estimates. It is also of interest that the distribution of leukemia cases is skewed to the right, as in single-source common-vehicle epidemics of infectious diseases. The skewness in the ankylosing spondylitis data may partially reflect the number of patients who had multiple exposures over a period of several years.

An example of similar reasoning is the analysis of the changing pattern of mortality from leukemia among children under five years old in England and Wales between 1931 and 1953 (Hewitt, 1955). Hewitt noted the similarity between the shape of the mortality curve and the curves usually observed in

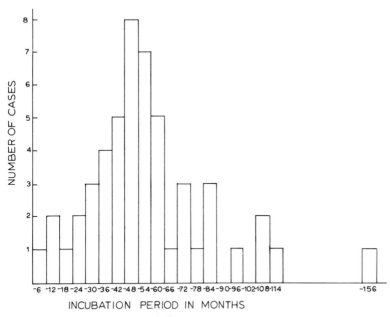

Figure 3–6.   Distribution of incubation periods of leukemia cases following irradiation for ankylosing spondylitis. *Source:* Cobb, Miller, and Wald (1959).

incubation periods of infectious diseases. He also noted an increasing peak of mortality during this period at about three to four years of age (Figure 3–7). He postulated that the increased use of X-rays during this period, which were known to be leukemogenic, was one possible explanation. This analysis provided the basis for a field investigation of the possible influence of prenatal and postnatal X-rays and other procedures on the occurrence of childhood leukemia (Stewart, Webb, and Hewitt, 1958). Their finding of a connection between intrauterine radiation (mainly X-ray pelvimetry) and childhood leukemia stimulated many others to investigate this relationship (Diamond, Schmerler, and Lilienfeld, 1973; Graham et al., 1966; Kato, 1971; MacMahon, 1962). Several of these studies suggested that although the entire increase in death rates could not be explained by intrauterine radiation, a part of the increase could be so explained (Diamond, Schmerler, and Lilienfeld, 1973; Graham et al., 1966; MacMahon, 1962). It must be admitted, however, that there are still differences of opinion among those who have investigated the problem (Kato, 1971).

Armenian and Lilienfeld (1974, 1983) analyzed the incubation periods of certain neoplastic diseases, including several with known etiological factors and specific exposure times such as thyroid adenomas, cancers following childhood exposure to radiation, bronchogenic carcinoma in asbestos workers, and bladder tumors among dyestuff workers. Figure 3–8 shows the distribution of incubation

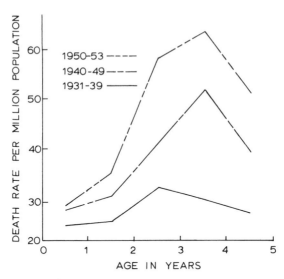

Figure 3–7. Age-specific death rates from leukemia among children under five years old, England and Wales, 1931–1953. *Source:* Hewitt (1955).

periods for 281 cases of bladder tumors that occurred among dyestuff workers. The shape of the distribution is skewed to the right and was demonstrated to be log-normal with a median incubation period of about seventeen years. Similarly, Armenian and Khoury (1981) analyzed the distribution of the ages at onset for various inherited conditions, such as familial hypercholesterolemia, and found that these distributions were log-normal; for diseases of known multifactorial etiology, the distribution of the age at onset was not log-normal (Armenian and Lilienfeld, 1983).

If, in infectious diseases, the incubation period reflects the multiplication of an organism and its interaction with host defenses, it is interesting to speculate on the biological model that underlies the incubation period (or "latency" period, as investigators have called it) when exposure to a chemical carcinogenic agent is the etiologic factor. Doll and Pike have each postulated that the neoplastic transformation of a number of individual cells is necessary in order to produce a "nest" of transformed cells that constitute the beginning of a tumor (Doll, 1971; Pike, 1966). It is also possible that a carcinogenic agent initiates a malignant transformation that requires an additional promoting agent for further specific growth of the malignancy. Thus, an individual is exposed at a specific point in time to an initiating agent that transforms the cell, and only after an interval of years does exposure to a promoting agent occur, which stimulates growth leading to a malignant tumor (Armenian, 1987; Berenblum, 1941). To these concepts must be added the potentially important roles of oncogenes and immunogenetics

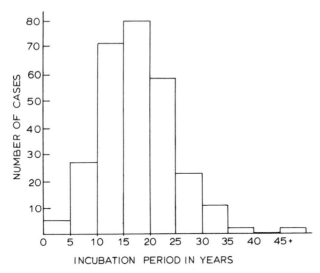

Figure 3–8. Distribution of incubation periods for 281 cases of bladder tumors among dyestuff workers. *Source:* Case et al. (1954).

in the genesis of cancer (Nowell, 1991). In cancer, the incubation period may result from the interaction between the growth of neoplastic cells and the development of immune responses by the host.

THE SPECTRUM OF DISEASE

The spectrum of disease may be defined as the sequence of events that occurs in the human organism from the time of exposure to the etiological agent until death, as shown in Figure 3–9 (Reimann, 1960). It has two broad components, subclinical and clinical. Whether an individual with the disease progresses through the entire spectrum depends upon the availability and efficacy of preventive and/or therapeutic measures that, if introduced at a particular point of the spectrum, will completely prevent or retard any further development of the disease. In the case of cancer of the cervix, the spectrum might consist of three main stages: dysplasia, carcinoma in situ, and invasive carcinoma. Similarly, cerebrovascular disease may have the following stages: atherosclerotic changes in carotid arteries, transient ischemic attacks, and stroke. The atherosclerotic changes in the carotid arteries are subclinical and can be ascertained only by special diagnostic tests such as carotid Doppler studies.

   In infectious diseases, this spectrum is usually known as the "gradient of infection," which refers to the sequence of manifestations of illness that reflect

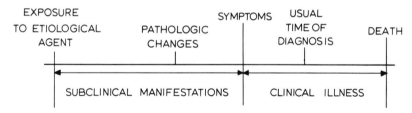

Figure 3–9.   Spectrum of disease.

the host's response to the infectious agent. This extends from ''inapparent infections'' at one extreme to death at the other (Figure 3–10). The frequency with which these different manifestations occur varies with the specific infectious disease. For example, in measles, the vast majority (over 90 percent) of infected persons exhibit clinical illness; in mumps, the proportion is somewhat less, approximately 66 percent; and in poliomyelitis, over 90 percent of the infections are not clinically apparent.

Clinicians and epidemiologists are usually only aware of a small part of the spectrum of a given disease or gradient of infection, the ''tip of the iceberg'' (Last, 1963). However, epidemiologists try to determine the entire range of the spectrum since it may provide a very different picture of a disease than that seen by clinicians in fully developed cases. Histoplasmosis is a case in point. From its first description in 1906 until the 1940s, histoplasmosis was regarded as a rare and usually fatal disease. Epidemiologic surveys by the Public Health Service in the 1940s, using the histoplasmosis skin test, completely changed this view. They revealed that most nonepidemic histoplasmosis infections produce no symptoms, or a mild influenzalike disorder, and rarely lead to a progressive systemic disease. In certain areas of the country (parts of Kentucky, Tennessee, Missouri, Indiana, Ohio, and Arkansas), the frequency of infection in the general population was found to be higher than 80 percent (Comstock, 1986). It should be emphasized that one of the major deterrents in elucidating the epidemiology of diseases of unknown etiology is the absence of methods to detect the subclinical state—the bottom of the ''iceberg.''

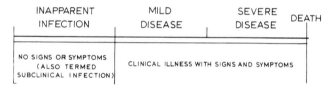

Figure 3–10.   Gradient of infection.

Inapparent infections are important because they play a role in the transmission of infectious agents. The spread of poliomyelitis, meningococcal meningitis, and other diseases can only be explained on this basis. To estimate the
number of individuals in the population who have become immune to the infectious agent, the frequency of these clinically inapparent infected persons must be
assessed by means of tests for antibodies or skin tests for a specific disease, if
available.

Epidemiologists have to consider the role of latent, as well as inapparent,
infections in the study of certain diseases, particularly viral diseases. Latent infection is distinguished from inapparent infection in that the host does not shed the
infectious agent, which lies dormant in the host cells. A viral disease may occur
early in life in one clinical form, and in later life, the dormant virus may produce
a different clinical disease due to some (as yet unknown) mechanism; these are
referred to as "slow virus diseases" (Fucillo, Kurent, and Sever, 1973; Gajdusek,
1977; Gajdusek and Gibbs, 1975). For example, investigations into the relationship of measles virus to subacute sclerosing panencephalitis suggest that the latter
may represent a late manifestation of measles infections and may be a slow virus
disease.

HERD IMMUNITY

Herd immunity is the resistance of a community to a disease (Last, 1990). Just
as individual immunity decreases the probability that an individual will develop
a particular disease when exposed to an infectious agent, "herd immunity" refers
to the decreased probability that a group or community will experience an epidemic after the introduction of an infectious agent, although some persons in the
group may be individually susceptible to the agent (Fox et al., 1971; Cliff et al.,
1981; Cliff and Haggett, 1984; Anderson and May, 1990). This concept is helpful
in understanding why an epidemic does not occur in a community and in explaining the periodic variation of some infectious diseases, particularly those that are
transmitted from one person to another. It also is useful in the formulation of
national vaccination policies. Herd immunity is measured in terms of the proportion of immune, or conversely, of susceptible, persons in a social group.
Clearly, the presence of a large proportion of immune individuals in a community
decreases the chances of contact between infected and susceptible persons. By
acting as a barrier between the two, the immune population decreases the rate of
spread of the infectious agent. The degree of herd immunity necessary to prevent
the development of an epidemic varies with the specific disease. It depends upon
such factors as the degree to which an infected individual is capable of transmit-

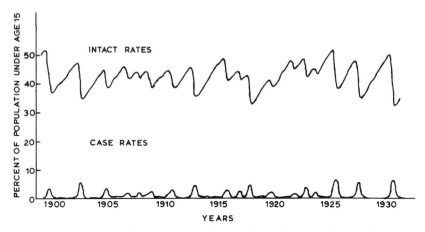

Figure 3-11. Estimated complete monthly attack rates from measles and intact rates (proportions not previously attacked for the population under fifteen, Old Baltimore, Md., July 1899–December 1931. *Source:* Hedrich (1933).

ting the infection, the length of time during which he is infectious, and the size and social behavior of the community.

The relationship between the proportion of susceptible individuals in a community and the periodicity of disease is illustrated by the analysis of case rates of measles in Baltimore for the period 1899–1931 (Figure 3–11) (Hedrich, 1933). The incidence of measles increases when the number of susceptible persons is highest and herd immunity is lowest. Mathematical models have shown that the smaller the community, the longer the interval between epidemics (Bartlett, 1957). (The smaller the community, the lower the probability of contact by a susceptible person with an infectious one.)

A very practical aspect of this concept of herd immunity is that an entire population (100 percent) does not have to be immunized to prevent the occurrence of an epidemic (Fox et al., 1971). For measles, for instance, Schlenker et al. (1992) suggested that transmission of the virus would stop if only 70 percent of the population were immunized. However, in the large metropolises of modern urban society, one must recognize that the interpersonal contacts necessary for the spread of an infectious agent occur in smaller neighborhood groups, not in the entire metropolis. Consequently, from the viewpoint of immunization and other public health practices, it is the herd immunity of these smaller groups that must be taken into consideration.

National differences in rubella vaccination policy illustrate the application of herd immunity. In the United States, girls and boys are vaccinated at around two years of age. This policy aims to block all transmission of the rubella virus and thereby prevent congenital rubella syndrome (CRS). However, there is no boosting of immunity by reexposure to the virus in the community. This policy is effective only if high levels of immunization are achieved (80–85 percent); in the United States, such high levels are met by requiring vaccination for school entry (Anderson and Nokes, 1991). Since 1964, when nationwide vaccination began, measles incidence has declined by more than 90 percent. CRS incidence has simlarly declined. In the United Kingdom, many other European countries, and Australia, a different approach has been taken: Girls are vaccinated at age 12 years. The result is natural immunity among children less than 12 years old and continued circulation of the virus in the community, allowing immunity to be boosted. Since the girls are vaccinated before menarche, CRS will presumably be prevented. This policy should be more effective at preventing CRS if the proportion of persons in the population who have been vaccinated is low (less than 60 percent), as was the case in the United Kingdom.

SUMMARY

The occurrence of disease reflects the interaction of the **agent,** the **host,** and the **environment.** The interaction may reflect a single exposure of a population to the agent, resulting in a **common-vehicle** outbreak. Another possibility is a disease spread by serial transfer of the agent from an affected individual to a susceptible host. Once the agent has been introduced to a susceptible host, a series of biological events takes place leading to either subclinical or clinically apparent disease. The gradient between a subclinical event and a severe clinical event (perhaps resulting in death) is the spectrum of disease. The time period from exposure to the agent until the appearance of clinical disease is the incubation period. Each disease has a characteristic incubation period. In the case of single-vehicle outbreaks, the incubation period is defined as the median time period from exposure to the agent until occurrence of the disease among all cases. The distribution of such time periods is known as the epidemic curve. It is log-normally distributed, regardless of whether the agent is infectious or noninfectious.

The concept of **herd immunity** provides a basis for population-based vaccination activities. As the proportion of the population immunized (either by previous exposure to the agent or by vaccination) increases, the opportunity for transmission of the agent within that population declines. For many infectious agents, the level of immunization within the population at which transmission ceases is less than 100 percent; it is as low as 70 percent in the case of measles. Herd immunity is one of the bases for current rubella vaccination policies in both the United Kingdom and the United States. The policy differences between these two countries reflect different levels of attained immunization in their respective populations.

STUDY PROBLEMS

1. Define the latency period for a non-infectious disease, such as ischemic heart disease or chronic obstructive lung disease. Give an example of a latency period.

2. Contrast the epidemic curves encountered in:
   (a) a common-vehicle single-exposure outbreak,
   (b) a common-vehicle continuous-exposure outbreak,
   (c) a serial-transfer propagated epidemic,
   (d) an outbreak resulting from a slow-virus disease.

3. Of what importance is the concept of herd immunity to the public health administrator?

4. Subclinical cases have always posed a problem in investigating the etiology of both infectious and noninfectious diseases. Discuss the reasons for this.

5. Hall and Barker (1984) noted that the distribution of the age of onset of Legg-Perthes disease (avascular necrosis of the head of the femur in children) in several case series was a log-normal one. What does this observation imply about the causal agent?

6. One often hears that there is a sexually transmitted disease epidemic in the United States today. Into what category (e.g., common vehicle, serial transfer) would you classify this epidemic?

7. A local health officer in a small community received reports from three physicians that they were taking care of persons who had diarrhea, abdominal cramps, vomiting, chills, and fever. From stools collected from several patients, a strain of salmonella (S. typhimurium) was isolated. A total of 119 patients were identified and the times of onset of the disease in this group were tabulated as follows:

JANUARY 7		JANUARY 8		JANUARY 9	
TIME	NO. OF ILL PERSONS	TIME	NO. OF ILL PERSONS	TIME	NO. OF ILL PERSONS
6–7 A.M.	2	12–1 A.M.	5	12–1 A.M.	3
8–9 A.M.	5	2–3 A.M.	3	2–3 A.M.	2
10–11 A.M.	11	4–5 A.M.	3	4–5 A.M.	0
12–1 P.M.	18	6–7 A.M.	3	6–7 A.M.	1
2–3 P.M.	10	8–9 A.M.	4	8–9 A.M.	0
4–5 P.M.	7	10–11 A.M.	6	10–11 A.M.	1
6–7 P.M.	5	12–1 P.M.	8	12–1 P.M.	0
8–9 P.M.	4	2–3 P.M.	4	2–3 P.M.	0
10–11 P.M.	4	4–5 P.M.	3		

JANUARY 7		JANUARY 8		JANUARY 9	
TIME	NO. OF ILL PERSONS	TIME	NO. OF ILL PERSONS	TIME	NO. OF ILL PERSONS
		6–7 P.M.	3		
		8–9 P.M.	2		
		10–11 P.M.	2		

(a) Make a graph of the epidemic curve.

(b) What type of outbreak does this curve resemble? Why?

(c) What are the possible reasons for the bimodality of this epidemic curve?

(d) Describe the investigation that the health officer should conduct.

8. Rose (1982) has noted that strong correlations could be found between serum cholesterol concentrations and systolic blood pressure measurements in 1958–1964 in men, ages 40–59, in population samples from Finland, Greece, Italy, Japan, the Netherlands, the United States, and Yugoslavia, and subsequent national mortality from coronary heart disease 10 years later. Both serum cholesterol concentration and systolic blood pressure are known risk factors for coronary heart disease. What does this finding imply about the latency period of coronary heart disease? What would be the next step in such an investigation?

REFERENCES

Anderson, R. M., and May, R. M. 1990. "Immunisation and herd immunity." *Lancet* 335: 641–645.

Anderson, R. M., and Nokes, D. J. 1991. "Mathematical models of transmission and control." In *Oxford Textbook of Public Health.* Second Edition. W. W. Holland, R. Detels, and G. Knox, eds. Oxford: Oxford University Press.

Armenian, H. K., 1987. "Incubation periods of cancer: old and new." *J. Chron. Dis.* 40(Suppl 2):9S–15S.

Armenian, H. K., and Khoury, M. J. 1981. "Age at onset of genetic diseases." *Am. J. Epidemiol.* 113:596–605.

Armenian, H. K., and Lilienfeld, A. M. 1974. "The distribution of incubation periods of neoplastic diseases." *Amer. J. Epid.* 99:92–100.

———. 1983. "Incubation period of disease." *Epi. Rev.* 5:1–15.

Bartlett, M. S. 1957. "Measles periodicity and community size." *J. Roy. Stat. Soc.* 120: 48–70.

Benenson, A. S. 1990. *Control of Communicable Diseases in Man.* 15th Edition. New York: American Public Health Association.

Berenblum, I. 1941. "The mechanism of carcinogenesis. A study of the significance of cocarcinogenic action and related phenomena." *Cancer Res.* 1:807–814.

Burnet, M., and White, D. O. 1972. *Natural History of Infectious Disease.* 4th Edition. Cambridge, England: Cambridge University Press.

Case, R.A.M., Hosker, M. E., McDonald, D. B., and Pearson, J. T. 1954. "Tumours of the urinary bladder in workmen engaged in the manufacture and use of certain dyestuff intermediates in the British industry. Part I. The role of aniline, benzidine, alphanapthylamine and beta-naphthalamine." *Brit. J. Ind. Med.* 11:75–104.

Cliff, A., and Haggett, P. 1984. "Island epidemics." *Sci. Am.* 250(5):138–147.

Cliff, A. D., Haggett, P., Ord, J. K., and Versey, G. R. 1981. *Spatial Diffusion. An Historical Geography of Epidemics in an Island Community.* Cambridge: Cambridge University Press.

Cobb, S., Miller, N., and Wald, N. 1959. "On the estimation of the incubation period in malignant disease." *J. Chron. Dis.* 9:385–393.

Comstock, G. W. 1986. "Histoplasmosis." In *Maxcy-Rosenau Preventive Medicine and Public Health.* 10th Edition. J. Last, ed. New York: Appleton-Century-Crofts.

Diamond, E. L., Schmerler, H., and Lilienfeld, A. M. 1973. "The relationship of intrauterine radiation to subsequent mortality and development of leukemia in children: a cohort study." *Amer. J. Epidemiol.* 97:283–313.

Doll, R. 1971. "The age distribution of cancer: implications for models of carcinogenesis." *J. Roy. Stat. Soc.* 134:133–166.

Fox, J. P., Elveback, L., Scott, W., Gatewood, L., and Ackerman, E. 1971. "Herd immunity: basic concept and relevance to public health immunization practices." *Amer. J. Epidemiol.* 94:179–189.

Fracasatoro, H. 1930. *De contagione et contagiosis morbis et eorum curatione, Libri III.* Translation and notes by W. C. Wright. New York: G. P. Putnam and Sons.

Fucillo, D. A., Kurent, J. E., and Sever, J. L. 1974. "Slow virus diseases." *Ann. Rev. Microbiol.* 28:231–264.

Gajdusek, D. C. 1977. "Unconventional viruses and the origin and disappearance of kuru." *Science* 197:943–960.

Gajdusek, D. C., and Gibbs, C. J. 1975. "Slow virus infections of the nervous system and the laboratories of slow, latent, and temperate virus infections." In *The Nervous System, Vol. 2,* D. B. Tower, ed. New York: Raven Press, pp. 113–135.

Graham, S., Levin, M. L., Lilienfeld, A. M., Schuman, L. M., Gibson, R., Dowd, J. E., and Hempelman, L. 1966. "Preconception, intrauterine, and postnatal irradiation as related to leukemia." In *Epidemiological Approaches to the Study of Cancer and Other Chronic Diseases.* W. Haenszel, ed. National Cancer Institute Monograph No. 19. Washington, D.C.: United States Government Printing Office.

Hall, A. J., Barker, D.J.P. 1984. "The age distribution of Legg-Perthes disease: an analysis using Sartwell's incubation period model." *Am. J. Epidemiol.* 120:531–536.

Hedrich, A. W. 1933. "Monthly estimates of the child population 'susceptible' to measles, 1900–1931, Baltimore, Md." *Amer. J. Hyg.* 17:613–636.

Hess, A. D., and Holden, P. 1958. "The natural history of the arthropod-borne encephalitides in the United States." *Ann. N.Y. Acad. Sci.* 70:294–311.

Hewitt, D. 1955. "Some features of leukemia mortality." *Brit. J. Prev. Soc. Med.* 9:81–88.

Kato, H. 1971. "Mortality in children exposed to A-bombs while *in utero,* 1945–1969." *Amer. J. Epidemiol.* 93:435–442.

Last, J. M. 1963. "The iceberg: completing the clinical picture in general practice." *Lancet* 2:28–31.

————. 1990. *Dictionary of Epidemiology,* 2nd ed. New York: Oxford University Press.

MacMahon, B. 1962. "Prenatal X-ray exposure and childhood cancer." *J. Nat. Cancer Inst.* 28:1173–1191.

Nowell, P. C. 1991. "How many cancer genes?" *J. Nat. Cancer Inst.* 83:1061–1064.

Pike, M. C. 1966. "A method of analysis of a certain class of experiments in carcinogenesis." *Biometrics* 22:142–161.

Polednak, A. P. 1974. "Latency periods in neoplastic diseases." *Amer. J. Epidemiol.* 100: 354–356.

Reimann, H. A. 1960. "Spectrums of infectious disease." *Arch. Int. Med.* 105:779–815.

Rose, G. 1982. "Incubation period of coronary heart disease." *Br. Med. J.* 284:1600–1601.

Sartwell, P. E. 1950. "The distribution of incubation periods of infectious disease." *Amer. J. Hyg.* 51:310–318.

————. 1966. "The incubation period and the dynamics of infectious disease." *Amer. J. Epid.* 83:204–216.

Schlenker, T. L., Bain, C., Baughman, A. L., Hadler, S. C. 1992. "The association of attack rates with immunization rates in preschool children." *JAMA* 267:823–826.

Stewart, A., Webb, J., and Hewitt, D. 1958. "A survey of childhood malignancies." *Brit. Med. J.* 1:1495–1508.

II

DEMOGRAPHIC STUDIES

Chapters 4, 5, 6, and 7 deal with the conduct and interpretation of **demographic studies.** Demographic studies, focused on the occurrence of disease in *populations,* search for associations between disease frequency and the presence or absence of possible etiologic agents in those populations. These studies address such issues as whether a disease is increasing or decreasing in the population and whether the disease occurs more often in populations that have greater exposure to a potential cause. Also, the means by which the epidemiologist can assess the health status of a population from the perspective of morbidity and mortality are encompassed in the demographic study. Since demographic studies often can be conducted by using readily available vital and health statistics, they are often inexpensive and may be used as the first test of an etiologic hypothesis. **Epidemiologic studies,** in contrast, concentrate on the occurrence of disease among *individuals* in relation to possible risk factors and therefore are generally more expensive than demographic studies.

Chapter 4 shows how mortality statistics are assembled and describes the advantages and problems of working with such data. The means by which epidemiologists contend with the difficulties are also discussed. Chapter 5 addresses the use of mortality data. Such issues as the validity of mortality data, the assessment of temporal information about mortality in the population, and the demographic characteristics (e.g., age, sex, and race) of those who die from the disease are discussed. Although mortality data are often of direct interest to the epidemiologist, they can also serve as proxies for morbidity information about a population.

Chapter 6 applies many of the ideas presented in Chapters 4 and 5 to morbidity statistics. The possible sources of morbidity data (e.g., surveillance) are reviewed, with an emphasis on the cross-sectional survey. Ongoing national surveys, which provide information on the health status of a population, are also described. The accuracy and validity of survey data are important considerations in their use. The concepts of sensitivity and specificity of diagnostic tests are considered, as are their positive and negative predictive value. These four measures of screening and diagnostic test performance are important to both the clinician and the epidemiologist. Another measure of test performance, kappa (K), provides information on inter- and intra-observer variability, two sources of error in the interpretation of clinical data.

The means of analyzing morbidity data are discussed in Chapter 7. Examples of how such data provide important clues to the etiology of various diseases are presented. Usually the epidemiologist focuses on time, place, and persons. Sometimes a disease may occur in a cluster, defined either by time or by place. Even when examining the occurrence of clusters, however, the epidemiologist must remember that demographic studies may only suggest a hypothesis regarding the cause of a disease or provide an initial test of a hypothesis. For a more definitive assessment of a hypothesis, an epidemiologic study (discussed in Part III), in which the association between disease occurrence and exposure to a possible agent is assessed in individuals, is necessary.

4

MORTALITY STATISTICS

> Anyone can stop a man's life, but no one his death; a
> thousand doors open on to it.
> SENECA, Phoenissae, 152

The study of mortality provides information that may prevent early and perhaps needless deaths. What are the leading causes of death? How do they differ around the world and what are the important determinants of early death? These are the kinds of questions epidemiologists ask in an effort to diagnose the health problems of the community and generate hypotheses about the causes of those diseases that are important contributors to premature mortality. As biologists we recognize the inevitability of death, but as medical scientists we strive to delay it and to improve the quality of the longer life we seek. The study of mortality patterns is a fruitful way to pursue these goals.

SOURCES OF MORTALITY DATA

Death certificates were introduced not for epidemiologic studies, but rather as legal documents. Graunt's use of the Bills of Mortality and Farr's adaptation of the Registration System to portray the health and social conditions of the population (Chapter 2) initiated the broad epidemiologic use of data that were regularly collected. Although this chapter deals with mortality statistics, it should be noted that these are only part of a system of vital records existing today in most developed countries. In addition to deaths, such vital events as births, marriages, and divorces are also recorded. Such reporting systems, however, are most highly developed for births and deaths.

National death registration has been legally mandated in England and Wales since 1837. Mortality data are now compiled by the Office of Population Censuses and Surveys (OPCS), which regularly reports the annual tabulations of deaths, their causes, and the demographic characteristics (e.g., age, gender, residence) of those who died.

In 1902 the collection of copies of death certificates by a permanent U.S. Bureau of Census began as an annual procedure in ten states and in several additional cities that had an adequate registration system, thereby creating a Death Registration Area (Cassedy, 1965). This Area was predominantly urban and included about 40 percent of the U.S. population (Dorn, 1966). By 1933, the Death Registration Area covered the entire United States, and when Alaska and Hawaii became states they also entered this data system. These changes in the denominator may have affected mortality statistics in the United States over this century.

CLASSIFICATION OF CAUSE OF DEATH

A standard death certificate developed by the National Center for Health Statistics has been adopted, with only minor modifications, by most states (Figure 4–1); there is a separate certificate for fetal deaths. Information is requested on demographic factors such as place of residence, occupation, national origin, age, and sex, as well as cause of death. The cause of death as stated on the certificate must be accepted with caution. Figure 4–1 shows that the immediate cause is entered first, then any intermediate conditions, and finally the underlying cause. A separate space allows for the inclusion of other significant conditions. (In other countries, a similar death certificate, modeled on one developed by the World Health Organization, is used.) In official tabulations, the cause of death is, in fact, the underlying cause, classified according to the International Statistical Classification of Diseases, Injuries and Causes of Death (ICD), which is revised about every eight or ten years by the World Health Organization. Changes in ICD classification or patterns of diagnosis can cause artifactual changes in mortality trends.

A problem develops when the physician enters two or more causes on the death certificate. Before 1949, a *Manual of Joint Causes of Death,* specifying rules for assigning priorities to various causes, was used to assure standardization for selecting the cause of death based on both the sequence of pathophysiologic events accepted at the time and the information required for public health programs. This manual was updated periodically but ended when the sixth ICD revision was adopted in 1949 and the physician became responsible for determining the underlying cause of death. These changing methods of tabulating causes of death have affected the mortality trends of certain diseases, such as diabetes; but, for most diseases, the effects have been small (Dunn and Shackley,

1945; Faust and Dolman, 1963; Faust, 1964, 1965). Still, these facts must be kept in mind when interpreting mortality statistics.

The use of a single cause of death for routine statistical tabulations has been criticized as not providing a complete representation of events (Krueger, 1966). It has been suggested that epidemiologists should really be interested in "those diseases that one dies with as well as from," i.e., a listing of multiple causes of death. Since 1978, multiple cause-of-death data have been available for all recorded deaths in the United States after 1968. Table 4–1 shows the number of deaths in the United States in 1979 in which selected causes of death were stated. For some diseases, such as hypertension, angina pectoris, and nutritional deficiencies, the condition is more often reported as a nonunderlying cause than as an underlying one. Other diseases, however, are mentioned on the death certificate more frequently as an underlying cause. In other countries, multiple cause-of-death data have recently been made available, i.e., for the years 1985 and 1986 in England and Wales.

Because the physician completing the death certificate may not have been the attending physician and therefore would be unfamiliar with the deceased's medical history, the reliability of statements of causes of death can be less than optimal. Even if an autopsy is performed, the results may not be available in time to be entered on the death certificate (which is required for burial).

Many studies have been conducted to evaluate the accuracy of the cause-of-death statements on the certificate (James et al., 1955; Moriyama et al., 1958; Moriyama et al., 1966; Pohlen and Emerson, 1942; Pohlen, 1943). With AIDS, for example, underreporting of the underlying cause of death on the death certificate has been noted (Hardy et al., 1987). On the other hand, overreporting occurs for stroke. In about 40 percent of deaths attributed to stroke in one study in Framingham, Massachusetts, no evidence of a stroke could be found (Corwin et al., 1982). Other studies have shown that differences among physicians in evaluating the same case histories lead to variation in the underlying cause of death stated on the death certificate (Moriyama, 1989; Moussa et al., 1990; Benavides et al., 1989).

Mortality data may be collected from sources other than death certificates such as autopsy, hospital, occupational, and financial records (e.g., insurance, pension funds). Death certificates can be linked to other data bases to form records that contain information about occupational history, outpatient pharmaceutical use, parental background, or hospital treatment before death. The National Death Index (NDI) is a computer file of all deaths in the United States and it can be linked to other databases through combinations of the Social Security number, name, and date of birth. This system began in 1979, but mortality databases have existed in other countries for decades; the Canadian mortality database was founded in 1950 (Last, 1987). All infant death certificate records (deaths occurring

STATE OF MARYLAND / DEPARTMENT OF HEALTH AND MENTAL HYGIENE
CERTIFICATE OF DEATH

REG. NO.

FOR STATE REGISTRAR

1 -

TO BE COMPLETED BY FUNERAL DIRECTOR

1. DECEDENT'S NAME (First, Middle, Last)

2. DATE OF DEATH MONTH DAY YEAR

3. TIME OF DEATH M

4. SOCIAL SECURITY NUMBER

5. SEX 1 ☐ M 2 ☐ F

6. AGE (In yrs. last birthday) YRS.

IF UNDER 1 YEAR MONTHS DAYS

IF UNDER 24 HRS. HOURS MIN.

7. DATE OF BIRTH (Month, Day, Year)

8. BIRTHPLACE (State or Foreign Country)

9a. FACILITY NAME (If not institution, give street and number)

9b. CITY, TOWN OR LOCATION OF DEATH

9c. COUNTY OF DEATH

RESIDENCE OF DECEDENT

10a. STATE

10b. COUNTY

10c. CITY, TOWN OR LOCATION

10d. INSIDE CITY LIMITS? 1 ☐ YES 2 ☐ NO

10e. STREET AND NUMBER

10f. ZIP CODE

10g. CITIZEN OF WHAT COUNTRY?

11. MARITAL STATUS
1 ☐ Never Married 2 ☐ Married
3 ☐ Widowed 4 ☐ Divorced

12. WAS DECEDENT EVER IN U.S. ARMED FORCES? 1 ☐ YES 2 ☐ NO
IF YES, GIVE WAR OR DATES

13. WAS DECEDENT OF HISPANIC ORIGIN? (Specify Yes or No—If yes, specify Cuban, Mexican, Puerto Rican, etc.)
1 ☐ YES 2 ☐ NO Specify

14. RACE — American Indian, Black, White, etc.
Specify

15. DECEDENT'S EDUCATION (Specify only highest grade completed)
Elementary/Secondary (0-12)   College (1-4 or 5 +)

16a. DECEDENT'S USUAL OCCUPATION (Give kind of work done during most of working life. Do NOT use retired.)

16b. KIND OF BUSINESS/INDUSTRY

17. FATHER'S NAME (First, Middle, Last)

18. MOTHER'S NAME (First, Middle, Maiden Surname)

19a. INFORMANT'S NAME (Type/Print)

19b. MAILING ADDRESS (Street and Number or Rural Route Number, City or Town, State, Zip Code)

20a. METHOD OF DISPOSITION
1 ☐ Burial 2 ☐ Cremation 3 ☐ Removal from State
4 ☐ Donation 5 ☐ Other (Specify)

20b. PLACE OF DISPOSITION (Name of cemetery, crematory or other place)

20c. LOCATION — City or Town, State

21. SIGNATURE OF FUNERAL SERVICE LICENSEE

22. NAME AND ADDRESS OF FACILITY

▲

62

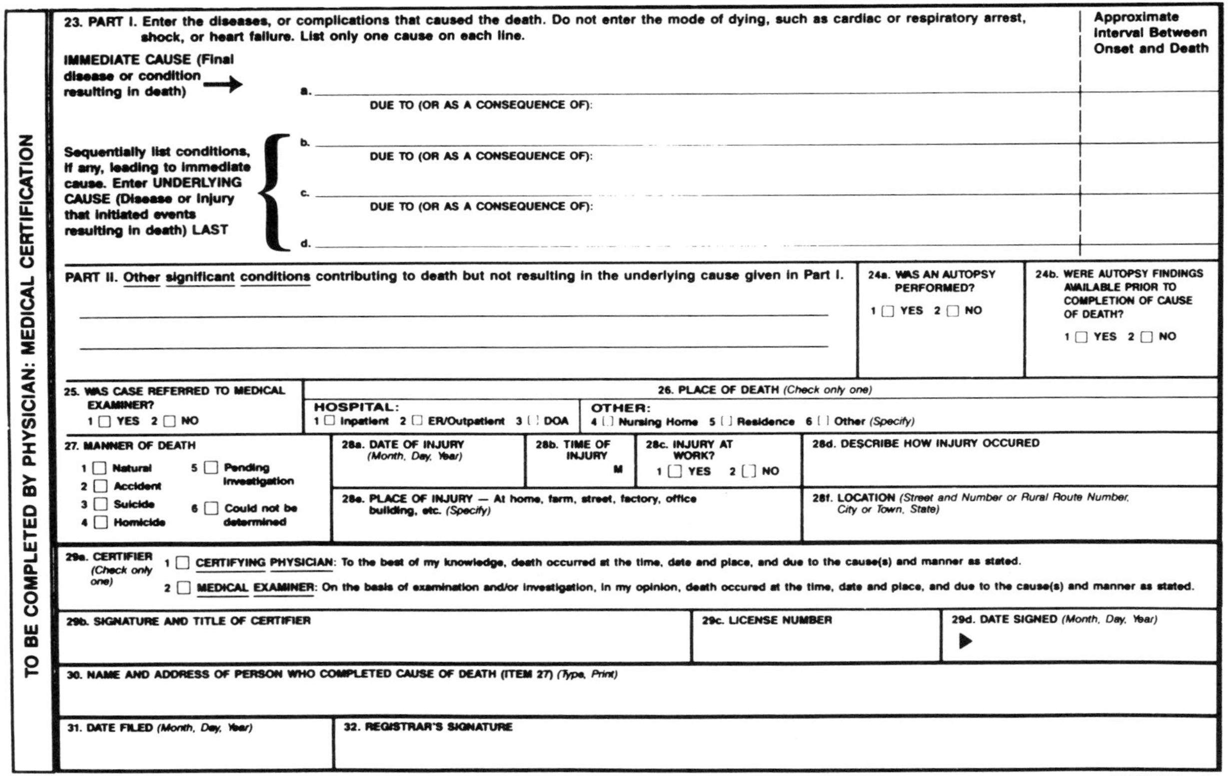

23. PART I. Enter the diseases, or complications that caused the death. Do not enter the mode of dying, such as cardiac or respiratory arrest, shock, or heart failure. List only one cause on each line.

Approximate interval Between Onset and Death

IMMEDIATE CAUSE (Final disease or condition resulting in death) →

a. _____ DUE TO (OR AS A CONSEQUENCE OF):

Sequentially list conditions, if any, leading to immediate cause. Enter UNDERLYING CAUSE (Disease or injury that initiated events resulting in death) LAST

b. _____ DUE TO (OR AS A CONSEQUENCE OF):

c. _____ DUE TO (OR AS A CONSEQUENCE OF):

d. _____

PART II. Other significant conditions contributing to death but not resulting in the underlying cause given in Part I.

24a. WAS AN AUTOPSY PERFORMED?
1 ☐ YES   2 ☐ NO

24b. WERE AUTOPSY FINDINGS AVAILABLE PRIOR TO COMPLETION OF CAUSE OF DEATH?
1 ☐ YES   2 ☐ NO

25. WAS CASE REFERRED TO MEDICAL EXAMINER?
1 ☐ YES   2 ☐ NO

26. PLACE OF DEATH (Check only one)
HOSPITAL:
1 ☐ Inpatient   2 ☐ ER/Outpatient   3 ☐ DOA
OTHER:
4 ☐ Nursing Home   5 ☐ Residence   6 ☐ Other (Specify)

27. MANNER OF DEATH
1 ☐ Natural
2 ☐ Accident
3 ☐ Suicide
4 ☐ Homicide
5 ☐ Pending investigation
6 ☐ Could not be determined

28a. DATE OF INJURY (Month, Day, Year)

28b. TIME OF INJURY
M

28c. INJURY AT WORK?
1 ☐ YES   2 ☐ NO

28d. DESCRIBE HOW INJURY OCCURRED

28e. PLACE OF INJURY — At home, farm, street, factory, office building, etc. (Specify)

28f. LOCATION (Street and Number or Rural Route Number, City or Town, State)

29a. CERTIFIER (Check only one)
1 ☐ CERTIFYING PHYSICIAN: To the best of my knowledge, death occurred at the time, date and place, and due to the cause(s) and manner as stated.
2 ☐ MEDICAL EXAMINER: On the basis of examination and/or investigation, in my opinion, death occurred at the time, date and place, and due to the cause(s) and manner as stated.

29b. SIGNATURE AND TITLE OF CERTIFIER

29c. LICENSE NUMBER

29d. DATE SIGNED (Month, Day, Year)

30. NAME AND ADDRESS OF PERSON WHO COMPLETED CAUSE OF DEATH (ITEM 27) (Type, Print)

31. DATE FILED (Month, Day, Year)

32. REGISTRAR'S SIGNATURE

TO BE COMPLETED BY PHYSICIAN: MEDICAL CERTIFICATION

DHMH-16 Rev 1/89

Figure 4–1. Maryland Certificate of Death.

Table 4-1. Number of Deaths with Any Mention of Specified Causes, with Specified Causes as Underlying Cause of Death, and Ratio of Reported to Underlying Cause in the United States, 1979 (examples from the National Center for Health Statistics "List of 72 Selected Causes of Death")

CAUSE OF DEATH (ICD–9 CODES)*	DEATHS WITH ANY MENTION OF SPECIFIED CAUSE	SELECTED AS UNDERLYING CAUSE	RATIO OF ANY MENTION TO UNDERLYING CAUSE
Septicemia (038)	52,154	8,024	6.50
Syphilis (090–097)	565	180	3.14
Malignant neoplasms of all other and unspecified sites (170–173, 190–199)	199,546	48,591	4.11
Diabetes mellitus (250)	128,373	33,192	3.87
Nutritional deficiencies (260–269)	22,111	2,210	10.00
Anemias (280–285)	27,465	3,171	8.66
Hypertension with and without heart disease ((401,403)	77,819	7,275	10.70
Angina pectoris (413)	4,113	500	8.23
All other forms of heart disease (415–423, 425–429)	675,733	142,942	4.73
Cerebral embolism (434.1)	3,314	850	3.90
Atherosclerosis (440)	160,086	28,801	5.56
Acute bronchitis and bronchiolitis (466)	1,846	554	3.33
Pneumonia (486)	147,089	44,426	3.31
Hernia of abdominal cavity and intestinal obstruction without mention of hernia (550–553, 560)	19,397	5,349	3.63
Hyperplasia of prostate (600)	4,096	810	5.06

*International Classification of Diseases, Ninth Revision.

Source: Israel et al., 1986.

in the first year of life) are linked to birth records in the United States and in many other countries to produce a set of data on maternal characteristics (i.e., age and pregnancy history), infant characteristics at birth (birth weight and other data), and cause of death.

Autopsy data, hospital records, and other sources of mortality data may provide accurate information about details omitted from death certificates, but they may not represent the general population. For example, autopsy series are selected from a hospital population but are not representative of that population or of the general population (Mainland, 1953; McMahan, 1962; Waife et al., 1952).

In view of such bias in selection, it may be impossible to correlate an autopsy series with any well-defined population at risk and therefore impossible to use such data to estimate the frequency of a disease. Despite the limitations of autopsy series for determining the frequency of a disease in a population, inferences made from an analysis of autopsy series may provide useful leads for more refined epidemiologic studies. For example, the observation that the relative proportion of lung cancer in different series of autopsies was increasing with time, and that the ratio of squamous cell carcinoma to adenocarcinoma was also increasing (while the proportion of adenocarcinoma remained fairly constant), led to the hypothesis that the total increase of lung cancer might be limited to squamous cell carcinoma (Cornfield et al., 1959; Kreyberg, 1954, 1962). Subsequent mortality and morbidity studies confirmed this.

MEASURES OF MORTALITY

Mortality Rates

The most frequently used measure of mortality is the mortality rate or death rate, which has three essential elements:

1. A specifically defined population group—the denominator.
2. A time period.
3. The number of deaths occurring in that population group during that time period—the numerator.

The numerator of the rate is the number of deaths that occurred in the specified population and the denominator is obtained either from a census or from estimates of that population:

$$\begin{array}{l}\text{Annual death rate} \\ \text{from all causes} \\ \text{(per 1,000} \\ \text{population)}\end{array} = \dfrac{\begin{array}{l}\text{Total number of deaths during} \\ \text{a specified twelve-month period}\end{array}}{\begin{array}{l}\text{Number of persons in the} \\ \text{population at the middle of the} \\ \text{period}\end{array}} \times 1,000$$

The numerator and denominator are related to each other in that the numerator represents those individuals who died, and the denominator those who were at risk of death. For example, in 1988, in the United States there were 2,167,999 deaths in a population of 245,807,000. Thus:

$$\begin{array}{l}\text{Annual death rate} \\ \text{in 1988 (per} \\ \text{1,000 population)}\end{array} = \dfrac{\text{2,167,999 deaths during 1988}}{\begin{array}{l}\text{245,807,000 persons estimated} \\ \text{alive on July 1, 1988}\end{array}} \times 1,000 = \begin{array}{l}\text{8.8 deaths per} \\ \text{1,000 population}\end{array}$$

The "crude" or unadjusted death rate is expressed in terms of a single year and a population of 1,000. The unit of time or the population can be selected by the investigator, but they should be specified. These rates can be made explicit for a variety of characteristics, such as age, gender, marital status, ethnicity, and specific causes. Two examples are shown below.

$$\begin{array}{l}\text{Annual age-specific death} \\ \text{rate from all causes for} \\ \text{those less than 1 yr of age in} \\ \text{1988 (per 1,000 population)}\end{array} = \dfrac{\begin{array}{l}\text{Number of deaths of individuals less than} \\ \text{1 yr of age in 1988}\end{array}}{\begin{array}{l}\text{Number of individuals in the} \\ \text{population less than 1 on July 1, 1988}\end{array}}$$

$$= \dfrac{\text{38,910 deaths}}{\text{3,859,000 persons}} \times 1,000$$

$$= 10.1 \text{ deaths per 1,000 population less than 1} \\ \text{year of age}$$

$$\begin{array}{l}\text{Annual death rate from lung} \\ \text{cancer in 1989 (per 100,000} \\ \text{population)}\end{array} = \dfrac{\text{Number of deaths from lung cancer in 1989}}{\begin{array}{l}\text{Number of persons in the population on} \\ \text{July 1, 1989}\end{array}}$$

$$= \dfrac{\text{133,284 deaths}}{\text{245,807,000 persons}} \times 100,000$$

$$= 54.2 \text{ deaths per 100,000 population}$$

Another type of rate, frequently and incorrectly termed a "mortality rate" in the clinical literature, is the "case-fatality rate":

$$\text{Case fatality rate} \atop \text{(percent)} = \frac{\begin{array}{l}\text{Number of individuals dying during a} \\ \text{specified period of time after} \\ \text{disease onset or diagnosis}\end{array}}{\begin{array}{l}\text{Number of individuals with the} \\ \text{specified disease during that} \\ \text{period of time}\end{array}} \times 100$$

This rate represents the risk of dying during a defined period of time for those individuals who have a particular disease. Again, the period of time during which the deaths occurred should be specified. Case-fatality rates can also be made specific for age, gender, severity of disease, and any other factors of clinical and epidemiologic importance.

The proportionate mortality rate or ratio (PMR), which represents the proportion of total deaths that are due to a specific cause, is also frequently used:

$$\text{Proportionate U.S. mortality} \atop \text{rate from cardiovascular} \atop \text{diseases in 1993} = \frac{\begin{array}{l}\text{Number of U.S. deaths from} \\ \text{cardiovascular diseases in 1993}\end{array}}{\text{Total U.S. deaths in 1993}} \times 100$$

This rate is often multiplied by one hundred and expressed as a percentage, but it may also be expressed as a decimal fraction.

The proportionate mortality rate does not directly measure the risk or probability that a person in a population will die from a specific disease, as does a cause-specific mortality rate. To illustrate its limitation, let us assume that there are two countries, A and B, each with a population of one million. Furthermore, Country A had a death rate from all causes of death of 30 per 100,000 population in 1993, representing 300 deaths, and Country B had an all-cause death rate of 10 per 100,000 in 1993, representing 100 deaths. Each country had the same death rate from cardiovascular diseases of 5 per 100,000, representing 50 deaths, and a person's risk of dying from cardiovascular disease in each country was therefore the same. The proportionate mortality rates expressed as the percentage of all deaths from cardiovascular diseases in each country would then be as follows:

$$\text{Country A:} \quad \frac{50}{300} = 17 \text{ percent}$$

$$\text{Country B:} \quad \frac{50}{100} = 50 \text{ percent}$$

Clearly, this difference in proportionate mortality rates does not reflect the risk of dying from cardiovascular diseases in these countries—which is the same— but the difference in mortality from *other* causes of death. However, the proportionate mortality rate shows *within* any population group the relative importance of specific causes of death in the total mortality picture. This rate is useful to the epidemiologist in selecting areas for further study and to the health administrator in determining priorities for planning purposes.

Age Adjustment of Mortality Rates

Age is one of the main determinants of mortality (Figure 4–2). The age composition of a population will influence the total mortality rate; thus it is preferable to compare age-specific mortality rates in different geographical areas, population groups, or time periods. However, it is often useful to have a summary statistic of such comparisons that takes into account the differences in the age distribution of the population. This is accomplished by ''age adjustment'' or ''age standardization.'' Of the several summary statistics that are available, two will be described here: the *direct* method of age adjustment, and the *indirect* method, the Standardized Mortality Ratio (SMR). Although age adjustment and standardization were originally developed to analyze and present mortality statistics and still are frequently used for this purpose, they can be applied to other types of rates such as morbidity or fertility rates. The same methods of adjustment can be used for taking into account other factors such as age, gender, social class, number of cigarettes smoked, or size of family.

An Example of Age Adjustment: Mortality Rates in Alaska and Florida

The overall or ''crude'' (not adjusted for age) mortality rates for Florida and Alaska in 1988 were 1,062.4 and 393.9 per 100,000, respectively (Table 4–2), and one's first conclusion is that the forces of mortality are stronger in Florida than in Alaska. The two states have very different age distributions, however (Figure 4–3); Florida is a retirement state for many elderly people, and Alaska draws many young people.

In the direct method of standardization, one applies the age-specific death rates from two populations with different age structures (Florida and Alaska) to a third ''standard'' population (e.g., the 1988 U.S. population). One multiplies the age-specific death rates from Florida and Alaska by the numbers in that age group for the U.S. population to produce an expected number of deaths in the standard population. The expected numbers of deaths are totaled and divided by the total standard population, in this case the total U.S. population, to produce a

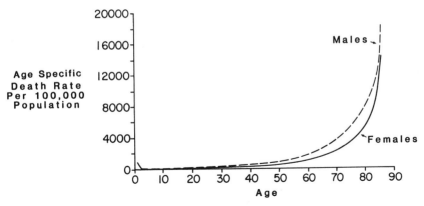

Figure 4–2. Age-specific death rates by sex, United States, 1987. *Source:* Vital Statistics of the United States (1990).

summary rate (the age-adjusted mortality rate) that would represent Florida and Alaska if each had the same age structure as the standard population. In this example, Florida would have an overall death rate of 812.0 per 100,000 population, not much different from Alaska's 764.4 or the U.S. overall rate of 882.0 (Table 4–3). Thus, the effect of the different age distributions is "adjusted" between the two states.

To use the indirect method of standardization, one applies the age-specific death rates from a standard population (here we used the death rates for the 1988 U.S. population) to the age-specific populations for Florida and Alaska. Multiplying death rates by population totals, one calculates the number of deaths in Florida and Alaska that might be expected if their populations were subjected to the same mortality experience as that of the standard population. Then one totals the age-specific expected deaths and compares them to the observed deaths; the expected number divided by the observed number multiplied by 100 produces the standardized mortality ratio (SMR). If the observed mortality is the same as expected, the SMR will be 100. An SMR greater than 100 indicates that mortality is higher than expected, and an SMR less than 100 indicates the opposite. In this

Table 4–2.   Crude Mortality Rates in Florida and Alaska in 1988

	FLORIDA	ALASKA
Number of deaths	131,044	2,064
Total population	12,335,000	524,000
Crude (or overall) mortality rates	1,062.4 deaths per 100,000	393.9 deaths per 100,000

Source: Vital Statistics of the United States (1991).

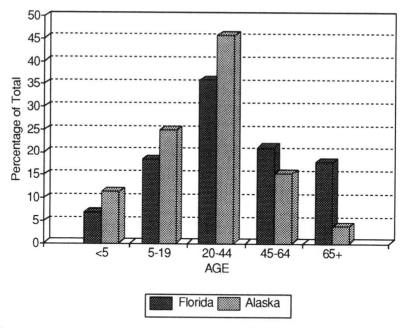

Figure 4–3. Percentage distribution of age groups in the Florida and Alaska populations, 1988. *Source:* Vital Statistics of the United States (1991)

Table 4–3. Age-Adjusted Mortality Rates for Florida and Alaska, 1988, Calculated by Direct Method

| | AGE-SPECIFIC DEATH RATES/100,000 | | U.S. POP. | EXPECTED NUMBER OF DEATHS | |
AGE GROUPS	FLORIDA	ALASKA	(MILLIONS)	FLORIDA	ALASKA
<5	284	274	18.3	52,000	50,000
5–19	57	65	52.9	30,000	34,000
20–44	198	188	98.1	194,000	184,000
45–64	815	629	46.0	375,000	289,000
>65	4425	4350	30.4	1,345,000	1,322,000
			Total 245.7	1,996,000	1,879,000

$$\text{Expected death rate} = \frac{\text{Total expected deaths}}{\text{Total in standard population}} \times 100{,}000$$

$$\text{Expected death rate, Florida} = \frac{1{,}996{,}000}{245{,}800{,}000} \times 100{,}000 = 812.0$$

$$\text{Expected death rate, Alaska} = \frac{1{,}879{,}000}{245{,}800{,}000} \times 100{,}000 = 764.4$$

Source: Vital Statistics of the United States (1991).

example, Florida has an SMR of 110 and Alaska has an SMR of 111 (Table 4–4). They are virtually identical, and the mortality rate is not much higher than the overall U.S. mortality rate.

The crude rates, the direct adjusted rates, and the SMRs (indirect) for Florida and Alaska are shown in Table 4–5. Each method has advantages and disadvantages; the choice depends on the research question. An obvious disadvantage of the SMR is that it produces a ratio instead of a rate. It gives relative information but does not *describe* the mortality in the population. Both methods of adjustment depend on the choice of the standard population, and this is sometimes problematic. Texts are available that describe in more detail the technical methods used in age adjustment (Mausner and Bahn, 1974; Fleiss, 1981; Selvin, 1991). In our example, both methods show that the crude differences in mortality between Florida and Alaska are explained by differences in the age structure of the two populations. The direct age-adjusted mortality rates for both states are similar, and the SMRs are similar, demonstrating that mortality rates in Florida and Alaska are similar after adjusting for the differences in the age structures of the two states.

Both methods of adjustment can be used for other types of rates or variables. Studies of infant mortality often adjust for birth weight because birth weight distributions vary and birth weight is a strong predictor of infant deaths. Studies of pregnancy outcomes often adjust for the age of the mother because maternal age is a predictor of many birth outcomes.

Table 4–4. Calculations of Standardized Mortality Ratios (SMRs) for Florida and Alaska, 1988

| AGE GROUPS | U.S. DEATH RATES* | POPULATION (MILLIONS) | | EXPECTED DEATHS | |
		FLORIDA	ALASKA	FLORIDA	ALASKA
<5	251.1	.85	.06	2,134	151
5–19	47.2	2.28	.13	1,076	61
20–44	161.8	4.41	.24	7,135	388
45–64	841.9	2.60	.08	21,889	674
>65	5,104.8	2.20	.02	112,305	1,021
		Total expected		144,539	2,295
		Total observed (from Table 4–2)		131,044	2,064
		SMR (ratio of expected to observed multiplied by 100)		110	111

*Per 100,000 population.

Source: Vital Statistics of the United States (1991).

Table 4–5. Crude Death Rates and Age-Adjusted Rates for
Florida and Alaska, 1988

	FLORIDA	ALASKA
Crude death rates per 100,000	1062.4	393.9
Age-adjusted death rate per 100,000	812.0	764.4
Standardized mortality ratio	110	111

Source: Vital Statistics of the United States (1991).

Survival Analysis

Survival analysis (or life table analysis), as its name suggests, originated with studies of survivorship in actuarial populations for use by insurance companies to predict survivorship and set premium charges. It is used to make demographic predictions and to analyze data in clinical trials. Data describing the time from entry into the study until death or withdrawal from the study are collected for each patient or subject. The method allows one to compare groups and calculate a relative risk even when people are observed for different lengths of time. Survival analysis is commonly used in clinical trials to compare treatments, but it can be used in any study that measures time to a particular event. There are many texts describing the technique (Elandt-Johnson & Johnson, 1980; Lee, 1980) and computer programs to carry out the analysis. As with the other measures discussed above, it can be applied to data with endpoints other than death.

SUMMARY

Death certificate data are readily available, comprehensive, relatively uniform, and generally reliable. They constitute a major source of information for epidemiologists. Even so, trends in mortality data may be artifactual, reflecting changes in coding practices (e.g., ICD revisions, training of physicians), diagnostic capabilities (e.g., new tests, procedures for assigning diagnoses), and the denominator population (changing geographic coverage or census inaccuracies).

Mortality data are most often expressed as a rate, the number of deaths occurring in a given population over a specified period of time, and these rates can be specific for cause of death, for demographic characteristics such as age, gender, social class, residence, race, and ethnicity, or for any other variable of interest. Statistical techniques such as standardization (adjustment) can be used to adjust for differences in age or other variable distributions among populations. Epidemiologists can use mortality rates to develop and support hypotheses in mortality studies, the subject of Chapter 5.

STUDY PROBLEMS

Problems 1–5 refer to this table.

AGE GROUP	U.S. 1987 POPU-LATION	U.S. 1987 DEATHS FROM MALIG-NANT NEO-PLASMS	U.S. 1987 DEATHS FROM ACCI-DENTS	ALASKA 1987 POPU-LATION	ALASKA 1987 DEATHS FROM MALIG-NANT NEO-PLASMS	ALASKA 1987 DEATHS FROM ACCI-DENTS	FLORIDA 1987 POPU-LATION	FLORIDA 1987 DEATHS FROM MALIG-NANT NEO-PLASMS	FLORIDA 1987 DEATHS FROM ACCI-DENTS
<5	18,250,000	469	3,871	60,000	0	13	812,000	24	260
5–44	150,020,000	17,082	50,377	368,000	52	242	6,543,000	1,077	2,584
45–64	42,300,000	103,488	14,807	78,000	180	50	2,528,000	7,464	794
65+	29,840,000	242,617	25,838	19,000	210	15	2,140,000	21,599	1,482
Total	243,400,000	363,656	94,893	525,000	442	320	12,023,000	30,164	5,120

1. Calculate the death rate from all accidents in the age group 5–44 for the United States, Alaska, and Florida.
2. Calculate the death rate from all malignant neoplasms in the age group 65 and older for the United States, Alaska, and Florida.
3. Calculate the unadjusted death rates for the United States, Alaska, and Florida for (a) deaths from malignant neoplasms and (b) deaths from accidents.
4. Use the direct method of age adjustment to calculate mortality rates in Alaska and Florida for malignant neoplasms. The table below provides age-specific death rates from malignant neoplasms.

AGE GROUPS	AGE-SPECIFIC DEATH RATE FROM MALIGNANT NEOPLASMS PER 100,000 ALASKA	AGE-SPECIFIC DEATH RATE FROM MALIGNANT NEOPLASMS PER 100,000 FLORIDA	U.S. POPULATION	EXPECTED NUMBER OF DEATHS ALASKA	EXPECTED NUMBER OF DEATHS FLORIDA
<5	0	3.0	18,250,000		
5–44	16.5	14.1	150,020,000		
45–64	295.3	230.8	42,300,000		
65+	1009.3	1105.3	29,840,000		
Total			243,400,000		

5. Use the indirect method of age adjustment to calculate SMRs for Alaska and Florida deaths from accidents. The table below provides U.S. death rates.

	U.S. DEATH RATE PER 100,000	POPULATION		EXPECTED DEATHS	
		ALASKA	FLORIDA	ALASKA	FLORIDA
<5	21.2	60,000	812,000		
5–44	33.6	368,000	6,543,000		
45–64	35.0	78,000	2,528,000		
65+	86.6	19,000	2,140,000		
Total	39.0	525,000	12,023,000		

6. The crude (unadjusted) rates of death (per 100,000) from malignancies in Alaska and Florida are presented below. Compare them to the age-adjusted rates calculated in problem 4.

   Alaska 84.2

   Florida 250.8

7. The crude (unadjusted) rates of death (per 100,000) from accidents in Alaska and Florida are presented below. Compare them to the SMRs calculated in problem 5.

   Alaska 61.0

   Florida 42.6

8. Why is age adjustment especially useful in comparing patterns of mortality from malignancies and accidents in Alaska and Florida?

REFERENCES

Benavides, F. G., Bolumar, F., Peris, R. 1989. "Quality of death certificates in Valencia, Spain." *Am. J. Pub. Health* 79:1352–1354.

Cassedy, J. H. 1965. "Registration area and American vital statistics: Development of a health research resource, 1885–1915." *Bull. Hist. Med.* 39:221–231.

Cornfield, J., Haenszel, W., Hammond, E. C., Lilienfeld, A. M., Shimkin, M. B., and Wynder, E. L. 1959. "Smoking and lung cancer: Recent evidence and a discussion of some questions." *J. Natl. Cancer. Inst.* 22:173–203.

Corwin, L. I., Wolf, P. A., Kannel, W. B., McNamara, P. M. 1982. "Accuracy of death certification of stroke: the Framingham Study." *Stroke* 13:818–821.

Dorn, H. F. 1966. "Mortality." In *Chronic Diseases and Public Health.* A. M. Lilienfeld and A. J. Gifford, eds. Baltimore: The Johns Hopkins Press, pp. 23–54.

Dunn, H. L., and Shackley, W. 1945. "Comparison of cause of death assignments by the 1929 and 1938 revisions of the International List: Deaths in the United States, 1940." Vital Statistics—Special Reports 19:153–277, 1944. Washington, D.C.: United States Department of Commerce, Bureau of the Census.

Elandt-Johnson, R. C., and Johnson, N.L. 1980. *Survival Models and Data Analysis.* New York: John Wiley and Sons.

Faust, M. M., and Dolman, A.B. 1963. "Comparability of mortality statistics for the fifth and sixth revisions: United States, 1950." Vital Statistics—Special Reports, Selected

Studies 51: No. 2:133–178. Washington, D.C.: U.S. Government Printing Office, United States Department of Health, Education and Welfare, Public Health Services.

Faust, M. M. 1964. "Comparability ratios based on mortality statistics for the fifth and sixth revisions: United States, 1950." Vital Statistics—Special Reports, Selected Studies 51: No. 3:181–245. Washington, D.C.: United States Department of Health, Education and Welfare, Public Health Service.

———. 1965. "Comparability of mortality statistics for the sixth and seventh revisions: United States, 1958." Vital Statistics—Special Reports, Selected Studies 51: No. 4: 248–297. Washington, D.C.: United States Department of Health, Education and Welfare, Public Health Service.

Fleiss, J. L., 1981. *Statistical Methods for Rates and Proportions.* John Wiley & Sons, New York.

Hardy, A. M., Starcher II, E. T., Morgan, W. M., Druker, J., Kristal, A., Day, J. M., Kelley, C., Ewing, E., Curran, J. W. 1987. "Review of death certificates to assess completeness of AIDS case reporting." *Pub. Health Rep.* 102:386–391.

Israel, R. A., Rosenberg, H. M., and Curton, L. R. 1986. "Analytical potential for multiple cause of death data." *Am. J. Epid.* 124:161–179.

James, G., Patton, R. E., and Heslin, A. S. 1955. "Accuracy of cause-of-death statements on death certificates." *Pub. Health Rep.* 70:39–51.

Kreyberg, L. 1954. "The significance of histological typing in the study of the epidemiology of primary epithelial lung tumours: A study of 466 cases." *Brit. J. Cancer* 8: 199–208.

———. 1962. *Histological Lung Cancer Types: A Morphological and Biological Correlation.* Oslo, Norway: Norwegian Universities Press.

Krueger, D. E. 1966. "New enumerators for old denominators—multiple causes of death." In *Epidemiological Approaches to the Study of Cancer and Other Chronic Diseases.* W. Haenszel, ed. Natl. Cancer Inst. Monogr. No. 19. Washington, D.C.: United States Government Printing Office, pp. 431–443.

Last, J. M. (1987). *Public Health and Human Ecology.* Connecticut: Appleton and Lange.

Lee, E. T. 1980. *Statistical Methods for Survival Data Analysis.* Belmont, California: Lifetime Learning Publications.

Mainland, D. 1953. "Risk of fallacious conclusions from autopsy data on incidence of diseases with applications to heart disease." *Amer. Heart J.* 45:644–651.

Mausner, J .S. and Bahn, A. K. 1974. *Epidemiology: An Introductory Text.* Philadelphia, Pa.: W. B. Saunders.

McMahan, C. A. 1962. "Age-sex distribution of selected groups of autopsied cases." *Arch. Path.* 73:40–47.

Moriyama, I. M. 1989. "Problems in measurement of accuracy of cause-of-death statistics." *Am. J. Pub. Health,* 79:1349–1350.

Moriyama, I. M., Baum, W. S., Haenszel, W. M., and Mattison, B. F. 1958. "Inquiry into diagnostic evidence supporting medical certification of death." *Amer. J. Pub. Health* 48:1376–1387.

Moriyama, I. M., Dawber, T. R., and Kannel, W. B. 1966. "Evaluation of diagnostic information supporting medical certification of deaths from cardiovascular diseases." In *Epidemiological Approaches to the Study of Cancer and Other Chronic Diseases.* W. Haenszel, ed. Natl. Cancer Inst. Monogr. No. 19, Washington, D.C., United States Government Printing Office, pp. 405–419.

Moussa, M. A. A., Shafie, M. Z., Khogali, M. M., El-Sayed, A. M., Sugathan, T. N.,

Cherian, G., Abdel-Khalik, A. Z. H., Garada, M. T., Verma, D. 1990. "Reliability of death certificate diagnoses." *J. Clin. Epid.* 43:1285–1295.

Pohlen, K., and Emerson, H. 1942. "Errors in clinical statements of causes of death." *Amer. J. Pub. Health,* 32:251–260.

Pohlen, K. 1943. "Errors in clinical statements of causes of death: second report." *Amer. J. Pub. Health.* 33:505–516.

Selvin, S. 1991. "Statistical analysis of epidemiologic data." New York: Oxford University Press.

Szreter, S. 1991. "Introduction: the GRO and the Historian." *Soc. His. Med.* 4:401–414.

Vital Statistics of the United States. 1987. Volume II—Mortality, Part A. U.S. Department of Health and Human Services, Public Health Service, Centers for Disease Control, National Center for Health Statistics, Hyattsville, Maryland, 1990.

Vital Statistics of the United States. 1988. Volume II—Mortality, Part A. U.S. Department of Health and Human Services, Public Health Service, Centers for Disease Control, National Center for Health Statistics, Hyattsville, Maryland, 1991.

Waife, S. O., Lucchesi, P. F., and Sigmond, B. 1952. "Significance of mortality statistics in medical research: analysis of 1,000 deaths at Philadelphia General Hospital." *Ann. Intern. Med.* 37:332–337.

5

MORTALITY STUDIES

DISTRIBUTION OF MORTALITY IN POPULATIONS

Mortality statistics are routinely collected in many countries. They provide a readily available indicator of the frequency of disease as it occurs in *time, place, and persons* and therefore are important to the epidemiologist's view of disease.

Time: Trends in Mortality Rates

Figure 5–1 shows the age-adjusted mortality rates for selected sites of cancer in the United States from 1930 to 1987. These trends reveal considerable differences: lung cancer shows a marked increase; stomach and uterine cancer, a marked decrease; and primary liver cancer, a moderate but continuous decline. Slight but consistent increases are noted for pancreatic cancer and leukemia. Colon, rectum, and prostate cancer rates increased slightly until about 1950, after which the rates have remained essentially stable. Breast cancer mortality rates appear unchanged.

Trends over time are sometimes called *secular trends*. Epidemiologists constantly search for explanations of such trends. Table 5–1 provides a broad framework for considering possible reasons underlying changes in mortality trends.

One explanation to be considered immediately is that the trends may not be real, but rather artifactual—the result of errors in the numerator or denominator of the mortality rates. Improvements in medical services over any given period of time are reflected in improved diagnoses of disease and, in turn, in the accuracy of statements of the cause of death on death certificates. For example, the decline in mortality from primary liver cancer may have reflected diagnostic improve-

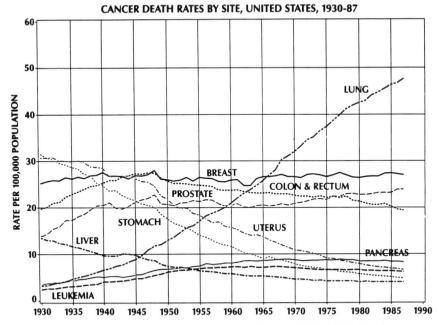

Figure 5–1. Cancer death rates by site, United States, 1930–1987. *Source:* American Cancer Society (1991).

Table 5–1. Outline of Possible Reasons for Changes in Mortality Trends of Disease

A. Artifactual
   1. Errors in the numerator due to
      (a) changes in the recognition of disease
      (b) changes in rules and procedures for classification of causes of death
      (c) changes in the classification code of causes of death
      (d) changes in accuracy of reporting age at death
   2. Errors in the denominator due to errors in the enumeration of the population

B. Real
   1. Changes in age distribution of the population
   2. Changes in survivorship
   3. Changes in incidence of disease resulting from
      (a) genetic factors
      (b) environmental factors

ments, since clinical experience indicates that many cancers spread to the liver from their primary sites. With improved diagnostic techniques, the original site will be diagnosed more frequently and the certifying physician will designate it as the underlying cause on the death certificate, even if metastases to other organs such as the liver have occurred. In order to determine the accuracy of site-specific cancer mortality statistics, Percy et al. (1974) investigated the extent to which the site of a malignancy was correctly listed on the death certificate. They ascertained cancer cases from the Third National Cancer Survey, a cancer incidence survey of ten population centers in the United States during 1969–1971. These workers found that in 65 percent of cancer deaths the site was accurately described on the death certificate. Death certificate information about the site of a malignancy tended to be less specific than hospital diagnosis information. If there is a marked change in a mortality trend, knowledge of specific diagnostic improvements in the disease category usually permits a judgment as to whether they are responsible for the change.

The International Classification of Diseases (ICD) is revised periodically to improve its efficiency in classifying causes of death. The revisions entail changes in code numbers and the addition of different disease entities to categories within a specific code. Special studies have been conducted to determine the effect of these changes, if any, on comparability of death rates in different years. When the United States National Center for Health Statistics began to use the Ninth Revision of the International Classification of Diseases in 1979, it investigated the effect of the change on the number of deaths coded to each cause. The procedure was to code the underlying cause of death for a sample of death certificates from 1976 (which had already been coded according to the Eighth Revision) using the Ninth Revision. The total number of deaths for each cause using the Ninth Revision would then be estimated from the sample. This number would then be divided by the number of deaths for that cause using the Eighth Revision to estimate the "comparability ratio." A comparability ratio of less than one indicates that the introduction of the Ninth Revision reduced the number of deaths coded to that cause; a ratio of more than one indicates the opposite. Some of the comparability ratios for the deaths coded to cardiovascular disease are shown in Table 5–2. For some causes (rheumatic heart disease, old myocardial infarction and other forms of chronic ischemic heart disease, and other diseases of arteries, arterioles, and capillaries), the comparability ratios are less than one, while those for other diseases (hypertensive heart disease, hypertensive heart and renal disease, and all other forms of heart disease) are greater than one. Fortunately, for acute myocardial infarction, angina pectoris, and cerebrovascular diseases, which are also common causes of death, the ratio is close to one. Although these differences are not large, they indicate that ICD revisions must be taken into account when evaluating mortality trends.

Table 5–2. Estimated Number of Deaths and Comparability Ratios for Selected Cardiovascular Diseases Using the Eighth and Ninth Revisions of the International Classification of Diseases, in 1976 in the United States

	NUMBER OF DEATHS		
	EIGHTH REVISION	NINTH REVISION	COMPARABILITY RATIO
Rheumatic heart disease	8,715	13,110	0.6648
Hypertensive heart disease	22,026	6,670	3.3022
Hypertensive heart and renal disease	4,872	4,020	1.2119
Acute myocardial infarction	319,562	319,477	1.0003
Other acute and subacute forms of ischemic heart disease	4,924	4,028	1.2224
Angina pectoris	195	186	1.0484
Old myocardial infarction and other forms of chronic ischemic heart disease	242,839	322,382	0.7533
Other diseases of the endocardium	5,154	4,195	1.2286
All other forms of heart disease	124,701	49,810	2.5035
Hypertension with or without renal disease	7,787	6,130	1.2703
Cerebrovascular diseases	189,553	188,623	1.0049
Atherosclerosis	31,273	29,366	1.0649
Other diseases of arteries, arterioles, and capillaries	19,583	26,432	0.7409
Total cardiovascular disease	981,184	974,429	1.0069

Source: Adapted from NCHS (1980).

Another approach to assessing the accuracy of mortality trends is to estimate whether an increase in mortality from one cause of death can be explained by a decline in another. For example, Gilliam (1955) attempted to determine whether the increase in death rates from lung cancer could be explained by errors in certification of deaths from other pulmonary diseases, such as tuberculosis. This hypothesis arose from the observation that during the period in which lung cancer mortality was increasing, mortality from tuberculosis was decreasing. Perhaps some of the deaths that had been attributed to tuberculosis in the earlier half of the twentieth century were actually due to lung cancer. Gilliam computed the degree of error in the certification of deaths from lung cancer, tuberculosis, and all respiratory diseases that would be necessary to produce the amount of the observed increase in lung cancer mortality from 1914 to 1950. He concluded that only a small part of the increase in mortality attributed to cancer of the lung since 1941 in the United States among white males and females could be accounted for by erroneous death certification of other respiratory diseases, ''without unreasonable assumptions of age and sex differences in diagnostic error.'' Since 1950, lung cancer mortality has continued to increase at a rate that is substantially greater than the decline in tuberculosis mortality, which confirms that earlier misdiagnoses could not explain the trend of increasing lung cancer mortality.

Another possibility is that artifacts in mortality trends may result from errors in the denominator of the rate, the population census, taken every ten years in the United States (Spiegelman, 1968). The degree of error in the census may differ from one decade to another. More important, however, is the observation that the errors in the census vary by age, sex, and race, and undoubtedly, other characteristics. This is illustrated in Table 5–3, which shows that young black males are more likely to be undercounted than any other subgroup. Thus, mortality rates among nonwhite males in this age group, assuming nearly complete death registration in the group, can be overestimated. If the degree of undercount changes in the different census years with no change in the quality of death certification, artifactual trends in mortality will result.

Other methods are available to evaluate trends. For example, one can determine whether the increases or decreases in mortality agree with the analyses of trends based on autopsies (Cornfield et al., 1959), or whether there is consistency between the sexes. If a mortality trend is real, it may be a result of changes in the age distribution of the population. It is preferable to make this assessment by analyzing the trends of age-specific death rates and then summarizing them by age adjustment. A decline in mortality might indicate an increase in survivorship, reflecting improvements in the treatment of a disease, or it might reflect a change in the incidence of the disease.

Once these possibilities of artifactual error are eliminated, two broad explanatory hypotheses for the trends must be considered in the search for the etiology of disease, namely, genetic and environmental causes. Environmental causes may

Table 5–3. Estimated Undercounting of the U.S. Population by Age, Sex, and Race for the 1980 Census, as a Percentage

AGE	WHITE MALE	WHITE FEMALE	BLACK MALE	BLACK FEMALE
<5	100%	100%	90%	91%
5–14	100	100	96	96
15–24	99	100	95	99
25–34	97	100	87	97
35–44	97	100	82	95
45–54	97	100	83	96
55–64	98	101	91	99
65–74	100	101	102	105

Source: Adapted from U.S. Bureau of the Census (1988).

include changes in personal living habits (e.g., smoking, diet), occupation, air and water pollution, and use of drugs.

Ordinarily, genetic factors, per se, do not produce marked mortality changes over a short period of time unless a specific genetic factor present in the population interacts with a newly introduced agent in the environment. Thus, large increases or decreases in mortality trends usually indicate that a new environmental agent has been introduced into or removed from the population undergoing the changing mortality. The pattern of mortality from AIDS illustrates the introduction into a specific population of a new virus that causes a fatal disease (Figure 5–2).

The relationship of asthma mortality to the use of pressurized aerosols is another example. Between 1959 and 1966, mortality attributed to asthma steadily increased in England and Wales, after remaining stable for a century (Figure 5–3) (Speizer et al., 1968). A detailed analysis led to the conclusion that the increase was not artifactual and that the mortality trend most likely resulted from a new method of treating asthma. A study of about 180 deaths attributed to asthma in persons 5–34 years old during 1966–1967 indicated that in 84 percent of the cases, pressurized aerosol bronchodilators were known to have been used, and probably in excess, whereas only about 66 percent had received corticosteroids (Speizer and Strang, 1968). The period of introduction of these bronchodilators, particularly isoprenaline, coincided with the increase in asthma mortality. These analyses confirmed previous clinical reports of several patients who died suddenly

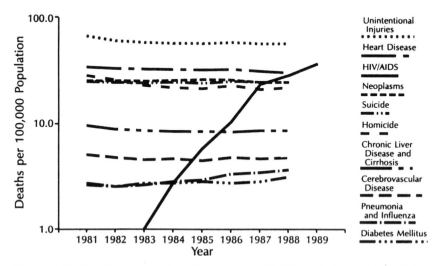

Figure 5–2. Leading causes of death among men 25–44 years of age, United States, 1981–1989. (The scale used for the y-axis, the death rate, is logarithmic. The slope of a line plotted on a logarithmic scale reflects percentage change. Hence, parallel lines in this graph reflect equivalent percentage changes.) *Source:* Centers for Disease Control (1991).

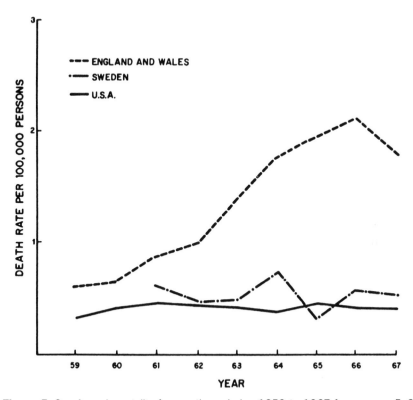

Figure 5–3. Annual mortality from asthma during 1959 to 1967 for persons 5–34 years old in England and Wales, the United States, and Sweden. *Source:* Stolley (1972).

following excessive use of aerosol inhalers (Greenberg, 1965; Greenberg and Pines, 1967; McManis, 1964). In June 1967, the Committee on Safety of Medicines issued a warning to all physicians in the United Kingdom, and in 1968 aerosols were made available by prescription only. Both deaths from asthma and aerosol sales declined and by 1969 asthma mortality had almost reached its earlier level (Inman and Adelstein, 1969). A further analysis of mortality rates from asthma in different countries, some showing a rise in asthma mortality and others not, strongly suggested a relationship between increased asthma mortality and high sales volume of a highly concentrated form of isoprenaline (isoproterenol) in pressurized aerosol nebulizers. The countries that did not show an increase in asthma mortality were those that had not licensed the concentrated nebulizers (Stolley, 1972). Subsequent pharmacologic studies provided information on the possible mechanism by which high concentrations of isoprenaline could result in asthma deaths (Conolly et al., 1971).

Mortality trends also provide a means of supporting hypotheses developed from other types of studies. A variety of epidemiologic studies, for example, showed a relationship between cigarette smoking and lung cancer (see Chapters

10 and 11). In light of the evidence of a marked increase in the consumption of cigarettes among males since 1920, one would expect to see a corresponding increase in lung cancer mortality, and this is shown in Figure 5–4.

Place

Mortality statistics from many countries are available for international comparisons in the compilations of national statistics that appear regularly in the World Health Organization Epidemiological and Vital Statistics Reports. With these data one may compare rates of diseases between countries. Figures 5–5 and 5–6 show the age-adjusted death rate for breast cancer in 15 different nations in 1987 and age-specific incidence of breast cancer in five different countries. In evaluating such reported international differences in mortality, one can follow the same sequence of reasoning that was used in evaluating mortality time trends (Table 5–1), substituting only the word "differences" for "changes." Again, one must determine whether the differences are artifactual, that is, due to distortions in the numerators and denominators of the mortality rates. International differences in the availability of medical services, diagnostic practices of physicians, and classification procedures may introduce distortions. Some countries do not conduct population censuses; also, it may be necessary to assess carefully the completeness of a census, particularly in a developing country.

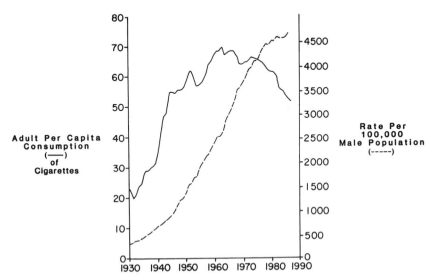

Figure 5–4. Adult per capita cigarette consumption and age-adjusted death rates from malignant neoplasms of the lung for males, United States, 1930–1980. *Source:* U.S. Department of Health and Human Services (1989).

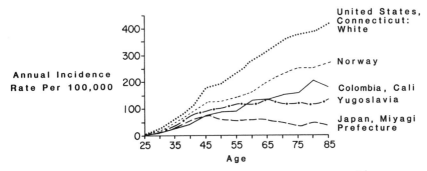

Figure 5–5. Age-adjusted death rates from malignant neoplasms of the breast among females in selected countries, latest available year, standardized to the 1989 world population. *Source:* World Health Organization (1989).

Comparability of coding practices is an example of the concerns an epidemiologist might have in comparing international death statistics. The degree of concern would depend on the disease being studied and the years and countries of interest. In work on ICD–9 and preparatory work on ICD–10 during the 1980s, the National Cancer Institute and the National Center for Health Statistics addressed the issue of cancer coding practices (Percy and Muir, 1989). They found a narrow range of variability in the coding of a sample of U.S. death certificates mentioning cancer when nine countries were given the opportunity to code them (see Table 5–4). The percentage of the sample coded for cancer as cause of death ranged from 87.2% in the United States to 95.8% in France.

If one can reasonably eliminate the possibility that mortality differences are artifactual and assume that they do reflect actual differences in disease frequency,

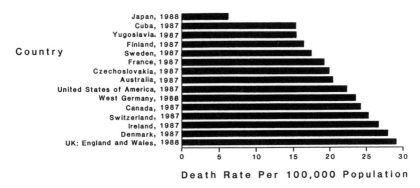

Figure 5–6. Average annual age-specific incidence rates of malignant neoplasms of the breast among females in selected countries, 1978–1982. *Source:* International Agency for Research on Cancer (1987).

Table 5–4. Percentage of 1,243 Death Certificates Listing Cancer, Circulatory, or
Other Diseases as Cause of Death That Mentioned Cancer

COUNTRY	CANCER %	CIRCULATORY DISEASES %	OTHER DISEASES %
United States	88.2	7.3	4.5
Canada	88.6	7.3	4.1
Federal Republic of Germany	91.6	5.7	2.8
New Zealand	90.5	6.6	2.9
England	91.6	5.5	2.9
France	95.8	3.0	1.2
Netherlands	90.9	6.1	3.0
USSR	90.1	7.5	2.1
Brazil	90.7	6.4	2.2

Source: Percy and Muir (1989).

it then becomes essential to resolve the issue of whether they are due to different environmental factors in the places studied or to different genetic compositions of the population. Migrant studies have been used for this purpose. These studies take advantage of the migration to one place by people from other places with different mortality experiences from many diseases. Comparisons are made between the mortality experience of the migrant groups and that of their place of origin and their current place of residence.

The rationale for these comparisons and the inferences derived from them can be stated in the following simplified form, where CO = country of origin, M = migrants, and CA = natives of the country of adoption.

1. If the change in environment is the explanation for an observed difference in death rates, one would expect that
   (a) CO rates would equal M rates and
   (b) M rates would approximate CA rates.
2. On the other hand, if genetic factors are of prime importance, one would expect that
   (a) CO rates would equal M rates and
   (b) CO and M rates will differ from CA rates.

Other factors that may influence these differences in mortality rates must also be taken into consideration:

1. *Premigration Environment.* If the premigration environment in the country of origin is of primary etiological importance, the mortality differences

would be erroneously interpreted as being genetically determined, according to the reasoning outlined above.

2. *Age at Time of Migration.* This may be significant since exposure to an etiological factor in the environment may occur, or be most likely, at a certain age or period of life. Such information would further determine whether genetic, premigration, or postmigration environmental factors are operating.

3. *Selective Factors.* Individuals who migrate may differ from those who remain in the country of origin in ways that influence the occurrence of disease. For example, the healthier and more physically fit would tend to migrate more often than those who are ill. Immigration laws of some countries may require potential migrants to pass a physical and mental examination.

Migration studies have been used within the United States to measure the effect of the environment on development of multiple sclerosis. This disease appears to vary with latitude; populations farther from the equator generally have higher incidences of multiple sclerosis than do populations closer to the equator (Kurland et al., 1965; Visscher et al. 1977). In a number of studies, researchers have shown that a migrating group can acquire the incidence rate in the geographic area to which they have migrated if they move at a young age, or can maintain the incidence rate of the place of origin if they move at an older age (about age 15 or over) (Alter et al., 1971; Dean, 1967). Detels et al. (1972) used death certificate data to compare age- and sex-adjusted death rates among four groups: migrants from high-risk areas of the United States (New England, Pacific, West–North Central, and East–North Central States) and migrants from low-risk areas of the United States (East–South Central and West–South Central) living in Washington (high risk) or California (low risk). These data, summarized in Table 5–5, show that migrants from high-risk areas have a higher death rate than

Table 5–5. Deaths from Multiple Sclerosis among Migrants to Washington and California

	CALIFORNIA		WASHINGTON	
	POPULATION AT RISK	AGE–SEX ADJUSTED RATE*	POPULATION AT RISK	AGE–SEX ADJUSTED RATE*
From northern areas:	3,597,993	0.81	784,897	1.35
From southern areas:	1,427,858	0.42	123,532	0.32

*Using the 1960 U.S. population, per 100,000.

Source: Detels et al., (1972).

migrants from low-risk areas when they move to either kind of area. Migrant studies help establish that there is an environmental contribution to a disease. Once an environmental effect is suggested, other studies are needed to measure and describe the effect.

There are geographical differences in mortality from many diseases, such as multiple sclerosis, coronary heart and cerebrovascular disease, anencephaly, and cancer of the esophagus (Gordon, 1966; Kmet and Mahboubi, 1972; Lilienfeld et al., 1972; Moriyama et al., 1971; Renwick, 1972; Tuyns, 1970). For some diseases, these regional differences within countries are as great as those between countries. Such a regional difference is illustrated by the reported mortality from cerebrovascular diseases in the United States (Figure 5–7).

This regional variation in cerebrovascular death rates may be artifactual. Inconsistency in coding cerebrovascular disease has been common historically (Table 5–6) but has been reduced by the development of more accurate diagnostic techniques. Between 1970 and 1980 computerized tomography improved the accuracy of the diagnosis of stroke. As part of the Minnesota Heart Survey, Iso et al. (1990) validated death certificate diagnosis of stroke in samples of deaths from 1970 and 1980. The proportion of death certificates that agreed with the independent review of medical records in assigning a diagnosis improved from 96 to 100 percent for the category of all types of stroke, from 59 to 82 percent for intracranial hemorrhage, and from 87 to 97 percent for nonhemorrhagic stroke (Table 5–7). Different areas of the country may have differed in the rate of access

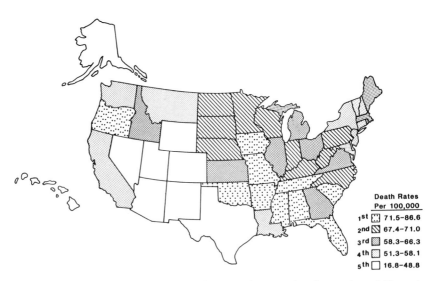

Figure 5–7.   Annual state death rates from cerebrovascular disease by quintile rank, United States, 1987. *Source:* Vital Statistics of the United States (1990).

Table 5–6. Estimated Number of Cerebrovascular Disease Deaths Coded on Death Certificates and Those Coded as Underlying Cause: United States, 1955

CAUSE OF DEATH	(ICD CODE)	TOTAL CODED CONDITIONS	CODED AS UNDERLYING CAUSE	
			NUMBER	PERCENT OF TOTAL
Cerebrovascular diseases (vascular lesions of the nervous system)	(330,334)	304,004	173,541	57.1
Subarachnoid hemorrhage	(330)	7,458	5,216	69.9
Cerebral hemorrhage	(331)	162,435	109,076	67.2
Cerebral embolism and thrombosis	(332)	67,308	41,326	61.4
Spasm of cerebral arteries	(333)	91	11	12.1
Other and ill-defined vascular lesions of the nervous system	(334)	66,712	17,912	26.8

Source: Vital Statistics of the United States (1965).

to diagnostic equipment and the rate with which physicians acquired new diagnostic skills. This would contribute to regional differences in the death rate from cerebrovascular disease.

Persons

The third general category that may influence the distribution of mortality consists of the characteristics of persons. In mortality data, the number of personal characteristics that can be analyzed is limited by the information available on death certificates. They include age, gender, ethnicity, occupation, marital status, and birth cohort (people born during specific years).

Age

Age is a major determinant of mortality. There is high mortality in the first year of life, a decline in mortality in ages 1–5, lowest mortality in ages 5–24, and

Table 5–7. Percentage of Death Certificates Agreeing with Independent Diagnoses, Minnesota Heart Survey, 1970 and 1980

YEAR	ALL TYPES OF STROKE	INTRACRANIAL HEMORRHAGE	NONHEMORRHAGIC STROKE
1970	96%	59%	87%
1980	100%	82%	97%

Source: Iso et al., (1990).

then a steady upward increase producing the well-known j-shaped curve (see Figure 4–2). Some diseases vary from the pattern of increasing mortality with age. AIDS, for example, affects young to middle-aged people more than elderly people because the behaviors leading to exposure occur more frequently in the young. Childbirth is another cause of death that is age-limited, occurring in women of child-bearing age but disappearing as women reach menopause.

Gender

Men have generally higher overall mortality than women at all ages and for many diseases. Figure 5–8 shows age-specific rates of mortality from ischemic heart disease on a semi-log scale for men and women aged 30–85 years. Even in the first year of life, male mortality is higher than female mortality, and this is found internationally, historically, for all ethnic groups, and throughout the first year of life (Table 5–8).

Of course, men and women experience different diseases and often die of different causes. Maternal mortality is a striking historical example of a gender-specific cause of death that has changed with time. United States maternal mortality declined from 1915–1919 rates of 727.9 per 100,000 live births to a 1949 rate of under 100, and to a 1988 rate of 8.4 per 100,000 live births (U.S. Vital Statistics, 1988). Antibiotics, sterile techniques and other technology have contributed to this decline, but so have changes in childbearing patterns. Changes in maternal mortality have affected overall female mortality rates and life expectancy.

In addition to biological factors, behavioral and occupational differences also affect mortality trends. The male mortality rate from accidents (motor vehicle

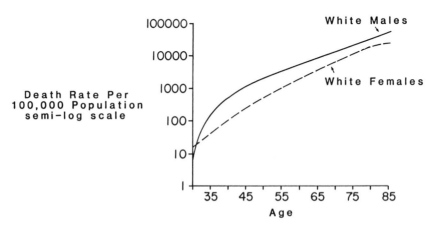

Figure 5–8. Annual age-specific death rates from ischemic heart disease by sex among whites, United States, 1987. *Source:* Vital Statistics of the United States (1990).

Table 5–8. Male and Female Infant Mortality by Ethnic Group and Age,
United States, 1988

ETHNIC OR RACIAL GROUP (PER 1000 LIVE BIRTHS)	MALE	FEMALE
White	9.5	7.4
Black	19.0	16.1
American Indian	9.5	8.6
Chinese	4.9	3.5
Japanese	4.2	3.5
Age at Death (per 100,000 live births)		
< 1 hour	112.1	95.6
1–23 hours	286.2	232.4
1–27 days	694.7	565.2
28–59 days	95.4	78.8

Source: Vital Statistics of the United States (1991).

and other) and homicides is twice as high as the rate for women (Table 5–9, Figure 5–9). Tendencies to be present where violent behavior is occurring and engaging in hazardous occupations may partially explain this difference. Behavioral variables such as seat belt use, driving speed, amount of time spent driving, and likelihood of driving while intoxicated may be gender-related and may contribute to mortality differences related to motor vehicle accidents.

Race and ethnicity

In the United States race is recorded on the death certificate, but in other nations indicators of ethnicity, national origin, or religion are sometimes recorded. These indicators serve as markers of both ''genetic background'' and social class characteristics, which are sometimes associated with particular diseases. Blacks are more likely than whites to carry the gene for sickle-cell anemia; Jews have a higher prevalence of the gene for Tay-Sachs disease than non-Jews.

In addition to genetic differences between ethnic or so-called racial groups,

Table 5–9. Death Rates per 100,000
Population for Accidents and Homicide by Sex,
1988, United States

CAUSE OF DEATH	MALE	FEMALE
Motor vehicle accidents	28.6	11.8
All other accidents	26.4	13.1
Homicide	14.0	4.2

Source: Vital Statistics of the United States (1991).

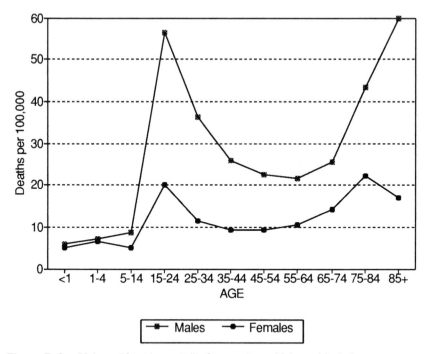

Figure 5–9. Male and female mortality from motor vehicle accidents by age groups, United States, 1988. *Source:* Vital Statistics of the United States (1991).

there are often differences in diet, life style, education, occupations, access to and use of health care, and many other characteristics. The interrelationship between these variables complicates the epidemiologist's effort to understand variations in mortality by race or ethnic group. Overall mortality in the United States is higher among blacks than among whites, as is infant mortality, maternal mortality, and mortality caused by malignant neoplasms, cardiovascular disease, diabetes, hypertension, and homicide (Table 5–10). These aggregate differences indicate the need for further investigation as it is quite unlikely that genetic explanations will account for much of the disparity.

Research on the relationship of race or ethnicity and social class to mortality has been insufficient. Social class may explain differences in mortality, but the definition of higher or lower social class may be different in specific racial or ethnic groups (Liberatos et al., 1988). There may also be an added stress related to membership in a minority that is subject to discrimination, and this stress may contribute to various illnesses, although solid evidence for this is lacking. Tyroler and James (1978) interpreted findings that darker skin color was associated with higher blood pressure among black males in Detroit (Harburg et al., 1978) to mean that ''skin color in the U.S. black population may be an indicator of psy-

Table 5–10. Some Mortality Differences between Blacks and Whites in the United States per 100,000 Population, 1988

CAUSE OF DEATH (ICD-9 CODE)	BLACK	WHITE
All causes	788.8	509.8
Malignant neoplasms (140–208)	171.3	130.0
Cardiovascular disease (390–488)	293.0	199.2
Diabetes (250)	21.2	9.0
Hypertension (401, 403)	5.7	1.5
Homicide (E960–E978)	34.1	5.3
Maternal mortality*	19.5	5.9
Infant mortality**	17.6	8.5

*Per 100,000 live births.
**Per 1,000 live births.
Source: Vital Statistics of the United States (1991).

chological processes. . . related to blood pressure.'' The same data however, can be interpreted differently, without invoking the stress hypothesis.

Social class

Socioeconomic status or social class has become a more important variable to study as epidemiologists have turned their attention to diseases with multiple causes and to the contribution that ''life style'' makes to disease. Social class may be considered as an independent risk factor or as a variable associated with other risk factors for the disease in question. Table 5–11 presents some variables associated with socioeconomic status that may affect health outcomes.

Socioeconomic status is difficult to measure and is not generally recorded on death certificates (Liberatos et al., 1988). Max Weber (1946) developed a model of social class that had three components: class, status, and power. In the United States, sociologists have commonly used occupation, education, and income as indicators of social class. Britain has used and updated an index of social class that was first developed by the British Registrar General in 1911. Its five social classes are categorized on the basis of occupation. The British have changed this categorization of social class every 10 years so that historical data may not be comparable, and time trends within a social class category may be artifactual. International comparisons can also be difficult if different nations use different measures, or if an occupation varies in its relative social standing, remuneration, and associated risks. Occupations with higher income or prestige in one country may be lower in another country. An example is the physician, who is well paid in the United States and was poorly paid in what was once the U.S.S.R.

Table 5–11.   Some Health-Related Outcomes That Vary with Social Class

COMMON INDICATORS OF SOCIOECONOMIC STATUS	INTERMEDIATE VARIABLES	HEALTH OUTCOMES
Wealth	Access to health care	Detection and treatment of illnesses
	Access to dietary choices	Obesity, blood pressure, cholesterol levels
Education	Knowledge, attitude and and behavior about diet, smoking, alcohol, exercise, sexual practices, illegal drug use, family planning, prenatal care	Changes in risk factors for heart disease, lung cancer, AIDS, low birth weight
Occupation	Exposure to hazards, psychological stresses, physical activity	Cancer, heart disease, accidents, miscarriages, birth defects, other conditions

The United States does not collect social class information on its death certificates. Occupation is described with two entries (usual occupation, kind of business or industry), and more recently some states have begun requesting information on highest education level. Shai and Rosenwaike (1989) compared accuracy of education reporting in a group of Utah and New York middle-aged men who participated in studies and self-reported their educational level, then died and had their educational level described on their death certificates by a spouse. There was agreement in 68 percent of cases, varying with educational level. It is necessary to link death certificates to other databases in order to study social class and a particular mortality outcome because of the lack or inaccuracy of information on death certificates regarding social class, education, and occupation.

Social class may explain some of the "racial" differences observed in mortality. A study by Bassett and Krieger (1986) is one of the few that have controlled for social class in examining breast cancer survival among black and white women. When race is the "risk factor" and the analysis adjusts for social class, the risk of dying is similar for both races. When the "risk factor" is social class and the analysis is adjusted for race, breast cancer mortality is elevated by 52 percent in the lower social class.

Birth cohort

Analysis of data by birth cohort sometimes provides supporting evidence for other observations. An initial finding of seven cases of adenocarcinoma of the

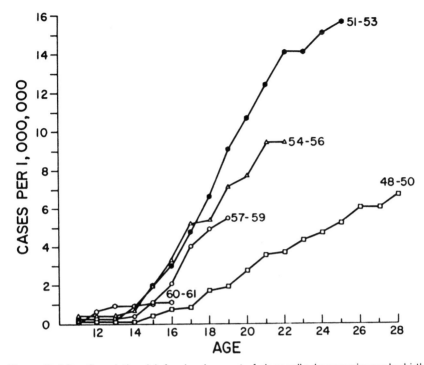

Figure 5–10.   Cumulative risk for development of clear-cell adenocarcinoma by birth cohort (white females born in the United States). *Source:* Herbst et al. (1971).

vagina in women under 25 years of age was so unusual that it led to a case-control study that identified in-utero exposure to diethylstilbestrol (DES) as a highly probable cause (Herbst and Scully, 1970; Herbst et al., 1971). In a birth-cohort analysis the mortality rate for adenocarcinoma was compared with DES sales (Figure 5–10). The risk was lowest for females born in 1948–1950 and highest for those born in 1951–1953, declining with subsequent cohorts. This pattern follows the sales figures for DES, which were highest in the years 1950–1952 and declined in the following years. This helped confirm the causal role of in-utero DES exposure.

SUMMARY

After ruling out artifact as an explanation of mortality patterns, one can ascribe changes in mortality to genetic or environmental agents. Environmental agents include everything in a person's environment—culture, geography, accidents, smoking, chemical hazards, new drugs, viruses, diet, and all other exposures. Comparisons of mortality by time, place, and persons have been useful in suggesting hypotheses about the causes of disease and in providing evidence to support or reject them. In this chapter we have given examples of studies that have shown changes in death patterns over time. Such studies often highlight directions for public health concerns. An increase in mortality from a disease may indicate the need for a change in health policy or research. Geographic comparisons of death rates and correlations with other factors that vary with geography such as culture, diet, behavior, climate, or ethnicity often suggest hypotheses for future research. Death certificates generally contain information about the person who died, including age at death, gender, ethnicity, occupation, marital status, and birth cohort. Comparisons by such characteristics provide much information about subgroups at risk for different causes of death and help target public health efforts. Death rates vary widely with these personal characteristics, and almost all epidemiologic research can be informed by available mortality data.

STUDY PROBLEMS

1. Temporal patterns of mortality can be seen over years, by season, or by the day of the week. For example, deaths from homicide occur most frequently on Friday and Saturday nights, suggesting that alcohol consumption might contribute to the increase in homicides.

   The numbers of deaths in 1987 caused by motor vehicle accidents are listed below by the day of the week on which death occurred. Suggest three hypotheses to explain the increased number of deaths on Fridays, Saturdays, and Sundays.

Sunday	Monday	Tuesday	Wednesday	Thursday	Friday	Saturday
8,056	5,825	5,660	5,646	6,230	7,481	9,391

   Be sure to consider the full range of epidemiologic thinking including chance, artifact, confounding, and causality.

2. Geographic variation is another clue used by epidemiologists to understand the causes of a disease. The death rates from HIV infection are the result of transmission of a retrovirus through contact with the blood or body fluids of an infected person, most frequently because of intravenous drug use associated with needle sharing, unprotected sex, blood transfusions, or mother-to-infant transmission. The death rates from HIV infection in 1987 are given on the next page for the top five and lowest five states.

TOP 5 HIV DEATH RATES		LOWEST 5 HIV DEATH RATES	
STATE	RATE PER 100,000	STATE	RATE PER 100,000
Washington, D.C.	28.8	South Dakota	.3
New York	19.2	North Dakota	.4
New Jersey	13.8	Montana	.5
California	9.6	Wyoming	.6
Florida	9.2	Idaho/Iowa	.8

(a) Suggest three hypotheses to explain the geographic distribution of high or low HIV rates.

(b) What might explain Washington, D.C.'s rate of 28.8, which is 50% higher than that of New York State?

3. Most Western countries have shown sharp declines in infant mortality since 1900. In the United States, infant mortality has declined for both whites and blacks, but differences between the races have persisted over time. Variations over time and between racial groups can give information about several causes of infant mortality.

Infant mortality rates in the United States (deaths under 1 year of age per 1,000 live births) are listed below by year and race (problems 4–6 also refer to this table).

Infant Mortality (deaths under 1
year per 1,000 live births)

	WHITE	BLACK
1915–1919	92.8	150.4
1920–1924	73.3	117.3
1930–1934	55.2	90.5
1940	43.2	72.9
1950	26.8	43.9
1960	22.9	44.3
1970	17.8	32.6
1980	11.0	21.4
1987	8.6	17.9

(a) What are some arguments that the time trends are real, not artifactual?

(b) What effect would improved birth registration have on these data?

(c) What effect would improved death registration have on these data?

4. What might explain the decline in infant mortality between 1915 and 1960?

5. What might explain the decline in infant mortality between 1960 and 1987?

6. What are three hypotheses that might explain the differences in infant mortality between whites and blacks?

REFERENCES

Alter, M., Okihiro, M., Rowley, W., and Morris, T. 1971. "Multiple sclerosis among Orientals and Caucasians in Hawaii." *Neurology* 21:122–130.

American Cancer Society. 1991. *Cancer Facts and Figures.* Atlanta: American Cancer Society, Inc.

Bassett, M. T., and Krieger, N. 1986. "Social class and black-white differences in breast cancer survival." *Am. J. Pub. Health* 76:1400–1403.

Centers for Disease Control. 1991. *Morbidity and Mortality Weekly Report* 40(3):41–44, January 25.

Conolly, M. E., Davies, D. S., Dollery, C. T., and George, C. F. 1971. "Resistance to β adrenoceptor stimulants: a possible explanation for the rise in asthma deaths." *Brit. J. Pharmacol.* 43:389–402.

Cornfield, J., Haenszel, W., Hammond, E. C., Lilienfeld, A. M., Shimkin, M. B., and Wynder, E. L. 1959. "Smoking and lung cancer: Recent evidence and a discussion of some questions." *J. Natl. Cancer. Inst.* 22:173–203.

Dean, G. 1967. "Annual incidence, prevalence, and mortality of multiple sclerosis in white South-African-born and in white immigrants to South Africa." *Brit. Med. J.* 2:724–730.

Detels, R., Brody, J. A., and Edgar, A. H. 1972. "Multiple sclerosis among American, Japanese and Chinese migrants to California and Washington." *J. Chron. Dis.* 25:3–10.

Gilliam, A. G. 1955. "Trends of mortality attributed to carcinoma of the lung: Possible effects of faulty certification of death to other respiratory diseases." *Cancer* 8:1130–1136.

Gordon, P. C. 1966. "The epidemiology of cerebral vascular disease in Canada: An analysis of mortality data." *Can. Med. Assoc. J.* 95:1004–1011.

Greenberg, M. J. 1965. "Isoprenaline in myocardial failure." (Letter). *Lancet* 2:442–443.

Greenberg, M. J., and Pines, A. 1967. "Pressurized aerosols in asthma." (Letter). *Brit. Med. J.* 1:563.

Harburg, E., Gleibermann, L., Roeper, P., Schork, M. A., and Schull, W. J. 1978. "Skin color, ethnicity and blood pressure I: Detroit blacks." *Am. J. Pub. Health* 68(12): 1177–1183.

Herbst, A. L., and Scully, R. E. 1970. "Adenocarcinoma of the vagina in adolescence." *Cancer* 25:745–757.

Herbst, A. L., Ulfelder, H., and Poskanzer, D. C. 1971. ''Association of maternal stilbes-terol therapy with tumor appearance in young women.'' *New Eng. J. Med.* 284(16): 878–881.

Inman, W.H.W., and Adelstein, A. M. 1969. ''Rise and fall of asthma mortality in England and Wales in relation to use of pressurized aerosols.'' *Lancet* 2:279–285.

International Agency for Research on Cancer. 1987. *Cancer Incidence in Five Continents, Average Annual Age-Specific Incidence Rates of Malignant Neoplasms of the Breast among Females in Selected Countries.* 1978–82. 5(88). Lyon: World Health Organization.

Iso, H., Jacobs, D. R., and Goldman, L. 1990. ''Accuracy of death certificate diagnosis of intracranial hemorrhage and non-hemorrhagic stroke.'' *Am. J. Epidemiol.* 132:993–998.

Kmet, J., and Mahboubi, F. 1972. ''Esophageal cancer in Caspian Littoral of Iran: Initial studies.'' *Science* 175:846–853.

Kurland, L. T., Stazio, A., and Reed, D. 1965. ''An appraisal of population studies of multiple sclerosis.'' *Ann. N.Y. Acad. Sci.* 122:520–541.

Liberatos, P., Link, B. G., and Kelsey, J. L. 1988. ''The measurement of social class in epidemiology.'' *Epidemiol. Rev.* 10:87–121.

Lilienfeld, A. M., Levin, M. L., and Kessler, I. I. 1972. *Cancer in the United States.* Cambridge, Mass.: Harvard University Press.

McManis, A. G. 1964. ''Adrenaline and isoprenaline: A warning.'' *Med. J. Aust.* 2:76.

Moriyama, I. M., Krueger, D. E. and Stamler, J. 1971. *Cardiovascular Diseases in the United States.* Cambridge, Mass.: Harvard University Press.

National Center for Health Statistics. 1980. Department of Health, Education and Welfare. Publication No. (PHS) 80-1120. Vol. 28, No. 11 Supplement, February 29.

Percy, C., and Muir, C. 1989. ''The international comparability of cancer mortality data.'' *Am. J. Epidemiol.* 129:934–946.

Percy, C., Garfinkel, L., Krueger, D. E., and Dolman, A. B. 1974. ''Apparent changes in cancer mortality. 1968.'' *Pub. Health Rep.* 89:418–428.

Renwick, J. H. 1972. ''Hypothesis: Anencephaly and spina bifida are usually preventable by avoidance of a specific but unidentified substance present in certain potato tubers.'' *Brit. J. Prev. Soc. Med.* 26:67–88.

Shai, D. and Rosenwaike, I. 1989. ''Errors in reporting education on the death certificate: Some findings for older male decedents from New York State and Utah.'' *Amer. J. Epidemiol.* 130:188–192.

Speizer, F. E., Doll, R., and Heaf, P. 1968. ''Observations on recent increase in mortality from asthma.'' *Brit. Med. J.* 1:335–339.

Speizer, F. E., and Strang, L. B. 1968. ''Investigation into use of drugs preceding death from asthma.'' *Brit. Med. J.* 1:339–343.

Spiegelman, M. 1968. *Introduction to Demography.* Rev. ed., Cambridge, Mass.: Harvard University Press.

Stolley, P. D. 1972. ''Asthma mortality: Why the United States was spared an epidemic of deaths due to asthma.'' *Am. Rev. Resp. Dis.* 105:883–890.

Tuyns, A. J. 1970. ''Cancer of the oesophagus: Further evidence of the relation to drinking habits in France.'' *Int. J. Cancer* 5:152–156.

Tyroler, H. A., and James, S. A. 1978. ''Blood pressure and skin color.'' *Am. J. Pub. Health* 68(12):1170–1172.

U.S. Bureau of the Census. "Current Population Reports." Series P-25, No. 985, as cited in section 7, Technical Appendix of Vital Statistics of the United States, 1988.

U.S. Department of Health and Human Services. *Reducing the Health Consequences of Smoking: 25 Years of Progress: A Report of the Surgeon General.* Department of Health and Human Services, Public Health Service, Centers for Disease Control, Off. Smoking and Health, DHHS Publ. 89-8411, 1989.

Visscher, B. R., Detels, R., Coulson, A. H., Malmgren, R. M., and Dudley, J. P. 1977. "Latitude, migration, and the prevalence of multiple sclerosis." *Am. J. Epidemiol.* 106:470–475.

Vital Statistics of the United States. 1965. 1955 Supplement: Mortality Data, Multiple Causes of Death. United States Department of Health, Education and Welfare, Public Health Service, National Center for Health Statistics, Washington, D.C.: U.S. Government Printing Office.

Vital Statistics of the United States, 1987, Volume II—Mortality, Part A., U.S. Department of Health and Human Services, Public Health Service, Centers for Disease Control, National Center for Health Statistics, Hyattsville, Maryland, 1990.

Vital Statistics of the United States, 1988, Volume II—Mortality, Part A., U.S. Department of Health and Human Services, Public Health Service, Centers for Disease Control, National Center for Health Statistics, Hyattsville, Maryland, 1991.

Weber, M. 1946. "Class, status and party." In *From Max Weber: Essays in Sociology.* Geith, H., Mills, C. W. eds. New York: Oxford University Press.

World Health Organization. 1989. World Health Statistics Annual. Geneva: World Health Organization.

6

MORBIDITY STATISTICS

SOURCES

The limitations of mortality statistics and the need to obtain information on various aspects of illness in the population stimulated the collection of morbidity statistics. Morbidity statistics are essential to health agencies attempting to control disease, especially communicable diseases. Various tax-financed public assistance programs and medical care plans require knowledge of morbidity of the population groups they serve for purposes of planning and evaluation of health and social services. Industry is concerned with the effect of morbidity on its employees, particularly as it affects absenteeism and productivity. The planning and evaluation of public health activities and health facilities require knowledge of the extent of morbidity in the population. Morbidity statistics are sometimes the by-products of societal activities such as conscription for the armed services and enrollment in retirement plans. In recent years, increased reliance has been placed on a variety of morbidity statistics to maintain surveillance of the quality of medical care and to measure the utilization of health care facilities and services.

Table 6–1 presents an overview of some sources of morbidity statistics. Detailed consideration of them can be found in books on demography or vital statistics (Spiegelman, 1968; Alderson, 1988). In assessing the utility of any of these sources for epidemiologic studies, one must be aware of two factors: (1) the variety of definitions of illness used, and (2) the composition of the population that has served as the source of information. The definition of illness used in a particular instance is influenced by the nature of the program or activity for which the data were collected (Table 6–1). These data serve many different administra-

Table 6–1. Various Sources of Morbidity Statistics

---

1. *Disease control programs*
   Disease reporting—communicable diseases; case registers of tuberculosis, cancer, cardiovascular disease, and other diseases; surveillance systems
   Case-finding programs in selected population groups
2. *Tax-financed public-assistance programs*
   Public assistance, aid to the blind, aid to the disabled
   State or federal medical care plans
   Armed forces, including preinduction records
   Department of Veterans Affairs
3. *Records of industrial and school absenteeism and preemployment and periodic physical examinations in industry and schools*
4. *Data accumulated as a by-product of insurance, prepaid medical care plans, and other health-related activities*
   Group health and accident insurance
   Prepaid medical care plans
   State disability insurance plans
   Life insurance companies
   Hospital insurance plans
   Railroad retirement board
   Selective Service records
   Clinics and hospitals
5. *Special research programs*
6. *Morbidity surveys on population samples for illness in general and for specific diseases*

---

tive purposes. Statistics derived from disability programs, for example, will vary according to the program's content and purpose (Lerner, 1974). Some programs are concerned with specific forms of disability such as blindness, whereas others consider a disabled person in terms of his physical or mental ability to support himself. Thus, disability may be defined with regard to specific types and/or according to a range from temporary and limited to permanent and total.

Determining whether a morbid condition or illness is present in an individual often depends upon the type and method of examination used. In a community case-finding program, for example, a single test such as an X-ray examination may be used to detect individuals with a high probability of having a specific disease, a process known as **screening.** Additional examinations would be necessary to determine whether they had the specific disease. Statistics derived from such programs provide information on presumptive diagnoses, whereas those obtained from hospitals and clinics usually represent the results of detailed examinations. Illness can also be determined by interview, i.e., by asking whether a person feels ill, or currently has or has had a specific disease. Thus, the various methods of determining the presence of illness will result in different definitions that must be considered in assessing the usefulness of such data for epidemiologic purposes.

Most sources of morbidity statistics, particularly items 2 to 5 in Table 6–1, only provide information on special population groups, i.e., the group covered by a particular health insurance plan or retirement program. In many instances, the population served by a facility, such as a hospital, is not even defined. Studies in the past have shown underreporting of communicable diseases (especially those transmitted sexually) by physicians. This, too, must be considered in evaluating the usefulness of such data (Schaffner et al., 1971; Sherman and Langmuir, 1952; Thacker and Berkelman, 1988). Underreporting of a variety of obstetrical conditions and congenital malformations on birth certificates has also been found (Milham, 1963; Lilienfeld et al., 1951). Case-finding programs have a similar limitation, and it has been particularly difficult to obtain even a 90 percent response to surveys for such chronic conditions as diabetes mellitus (McDonald et al., 1966; Colsher and Wallace, 1991; Nelson et al. 1990). Those who do respond to case-finding surveys may differ in important ways from those who do not. This may result in biased estimates of disease frequency in the population.

An approach that has proved extremely valuable in many areas of the United States and other countries is the population-based permanent or long-term registration system for a specific disease, such as cancer or one of the other chronic diseases (Bahn et al., 1965; Gordis et al., 1969; Gillum, 1978; Muir et al., 1987; Most and Peterson, 1969). A well-planned and well-operated registry can furnish a great deal of information on the frequency of a disease and can provide data for epidemiologic studies. An attempt is made through these registries to collect as much information as is practical on all newly recognized cases of the disease in a specific population. To achieve the desired degree of completeness, it is necessary to collect information from many sources, including hospitals, pathology laboratories, practicing physicians, and official death certificates.

Some registries require compulsory notification of cases by physicians; others depend on voluntary cooperation. In many instances, the reporting is limited to hospitalized cases (Most and Peterson, 1969; Gillum, 1978). If the registry is for a disease such as cancer where nearly all cases are hospitalized, registration is considered virtually complete.

The development of a case registry is costly. It is, therefore, essential to compare those costs and the benefits of having such data available with the costs and benefits for other methods of obtaining similar information, such as periodic population surveys. After its initiation, the survival of either a voluntary or compulsory case registry depends on maintaining the interest of cooperating physicians and hospitals. Interest in a registry generally can be sustained if the data collected are actually used as a basis for providing health and social services to patients or for research purposes.

SURVEILLANCE

The concept of surveillance derives from its French origins during the Napoleonic wars: to keep watch over a group of persons thought to be subversive (Eylenbosch and Noah, 1988). Until recently, epidemiologic surveillance focused on the identification of an infected individual, with the goal of isolation to minimize disease transmission (Langmuir, 1971; Thacker and Berkelman, 1988). In 1963, Langmuir shifted the focus to the status of a disease in a population, i.e., the "continued watchfulness over the distribution and trends of incidence through the systematic collection, consolidation and evaluation of morbidity and mortality reports and other relevant information" and the regular dissemination of such data to "all who need to know." An extension of epidemiologic surveillance is the use of data for disease prevention and control (Halperin and Baker, 1992). A surveillance system provides for the ongoing collection of data by a data center, the analysis of those data, the dissemination of the data and analyses, and the implementation of a response based upon the analyses.

There are three types of surveillance systems: *active, passive,* and *sentinel* (Table 6–2) (Eylenbosch and Noah, 1988; Thacker and Berkelman, 1988; Rut-

Table 6–2.   Advantages and Disadvantages of Different Types of Surveillance Systems

TYPE	CHARACTERISTIC	ADVANTAGES	DISADVANTAGES
Active	Regular periodic collection of case reports from health care providers or facilities	Data are more accurate than in other types of surveillance	Expensive
Passive	Reports of cases given by health care professionals at their discretion	Inexpensive	Data likely to underestimate the presence of disease in the population
Sentinel health event	Case report indicates a failure of the health care system or indicates that special problems are emerging	Very inexpensive	Applicable only for a select group of diseases

stein et al., 1976). **Active surveillance** depends on the periodic solicitation of case reports from health care providers or facilities. For example, the Connecticut Tumor Registry actively reviews hospital records throughout the state for new ("incident") cases of cancer and benign tumors (Heston et al., 1986). Hospitals outside the state are also under surveillance for such cases among Connecticut residents outside the state. Other cancer registries, in the United Kingdom for instance, exemplify active surveillance (Fraser et al., 1978; Muir et al., 1987).

In contrast, **passive surveillance** relies upon reporting of cases by health care professionals at their discretion. Reporting of cases of toxic shock syndrome in Wisconsin in the early 1980s exemplified this type of surveillance (Davis and Vergeront, 1982). Physicians and other community members (including patients) were asked to report cases to the state health department. One factor found to influence the level of reporting was media attention given to toxic shock syndrome.

In general, active surveillance requires more effort by the data collection center than does passive surveillance. It is therefore more expensive to maintain an active surveillance system than a passive one. On the other hand, active surveillance results in more complete and accurate data than does passive surveillance, because providers do not always report all cases to the data center. In an evaluation of active and passive surveillance systems for notifiable diseases in Vermont and in Pierce County, Washington, the physicians in the active system reported twice as many notifiable diseases per patient as did physicians in the passive one (Alter et al., 1987). Similar results have been reported by other researchers (Brachott and Mosley, 1972; Hinds et al., 1985; Thacker, et al., 1986; Marier, 1977; Vogt et al., 1983).

The third type of surveillance, **sentinel surveillance,** relies on reports of cases of disease whose occurrence suggests that the quality of preventive or therapeutic medical care needs to be improved (Rutstein et al., 1976; Rutstein et al., 1983). Such cases are termed "sentinel health events" since this occurrence serves as a warning to health officials. An example of a sentinel health event is a case of polio, which indicates the need for attention to immunization in the population. Similarly, the occurrence of malignant mesothelioma is a sentinel for past exposure to asbestos. Many European countries use sentinel surveillance systems to provide information on disease occurrence. Several developing countries have been encouraged by the Expanded Programme on Immunization of the World Health Organization to use sentinel surveillance systems for disease reporting (World Health Organization, 1985; World Health Organization, 1988). Although it is relatively inexpensive to maintain, sentinel surveillance lacks specificity regarding the cause of the disease and the risk factors to which the population has been exposed.

CROSS-SECTIONAL STUDIES

Cross-sectional studies, also known as "prevalence surveys," provide information on the frequency of disease in a population. Often the population is defined geographically, but it may also be defined by employment in a company or participation in a health care plan, for instance. In a cross-sectional study, the epidemiologist randomly selects a sample from the population of interest at one point in time (hence the name "cross-sectional"). Once the sample is selected, the epidemiologist determines the frequency of the disease(s) of interest in that population, as well as factors that may be associated with the presence or absence of the disease, such as age or gender (see Chapter 7).

When information on illness in a population is needed on a periodic or continuing basis, a morbidity survey, in which a cross-sectional study is repeatedly conducted in the same population, is established. Such surveys are also conducted because of the limitations of some of the sources of morbidity data mentioned above. This method was initiated on a large scale in continuous studies of all illnesses in a community by the United States Public Health Service in Hagerstown, Maryland, in 1921–1924 (Sydenstricker, 1974).

In general, community-wide morbidity surveys have collected information on population samples in two ways: by interview and by examination. Information obtained by interview can be elicited directly from the respondent or from a member of the household who reports the illnesses among all household members for a specified period of time. Information can be obtained by a complete physical examination or by examination of certain organ systems, e.g., cardiovascular, in a sample of the entire population or selected groups of the population, depending upon the purposes of the survey. Morbidity surveys can be carried out by a single visit to the household, a single examination of a person, or periodic visits or examinations.

Soon after the Hagerstown surveys, other national morbidity surveys were conducted in the United States for different purposes, but it was not until 1956 that a continuing program of surveying the health status of the United States population was begun. This was the United States National Health Survey, which is currently conducted by the National Center for Health Statistics (National Center for Health Statistics, 1963; Jekel, 1984). The National Health Survey includes three general programs of survey activities: the National Health Interview Survey (NHIS), the National Health and Nutrition Examination Survey (NHANES), and the National Health Record Survey (NHRS). National Center for Health Statistics findings from these surveys are reported in color-coded booklets, so that these reports have become popularly known as the "Rainbow Series" (Jekel, 1984).

The National Health Interview Survey is based on a sample of the noninstitutionalized population of the United States. It is conducted continuously by interviewing a sample of households each week and combining these findings to provide estimates of illness for longer periods of time. Among the specific items included in the NHIS are doctor visits and hospital stays, occurrence of reported acute and chronic conditions, health status indicators, and reported limitation of activities. Periodically, a supplemental set of questions is asked, such as knowledge and attitudes about AIDS, health promotion practices, and smoking habits (Chyba and Washington, 1990; Kovar, 1989; Jekel, 1984).

The National Health and Nutrition Examination Survey (NHANES) consists of examinations and a variety of physiological and psychological tests for specific diseases, carried out over a period of two or three years for a selected age group. Originally, the NHANES was organized as the National Health Examination Survey (NHES). The population groups examined in the three cycles of the NHES and the years that the examinations were conducted are shown in Table 6–3. In 1971, nutritional surveillance was added to the NHES and it became the National Health and Nutrition Examination Survey (Kovar, 1989). The sample is selected by methods similar to those of the Health Interview Survey, but it is much smaller. A special Hispanic Health and Nutrition Examination Survey (HHANES) was conducted in the 1980s to evaluate the health status of the Hispanic population in the United States (Kovar, 1989).

The Health Record Survey involves samples of institutions or facilities providing health or medical care services and is carried out on either a continuous or a periodic basis (Jekel, 1984; Kovar, 1989). Specifically, the National Hospital Discharge Survey, conducted annually since 1965, provides information about the diagnoses at discharge of a sample of patients admitted to short-stay hospitals. The complaints of patients and the diagnoses of physicians in their private offices are sampled by the National Ambulatory Medical Care Survey, conducted annually from 1974 to 1981 and then once every four years beginning in 1985.

Table 6–3. National Health Examination Surveys in the United States Since 1960

SURVEY	YEARS CONDUCTED	POPULATION SURVEYED
National Health Examination Survey		
NHES I	1960–1962	18–79 years of age
NHES II	1963–1965	6–11 years of age
NHES III	1966–1970	12–17 years of age
National Health and Nutrition Examination Survey		
NHANES I	1971–1974	1–74 years of age
NHANES II	1976–1980	6 months–74 years of age
NHANES III	1990–1993	6 months–74 years of age
HHANES	1982–1984	Hispanic Americans 6 months–74 years of age

Table 6–4. Annual Report Incidence Rates (per 100 population) of Fractures and Dislocations, and Sprains and Strains to the Musculoskeletal System,* United States, 1989

| AGE | PERCENTAGE INCIDENCE | | |
(YEARS)	FRACTURES AND DISLOCATIONS	SPRAINS AND STRAINS	TOTAL
<5	1.2	1.5	2.7
5–17	4.7	6.2	10.9
18–24	4.3	7.1	11.4
25–44	2.8	7.7	10.5
45–64	2.1	2.7	4.8
65+	2.6	2.9	5.5
All Ages	3.0	5.3	8.3

*Episodes associated with receipt of medical attention or with limitation of activity.
Source: Adams and Benson (1990).

In addition to these surveys, there is an ongoing program of data evaluation and methodological research as well as a program of analytical studies of epidemiologic and statistical problems. Table 6–4 and Figure 6–1 show some examples of the types of information provided by the National Health Survey Program (Adams and Benson, 1990).

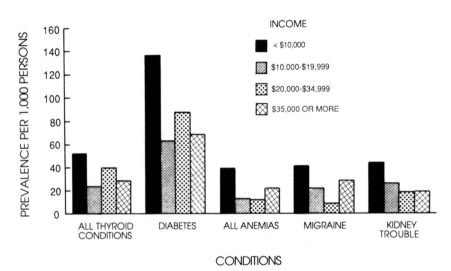

Figure 6–1. Prevalence of selected chronic conditions per 1,000 persons 65 years of age and older, by family income, National Health Survey, 1989. *Source:* Adams (1990).

A continuing program of health status surveys, similar to the United States National Health Survey, was begun in Japan in 1953 (Soda, 1965; Soda and Kosaki, 1975). The Office of Population Censuses and Surveys has conducted an annual General Household Survey in the United Kingdom since 1971; it provides information on the health status of the population similar to that of the NHIS (Office of Population and Censuses and Surveys, 1973; Alderson, 1988). Various types of continuing national health survey systems have also been developed by other European countries, e.g., the Netherlands since 1981 (Alderson, 1988).

MEASUREMENT OF MORBIDITY

To describe morbidity, two general types of rates are available: incidence and prevalence rates. They are defined as follows:

$$\text{Incidence rate per 1,000} = \frac{\text{Number of new cases of a disease occurring in the population during a specified period of time}}{\text{Number of persons exposed to risk of developing the disease during that period of time}} \times 1,000$$

$$\text{Prevalence rate per 1,000} = \frac{\text{Number of cases of disease present in the population at a specified period of time}}{\text{Number of persons at risk of having the disease at that specified time}} \times 1,000$$

The **incidence rate** is a direct estimate of the probability, or risk, of developing a disease during a specified period of time. This contrasts with the **prevalence rate,** which measures the number of cases that are present at, or during, a specified period of time. The prevalence rate (P) equals the incidence rate (I) multiplied by the average duration of the disease (D) or $P = I \times D$. For example, if the average duration of a disease is three years and its incidence rate is 10 cases per 1,000 persons per year, the prevalence rate would be 30 cases per 1,000 persons, i.e., $P = 3 \times 10$. The duration of disease is usually measured from the time of diagnosis to death. Although it would be highly desirable to measure the duration from the time of onset of a disease, it is usually difficult, if not impossible, to ascertain this for most diseases. The constant of 1,000 in the above rates was arbitrarily selected. One could use 1,000,000 instead of 1,000. For example, an incidence rate of 3,000 cases per 1,000,000 population per year is equivalent to an incidence rate of 3 cases per 1,000 population per year.

The two types of prevalence rates that are used by investigators are *point prevalence* and *period prevalence*. Point prevalence refers to the number of cases present at a specified moment of time; period prevalence refers to the number of cases that occur during a specified period of time—for example, a year. Period prevalence consists of the point prevalence at the beginning of a specified period of time plus all new cases that occur during that period. The distinction between these measures of prevalence (Figure 6–2) developed from practical considerations since it usually takes a period of time to conduct a prevalence survey and to ascertain all of the cases. Even if a survey does require some time for its execution, however, it is generally possible to estimate point prevalence.

The cases of disease that would be counted in an incidence rate during the annual period in Figure 6–2 would include case numbers 3, 4, 5, and 8. For measuring point prevalence as of January 1, case numbers 1, 2, and 7 would be included, and for point prevalence on December 31, one would include case numbers 1, 3, 5, and 8. Period prevalence from January 1 to December 31, 1992, would include case numbers 1, 2, 3, 4, 5, 7 and 8.

Clearly, the rates can vary depending upon the measure of morbidity that is used. In evaluating published data, it is important to keep in mind the measure used by the investigator (the two terms are often used erroneously in published reports). For example, the term "incidence" has been applied to data when prevalence is actually being measured. This creates some difficulties when rates from two different reports are compared.

The epidemiologist generally prefers to use incidence rates when comparing the development of disease in different population groups or attempting to determine whether a relationship exists between a possible etiological factor and a disease. This is because the incidence rate directly estimates the probability of developing a disease during a specified period of time. It permits the epidemiologist to determine whether the probability of developing a disease differs in

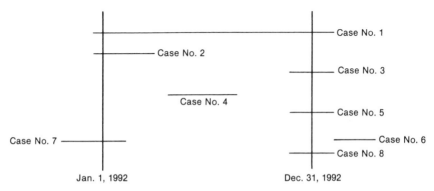

Figure 6–2. Number of cases of disease beginning, developing, and ending during a period of time, January 1, 1992–December 31, 1992. Length of each line corresponds to the duration of each case.

different populations or time periods or in relationship to suspected etiologic factors.

All forms of morbidity rates, including incidence, attack, and prevalence rates, can be made specific for age, gender, or any other personal characteristics that might be important and of interest. They also can be standardized in the same manner as mortality rates. It is important to distinguish between incidence and prevalence rates in comparing different population groups or different time periods. The incidence rates of a disease may be the same in these comparisons, but the prevalence rates may vary with the availability of curative medical services that influence duration of the disease. Thus, a higher prevalence rate does not necessarily reflect an increased probability of developing a disease but rather may reflect the lesser availability or efficacy of medical intervention.

Prevalence rates of disease are useful to the health service administrator in planning medical care services. In the absence of incidence rates, differences in prevalence rates between populations have also been useful in stimulating further epidemiologic studies. In some instances, they may be the only rates that are available for studying a particular disease. In persons with inflammatory bowel disease (Crohn's disease and ulcerative colitis), for instance, it is very difficult to determine accurately when the disorder began; often there are many years between the onset of symptoms and the time that a diagnosis is made.

A special form of incidence or attack rate, initially developed by C. V. Chapin to measure the spread of infection within a family or household following exposure to the first or primary case in the family, is the secondary attack rate (Frost, 1941). It is defined as follows:

$$\frac{\text{Secondary}}{\text{attack rate}}_{(\text{percent})} = \frac{\text{Number of exposed persons developing the disease within the range of the incubation period}}{\text{Total number of persons exposed to the primary case}} \times 100$$

This rate attempts to measure the degree of spread of a disease within a group that has been exposed to an agent by contact with a case. The numerator can be expressed in terms of clinical disease or any measurable component of the gradient of disease (such as those persons with rising antibody titers), providing the technical means are available to measure this component. The denominator consists of all persons who are exposed to (in contact with) the case. This can be more specifically defined to include those who are susceptible to the specific agent (if means are available to distinguish the immune from the susceptible persons). If the incubation period of a specific disease is unknown, the numerator can be expressed in terms of a specified time period. The primary case is excluded from both the numerator and denominator.

The secondary attack rate is usually applied to biological or social groups such as families, households, friends, or classmates, but it can be used with any closed aggregate of persons who have had contact with a case of disease. Meyer, for example, studied the occurrence of mumps in 170 families, each of which had at least two cases of the disease (Meyer, unpublished). Figure 6–3, taken from this study, presents the distribution of intervals between the day of onset of the first case in the family (designated as day "0") and that of one or more subsequent cases. The secondary cases are those occurring during the interval between 7–8 days and 29–30 days, which would approximate the range of the incubation period and, therefore, represents those cases developing as a result of contact with the first case. The cases that occur after this period are usually called "tertiary" cases and, for the most part, result from contact with secondary cases. They may also be produced by contact with cases outside the family. When the number of secondary cases has been determined and the total number of persons in the household is established, a secondary attack rate can be computed.

The secondary attack rate serves other purposes in addition to reflecting the degree of transmissibility of the agent, for instance, in evaluating the efficacy of a prophylactic agent. A study of an outbreak of infectious hepatitis among households in a municipal housing project illustrates this application (Lilienfeld et al., 1953). In this outbreak, some household members had received gamma globulin for prophylaxis at the city hospital nearby, and some had not. The gamma globulin was not administered to the household members in a systematic manner; as there was no formal protocol, its administration varied with the hospital staff member

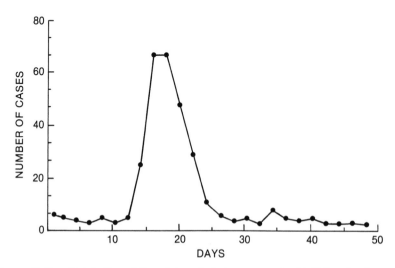

Figure 6–3. Distribution of time intervals between onset of initial and subsequent cases of mumps in 170 families with two or more cases. *Source:* Meyer (unpublished).

Table 6–5.   Age-Specific Secondary Attack Rates of Infectious Hepatitis among Total Number of Persons Exposed to a Case in a Household and among Those Receiving Gamma Globulin

AGE (YEARS)	NUMBER OF PERSONS EXPOSED TO A CASE	CASES OF HEPATITIS	
		NUMBER	PERCENT (SECONDARY ATTACK RATE)
Did Not Receive Gamma Globulin			
0–4	42	2	4.8
5–9	45	5	11.1
10–14	32	6	18.8
15–19	26	3	11.5
20+	83	4	4.8
Received Gamma Globulin			
0–4	17	1	6.0
5–9	21	0	0
10–14	13	0	0
15–19	3	0	0
20+	17	1	1.4

Source: Lilienfeld, Bross, and Sartwell (1953).

on duty. From the available data, it was possible to compute secondary attack rates for the household contacts of the primary case, according to whether or not they had received gamma globulin. Table 6–5 shows that the attack rates were lower among those contacts who had received gamma globulin than among those who had not.

Secondary rates are also used to determine whether a disease of unknown etiology is communicable and thus may indicate the possible etiological role of a transmissible agent. For example, they have been used by Beral and her colleagues to explore the hypothesis that Kaposi's sarcoma, a rare cancer associated with AIDS, may be a sexually transmitted disease (Beral et al., 1990). First, these investigators noted that the risk for Kaposi's sarcoma was ten times higher among homosexual and bisexual men with AIDS than in other HIV transmission groups (Beral et al., 1990). They then observed that the risk of this malignancy among AIDS patients in Britain was higher among those who had sexual partners from the United States or Africa (a secondary attack rate) than among those with partners from Britain or other areas (Beral et al., 1991). Further investigation of the specific behaviors associated with transmission are currently in progress. The agent, however, has not yet been isolated.

MORBIDITY STATISTICS—SOME ISSUES AND PROBLEMS

Although there are several advantages in obtaining information on illnesses from a specific population either by interview or examination, inaccuracy and variability of the information presents problems. These difficulties must be considered in assessing the findings from morbidity surveys, for they influence the methods used by epidemiologists in obtaining data and the inferences they derive from those data.

Validity of Interview Surveys

Several studies have addressed the issue of the validity or accuracy of the information obtained by interview about the presence of illness or about other characteristics (Jabine, 1987; Harlow and Linet, 1989). Generally, these investigations have compared interview-obtained information with that from a prepaid health insurance plan. Such studies have been undertaken in cooperation with the Health Insurance Plan of Greater New York (HIP) (in 1958), the Kaiser-Permanente Foundation Health Plan (KP) (in 1962–1963) and an unnamed plan in Michigan (in 1968) (Marquis et al., 1971; Woolsey et al., 1962; National Center for Health Statistics, 1968; Madow, 1967, 1973). The results of these studies, summarized in Table 6–6, show a consistent underreporting of conditions; in the HIP and KP studies, there was also significant overreporting of some conditions. Both underreported conditions and overreported conditions varied among the studies, and

Table 6–6. Estimates of the Underreporting and Overreporting of Conditions in Three Health Interview Surveys

	PERCENTAGE OF PHYSICIAN-REPORTED CONDITIONS NOT REPORTED IN SURVEY (UNDERREPORTING)	PERCENTAGE OF SURVEY-IDENTIFIED CONDITIONS NOT CONFIRMED BY PHYSICIAN REPORTS (OVERREPORTING)
Survey		
HIP (1958)	68.1	60.4
KP (1962–1963)	46.7	40.4
Michigan (1968)		
(Educational Level)		
≤11 years	35.1	7.9
12+ years	44.7	12.4

Source: Jabine (1987).

both have been found in smaller, more recent investigations, as reviewed by Harlow and Linet (1989). Some illnesses, such as chronic bronchitis or allergies, are less likely to be noted on the medical record than to be reported at interview, while other conditions, such as diabetes or heart disease, are more likely to be accurately reported at interview. Comparable results have been obtained in populations outside the United States as well (Alderson, 1984).

An investigation in the eastern and midwestern parts of the United States was carried out by the National Center for Health Statistics to determine whether a history of hospitalization was accurately reported (United States National Health Survey, 1961). Each of 1,505 persons who had been hospitalized during the previous year was asked to report hospitalizations for the year prior to the Sunday night of the week of the interview. The degree of underreporting of hospitalization is shown in Figure 6–4. It varied with the length of time between hospitalization

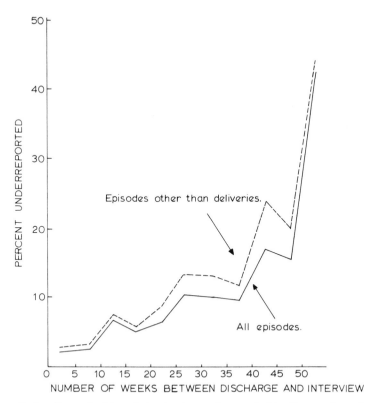

Figure 6–4. Percent of hospital episodes underreported by the number of weeks between the hospital discharge and interview, including and excluding deliveries. *Source:* United States National Health Survey (1961).

and interview; the longer the interval, the greater the degree of underreporting, ranging from 10 percent at about six months after hospitalization to about 35–45 percent at one year. Underreporting also varied with the length of stay in the hospital, the reason for hospitalization (whether for a delivery or a surgical or nonsurgical procedure), and other factors. Similar findings have been obtained outside the United States (Office of Population Censuses and Surveys, 1973).

Another method of validating interview surveys is to compare the information obtained by interview with that obtained by physical examination. Such comparisons were made in studies conducted in a rural and an urban area by the Commission on Chronic Illness (Commission on Chronic Illness, 1957, 1959).

The rural study was conducted during 1951–1955 in Hunterdon County, New Jersey. A sample of 13,113 persons (about 25 percent of the population) was interviewed. Of these, 1,202 persons were categorized into different strata, according to conditions reported on interview, and were invited to a medical center for a complete physical examination, including any indicated laboratory or diagnostic procedures. Seventy-two percent of those who were invited accepted. The proportions of match between interview-reported and clinically evaluated conditions are shown in Table 6–7 for both disabling and nondisabling

Table 6–7. Proportions of Match between Selected Interview-Reported Conditions and Clinically Evaluated Conditions

| | PERCENT MATCHING INTERVIEW-REPORTED CONDITIONS | |
DISEASE CLASSIFICATION	DISABLING	NONDISABLING
All conditions present during interview year	24	18
Infective; parasitic	22	8
Neoplasms (benign and malignant)	15	7
Allergic	57	12
Diabetes mellitus	63	100
Heart	38	54
Obesity	6	2
Anemias; other blood conditions	52	0
Mental, psychoneurotic, personality disorders	21	30
Nervous system	39	26
Injuries; poisonings	22	46
Genitourinary	7	16
Skin; cellular tissue	36	3
Dental; buccal cavity, and esophageal	15	2
Digestive, other than buccal cavity, and esophageal	23	64

Source: Adapted from Commission on Chronic Illness (1959).

conditions. The interview method clearly resulted in underreporting of clinically evaluated conditions. The degree of underreporting varied with the condition and was quite substantial for several disorders, such as neoplasms, obesity, and genitourinary conditions. On the other hand, many important conditions reported on interview were validated by clinical evaluation; for example, 80 percent of the reports of a heart condition and 85 percent of reported diabetes cases were validated. But for some conditions, such as gastrointestinal disorders, only 48 percent of the reports were clinically confirmed; some of these conditions, however, are not easily subject to clinical confirmation, conditions such as "spastic colitis" or "heartburn." It was of interest that gender and age did not influence the degree of difference. Those with less education and lower family incomes had a higher proportion of validated reports than those in the higher educational and income group. The urban study was conducted in Baltimore in a similar manner, with similar findings (Commission on Chronic Illness, 1957; Krueger, 1957). In both studies, approximately two-thirds of the interview-reported conditions were confirmed during physical examination and two-thirds of the conditions found during the examination were reported during the interview.

It can be seen that there are grounds for skepticism as to the accuracy of certain types of information obtained by interview (Alderson and Dowie, 1979; Alderson, 1984; Harlow and Linet, 1989; Jabine, 1987; Sanders, 1962). This issue is especially relevant in epidemiology, as the search for etiological factors often requires information concerning events that occurred many years in the past. The attempt to determine whether a relationship exists between alcohol consumption and esophageal cancer, for example, may involve interviewing esophageal cancer patients and controls who are mostly over 50 years old. They are asked about their alcohol consumption over a period of years. Thus, it is reasonable to question the validity of the information that is obtained. All this emphasizes the need to validate information obtained by interview with past medical or other records when conducting epidemiologic studies.

Accuracy and Reproducibility of Examinations

The uncertainty of information obtained by interview has stimulated a desire to use more objective methods of examination, laboratory tests, skin tests, or other markers of disease in measuring morbidity whenever possible. The procedure selected depends on the component of the disease spectrum (see Chapter 3) that the investigator is studying. Two aspects of these "objective" tests are important in epidemiology: (a) accuracy or validity, and (b) variability, reproducibility, or precision.

Assessment of accuracy or validity

Two indices are used to evaluate the accuracy of a test—**sensitivity** and **specificity.** These indices are usually determined by administering the test to one group of persons who have the disease and to another group who do not and then comparing the results. As indicated in Table 6–8, those who test positive and have the disease are called "true positives"; those who test positive but actually do not have the disease are called "false positives"; those who test negative and have the disease are called "false negatives"; and those who test negative and do not have the disease are called "true negatives." Using this terminology:

$$\text{Sensitivity} = \frac{\text{True positives}}{\text{True positives plus false negatives}} = \frac{\text{True positives}}{\text{All those with the disease}}$$

$$\text{Specificity} = \frac{\text{True negatives}}{\text{True negatives plus false positives}} = \frac{\text{True negatives}}{\text{All those without the disease}}$$

Sensitivity and specificity are not absolute values. The results of many laboratory tests, such as systolic blood pressure or serum lipoprotein concentrations, cannot be sharply categorized because they form a continuous spectrum. Figure

Table 6–8.   Indices to Evaluate the Accuracy of a Test or Diagnostic Examination: Sensitivity and Specificity

TEST OR EXAMINATION	DISEASE PRESENT	DISEASE ABSENT
Positive (indicating disease is probably present)	A (true positives)	B (false positives)
Negative (indicating disease is probably absent)	C (false negatives)	D (true negatives)
Totals	A + C	B + D

Sensitivity is defined as the percent of those who have the disease, and are so indicated by the test. Thus,

$$\text{Sensitivity (in percent)} = \frac{A}{(A + C)} \times 100$$

Specificity is defined as the percent of those who do *not* have the disease and are so indicated by the test. Thus,

$$\text{Specificity (in percent)} = \frac{D}{(B + D)} \times 100$$

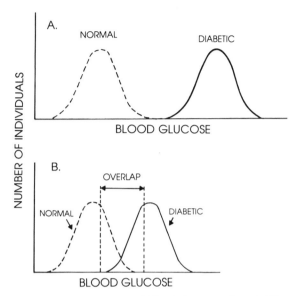

Figure 6–5. Hypothetical distribution of blood glucose values in (A) normal and diabetic population without any overlap and in (B) normal and diabetic populations with overlapping values.

6–5, for example, shows the hypothetical overlap between a normal and a diabetic population in the distribution of blood glucose levels. Table 6–9 presents data obtained from a two-hour postprandial blood test for glucose in a group of 63 true diabetics and 340 true nondiabetics (Wadena Health Study Group, unpublished). The percentage of diabetics so identified (sensitivity) and the percentage of nondiabetics so identified (specificity) are shown for varying levels of fasting blood glucose. An investigator who decides to use a blood sugar level of 5.6 mM as a division point for diabetes, for example, would identify 98.4 percent of the true diabetics and 63.2 percent of the true nondiabetics. In Table 6–10, these results are classified into the four categories of Table 6–8. The results are diagramatically presented in Figure 6–6, which also illustrates the effects of setting different upper limits of normal on blood glucose level. If the limit is set low, the blood glucose level becomes a very sensitive test, i.e., all diabetics have positive tests. However, this is done at the expense of mistakenly identifying many normal subjects as diabetic. If the limit is set high, the blood glucose level becomes a highly specific test for diabetes. However, many diabetics are erroneously diagnosed as nondiabetics. The intermediate choice minimizes both types of error—false positive and false negative.

Table 6–9. Sensitivity and Specificity of a Two-Hour Postprandial Blood Test for Glucose for 63 True Diabetics and 340 True Nondiabetics at Different Levels of Blood Glucose

REFERENCE VALUE (mg/dl)	BLOOD GLUCOSE (mM)	SENSITIVITY[1] (%)	SPECIFICITY[1] (%)
80	4.4	100.0 (63/63)	0.6 (2/340)
	5.0	100.0 (63/63)	19.7 (67/340)
	5.6	98.4 (62/63)	63.2 (215/340)
	6.1	95.2 (60/63)	93.5 (318/340)
115	6.4	95.2 (60/63)	97.4 (331/340)
	6.7	84.1 (53/63)	100.0 (335/340)
	7.2	74.6 (47/63)	100.0 (340/340)
140	7.8	66.7 (42/63)	100.0 (340/340)
	8.3	55.6 (35/63)	100.0 (340/340)
	8.9	44.4 (28/63)	100.0 (340/340)
	9.4	36.5 (23/63)	100.0 (340/340)
	10.0	33.3 (21/63)	100.0 (340/340)
	10.6	30.2 (19/63)	100.0 (340/340)
200	11.1	23.8 (15/63)	100.0 (340/340)

[1]Figures in parentheses are the number of diabetics with a two-hour postprandial blood glucose level at or above the specified level.

Source: Wadena City Health Study (unpublished).

Table 6–10. Sensitivity and Specificity of a Blood Glucose Level of 5.6 mM for Presumptive Determination of Diabetes Status

BLOOD GLUCOSE LEVEL (mM)	TRUE DISEASE STATUS	
	DIABETICS	NONDIABETICS
All those with level over 5.6 mM are classified as diabetics	62 (98.4 percent) (true positives)	215 (36.8 percent) (false positives)
All those with level under 5.6 mM are classified as nondiabetics	1 (1.6 percent) (false negatives)	125 (63.2 percent) (true negatives)
Total	63 (100.0 percent)	340 (100.0 percent)

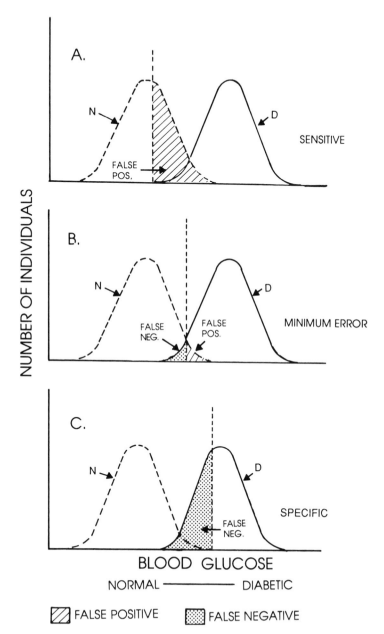

Figure 6–6. The effect of setting different blood glucose levels on false positives and false negatives: (A) a low limit results in a more sensitive test; (B) intermediate limit results in minimum total error; (C) a high limit results in a more specific test.

Predictive value

Although sensitivity and specificity provide information about the accuracy of a test, they do not provide information about the meaning of a positive or negative test result. The probability of the disease being present given a positive test result is the **positive predictive value:**

$$\text{Positive predictive value} = \frac{\text{True positives}}{\text{True positives plus false positives}} = \frac{\text{True positives}}{\text{All those with a positive test result}}$$

Negative predictive value is the probability of no disease being present given a negative test result:

$$\text{Negative predictive value} = \frac{\text{True negatives}}{\text{True negatives plus false negatives}} = \frac{\text{True negatives}}{\text{All those with a negative test result}}$$

For the data in Table 6–10, the positive predictive value is 22.3 percent (62/(62 + 215)), and the negative predictive value is 99.2 percent (125/(125 + 1)). See Table 6–11.

Unlike sensitivity and specificity, the positive and negative predictive values of a test depend on the prevalence rate of disease in the population. In Table 6–11, for example, the prevalence rate is 15.6 cases per 100 persons. Using the same test, if the prevalence rate were 45 cases per 100, then the positive predictive value would be 68.5 percent and the negative predictive value would be 97.9

Table 6–11. Positive and Negative Predictive Values of a Blood Glucose Level of 5.6 mM for Presumptive Determination of Diabetes Status with a Prevalence of 15.6 Cases per 100 Persons

BLOOD GLUCOSE LEVEL (mM)	TRUE DISEASE STATUS		TOTAL
	DIABETICS	NONDIABETICS	
All those with level over 5.6 mM are classified as diabetics	62 (22.3 percent) (true positives)	215 (77.7 percent) (false positives)	277 (100 percent) (all positive test results)
All those with level under 5.6 mM are classified as nondiabetics	1 (0.8 percent) (false negatives)	125 (99.2 percent) (true negatives)	126 (100 percent) (all negative test results)

percent (Table 6–12). For a test of given sensitivity and specificity, the higher the prevalence of the disease, the greater the positive predictive value and the lower the negative predictive value (Table 6–13).

In setting a test level at the point desired to identify those with a specific disease and to omit those without it, one must judge the relative costs of classifying persons as false negatives and false positives. The prevalence of the disease in the community, the cost of additional examinations that may be necessary, and the purpose for using the test must also be considered (Morrison, 1992).

Assessment of variability or precision

The problem of variability was initially brought into focus by Yerushalmy (1947) in his studies of the interpretation of chest X-ray films in the diagnosis of tuberculosis. He found two types of variability in interpretation:

1. *Interobserver* variability represents inconsistency of interpretation among different readers of the X-ray films.
2. *Intraobserver* variability reflects the failure of a reader to be consistent with himself in independent interpretations of the same set of films.

Both types of variability are illustrated by drawing on the results of an evaluation of cytologic diagnosis of human papillomavirus (HPV) infection. In this study, 87 cervicovaginal smears seen at a private cytology laboratory in Connecticut between 1973 and 1981 were examined for the presence or absence of HPV infection by two expert pathologists (Horn et al., 1985). A sample of 24 cytology specimens was then independently reexamined by these pathologists. The results show a 74 percent agreement among diagnoses between the two path-

Table 6–12. Positive and Negative Predictive Values of a Blood Glucose Level of 5.6 mM for Presumptive Determination of Diabetes Status with a Prevalence of 45 Cases per 100 Persons

BLOOD GLUCOSE LEVEL (mM)	TRUE DISEASE STATUS		TOTAL
	DIABETICS	NONDIABETICS	
All those with level over 5.6 mM are classified as diabetics	178 (68.5 percent) (true positives)	82 (31.5 percent) (false positives)	260 (100 percent) (all positive test results)
All those with level under 5.6 mM are classified as nondiabetics	3 (2.1 percent) (false negatives)	140 (97.9 percent) (true negatives)	143 (100 percent) (all negative test results)

Table 6–13.   Relation between the Prevalence of Disease in a Population and the Positive and Negative Predictive Value of a Test[1]

POPULATION PREVALENCE RATE (PER 100 PERSONS)	POSITIVE PREDICTIVE VALUE (PERCENT)	NEGATIVE PREDICTIVE VALUE (PERCENT)
15.6	22.3	99.2
30.0	53.4	98.8
45.0	68.5	97.9
60.0	80.2	97.1
75.0	89.0	94.1

[1]Test sensitivity = 98.4 percent and specificity = 63.2 percent

ologists (see Table 6–14). Pathologist A's diagnoses were more reproducible than were Pathologist B's.

It is possible that some proportion of the degree of agreement could have arisen by chance. In order to minimize the degree to which chance agreements affect the interpretation of such data, a measure of agreement has been developed that is known as **kappa, κ** (Cohen, 1960). Kappa represents the difference between the observed degree of agreement plus the degree of agreement expected to occur by chance, relative to the degree of agreement that would occur by chance alone (see the Appendix [p. 329] for a more detailed discussion of κ and its calculation). The interpretation of various values of κ is given in Table 6–15. Positive values of κ suggest agreement beyond what would be expected by chance, while negative values indicate that there is little agreement beyond what would occur by chance.

For the results shown in Table 6–14, the values of κ suggest that there was only fair agreement between the two pathologists' diagnoses. On the other hand, this level of agreement is greater than what would be expected by chance alone.

Table 6–14.   Reliability of the Cytologic Diagnosis of HPV Infection Made from Cervicovaginal Smears

TYPE OF RELIABILITY	NUMBER OF SLIDES	PERCENT AGREEMENT	κ (KAPPA)
Interobserver (Pathologist A vs. Pathologist B)	87	74	0.38
Intraobserver			
Pathologist A	23	96	0.89
Pathologist B	24	79	0.40

Source: Horn et al. (1985).

Table 6–15. Interpretation of Various Values of κ

κ	INTERPRETATION
<0	No agreement
0–0.19	Poor agreement
0.20–0.39	Fair agreement
0.40–0.59	Moderate agreement
0.60–0.79	Substantial agreement
0.80–1.00	Almost perfect agreement

Source: Landis and Koch (1977).

Not surprisingly, the measures for the reproducibility of each pathologist's own diagnoses reveal a greater agreement in diagnosis; for Pathologist A, a much higher level of agreement. These data suggest that while there are differences among pathologists in the cytological diagnosis of HPV infection, there is diagnostic agreement for many specimens. Similar results have been found for many diagnostic tests.

RECORD LINKAGE

Information on the characteristics of individuals from birth to death exists in the records of many institutions and agencies, private as well as governmental. At birth, a birth certificate is filled out and, when a person is hospitalized, a medical record of the hospitalization is initiated and usually maintained. A record in the Social Security system is filed at the beginning of employment; personnel records are maintained at the place of employment, school records are kept, including health as well as scholastic information; and at the time of death, a death certificate is completed. In Sweden and many other countries, employment censuses are conducted. Also, national medical insurance provides records of pharmaceutical and other medical therapeutics use in many countries.

Some of these records are combined on an *ad hoc* basis in many epidemiologic studies. The basis for this approach, known as record linkage, was stated by Dunn in 1946: "Each person in the world creates a book of life. This book starts with birth and ends with death. Its pages are made up of the records of the principal events in life. Record linkage is the name given to the process of assembling the pages of this book into a volume." A good example of the value of record linkage is the combined use of pharmaceutical and hospitalization billing records to investigate the role of nonsteroidal antiinflammatory drugs (NSAIDs) in the development of upper gastrointestinal hemorrhage (Strom, 1989). These studies found a strong relationship between the use of these agents and subsequent upper gastrointestinal bleeding.

Since the advent of the computer, it has become feasible to develop a systematic method of integrating all these records. This integration can be useful not only for epidemiologic research but also for genetic studies, the planning of medical care facilities, and determining the pattern of patient referrals to medical care in a community. A pioneering effort in record linkage was made by Newcombe (1969, 1974) in British Columbia for both population and genetic studies. He suggested that such a system could be valuable in the study of environmental carcinogenesis.

In 1962, the Oxford Record Linkage Study was initiated in Oxford, England, to determine the feasibility, cost, and methods of medical record linkage for an entire community. This system links morbidity and mortality information and provides the knowledge necessary for planning the allocation of various types of medical facilities as well as for facilitating clinical and epidemiological studies (Acheson, 1967). It is possible to use the system for a variety of inquiries into the etiology and natural history of different diseases. For instance, one of the first Oxford Record Linkage Study investigations focused on the relationship between prenatal events and respiratory morbidity during the first year of life (McCall and Acheson, 1968). Acheson (1987) has recently reviewed the results of this successful medical record linkage effort.

Other record linkage efforts have built upon the Oxford Record Linkage Study. For instance, all Scottish birth, death, hospitalization, cancer incidence, school medical examination, and handicapped children's records are linked (Heasman and Clarke, 1979). Similarly, the Office of Population Censuses and Surveys is conducting a longitudinal survey of one percent of the population of England and Wales alive in 1971, with linkage to cancer registration and mortality records (Office of Population Censuses and Surveys, 1978; Fox, 1981). Similar efforts have been initiated in the United States by the National Center for Health Statistics using data from the NHANES II survey (Jekel, 1984; Kovar, 1989; Feinleib, 1983). In many countries, medical billing data have been linked to hospitalization and other medical record datasets (Strom, 1989). Given the ease with which records can be linked by computers, it is likely that medical record linkage studies will be conducted with increasing frequency.

SUMMARY

Morbidity statistics provide information on the risk of developing disease (incidence) or of having disease (prevalence). Disease incidence is described by the incidence rate, the number of new cases of disease that occur in a population during a given time period divided by the number of persons in that population during that time period who were at risk of becoming a new case. A special type of incidence rate is the secondary attack rate, which is the incidence of disease among those persons exposed to a given case (the index case). Secondary attack rates are useful in studies of transmissibility of the causal agent and can also be used to evaluate the efficacy of a prophylactic agent.

Disease prevalence is described by the prevalence rate. For a given disease, the prevalence rate equals the incidence rate multiplied by the average duration of the disease. The prevalence rate can provide information about the frequency of disease in the community at a specified time (known as point prevalence) or during a period of time (period prevalence). Such data are available from a variety of sources, including the government, insurance companies, health care providers, and dedicated surveys of health status and disease occurrence. Undetected cases of disease can be discovered through screening programs designed to find asymptomatic but treatable individuals.

One means of obtaining morbidity statistics is through a surveillance system. Surveillance systems allow for the routine collection, analysis, and dissemination of information on disease occurrence in the community. If an increase in disease frequency is found, the health authorities are notified so that appropriate disease control activities can be implemented. Active surveillance relies upon routine review of health care records to ascertain new cases of disease. Passive surveillance depends upon reports of disease occurrence to ascertain incident cases. In sentinel surveillance, the occurrence of events indicative of specific health problems in the population is ascertained.

Cross-sectional studies provide information on the frequency of disease in a population. Repeated cross-sectional studies of the same population form a morbidity survey. These surveys are conducted to provide information on both disease occurrence and the correlates of disease in the community on a periodic or continuing basis. Such surveys are now conducted on a regular basis (usually annually) in a number of countries. Information on disease incidence and prevalence is usually gathered, depending on the type of survey. One must remember that the availability of morbidity survey data does not mean that the information itself is valid. Studies of validity suggest that these data must be viewed with some caution.

In order to provide a basis for understanding the validity of laboratory and other measures of health and disease, epidemiologists determine the sensitivity and specificity of a given test. Sensitivity measures the proportion of diseased persons detected by the test; specificity measures the proportion of those without the disease ascertained by the test. Positive predictive value measures the probability that someone with a positive test result actually has the disease, and negative predictive value, the probability that someone with a negative test result does not have the disease. The sensitivity and specificity of a test do not change from population to population. However, the predictive values of a test will vary among populations to the degree that the prevalence of disease varies. As prevalence increases, the positive predictive value increases and the negative predictive value decreases.

Another aspect of understanding such measures of disease is the variability inherent in their use. In X-ray readings, cytology examinations, physical examination findings, and other measures requiring judgment, such variability is present. This variability has two components, intraobserver and interobserver. A measure of of the degree of agreement for each component is κ, kappa. If κ is ≤ 0.0, then no more agreement is present than would be expected by chance. The closer κ is to 1.0, the stronger the agreement is compared with what would be expected by chance.

One approach to the assembly and use of morbidity information is the merger of various health records and personal identifiers into a single comprehensive record (record linkage). Such a unified record can be used for epidemiologic investigations and also benefits a patient who presents to a health care facility for diagnosis and treatment by providing a compilation of all examinations, laboratory findings, and therapeutics prescribed for the patient.

STUDY PROBLEMS

1. Why might clinical health care professionals find positive and negative predictive values more useful than sensitivity and specificity in evaluating a test?

2. The serologic test for past exposure to HIV is very sensitive and also very specific. In the early 1980s, during the first phase of the HIV epidemic, it was suggested that everyone in the United States be screened for past exposure to HIV. Why was this policy not followed?

3. What are the potential strengths and weaknesses of operating a registry for a disease in a community?

4. A colleague informs the local epidemiologist of a new screening test for the early detection of lung cancer. How might the test be assessed before it is used by the general medical community?

5. The World Health Organization MONICA project has established myocardial infarction registries around the world. What problems might attend the establishment of such registries?

6. Many academic medical centers maintain tumor registries. In what ways might such data be used by the epidemiologist? What are the limitations of such data?

7. A health officer has found that in a community of 100,000 persons, there are 250 new cases of osteoarthritis each year. The disease is present, on average, for 10 years. In planning for needed arthritis health care resources, one needs to know the prevalence of the disease. What is it?
8. The secondary attack rate was originally developed as a measure of the extent of familial aggregation of infectious diseases. Give at least four explanations for the observation of familial aggregation in a disease of unknown etiology.
9. Under what circumstances would it be desirable to minimize the percentage of individuals with false negative results on a test? Or with false positive results?

REFERENCES

Acheson, E. D. 1967. *Medical Record Linkage.* London: Oxford University Press.
———. 1987. "Introduction." In *Textbook of Medical Record Linkage.* J. A. Baldwin, E. D. Acheson, and W. J. Graham, eds. Oxford: Oxford University Press.
Adams, P. F., and Benson, V. 1990. "Current estimates from the National Health Interview Survey, 1989." National Center for Health Statistics. *Vital Health Stat* 10:176.
Alderson, M., and Dowie, R. 1979. *Health Surveys and Related Studies.* Oxford: Pergammon Press.
Alderson, M. R. 1984. "Health information resources: United Kingdom—health and social factors." In *Oxford Textbook of Public Health.* W. W. Holland, R. Detels, and G. Knox, eds. Oxford: Oxford University Press, pp. 21–51.
———. 1988. *Mortality, Morbidity and Health Statistics.* New York: Stockton Press.
Alter, M. J., Mares, A., Hadler, S. C., and Maynard, J. E. 1987. "The effects of underreporting on the apparent incidence and epidemiology of acute viral hepatitis." *Am. J. Epidemiol.* 125:133–139.
Bahn, A. K., Gorwitz, K., Klee, G. D., Kramer, M., and Tuerk, I. 1965. "Services received by Maryland residents in facilities directed by a psychiatrist." *Pub. Health Rep.* 80:405–416.
Beral, V., Bull, D., Jaffe, H., Evan, B., Gill, N., Tillet, H., and Swerdlow, A. J. 1991. "Is risk of Kaposi's sarcoma in AIDS patients in Britain increased if sexual partners came from United States or Africa?" *BMJ* 302:624–625.
Beral, V., Peterman, T. A., Berkelman, R. L., Jaffe, H. W. 1990. "Kaposi's sarcoma among persons with AIDS: a sexually transmitted infection?" *Lancet* 335:123–128.
Brachott, D., and Mosley, J. W. 1972. "Viral hepatitis in Israel: the effect of canvassing physicians on notifications and the apparent epidemiological pattern." *Bull. World Health Org.* 46:457–464.
Chyba, M. M., and Washington, L. R. 1990. "Questionnaires from the National Health Interview Survey, 1980–84." National Center for Health Statistics. *Vital Health Stat* 1:24.
Cohen, J. 1960. "A coefficient of agreement for nominal scales." *Educ. Psych. Meas.* 20:37–46.

Colsher, P. L., and Wallace, R. B. 1991. "Epidemiologic considerations in studies of cognitive function in the elderly: methodology and nondementing acquired dysfunction." *Epid. Rev.* 13:1–27.

Commission on Chronic Illness. 1957. *Chronic Illness in the United States Vol. IV, Chronic Illness in a Large City: The Baltimore Study.* Cambridge, Mass.: Harvard University Press.

———. 1959. *Chronic Illness in the United States Vol. III, Chronic Illness in a Rural Area: The Hunterdon Study.* Reported by R. E. Trussell and J. Elinson. Cambridge, Mass.: Harvard University Press.

Davis, J. P., and Vergeront, J. M., 1982. "The effect of publicity on the reporting of Toxic-Shock Syndrome in Wisconsin." *J. Infect. Dis.* 145:449–457.

Dunn, H. L. 1946. "Record linkage." *Am. J. Pub. Health* 36:1412–1416.

Eylenbosch, W. J., and Noah, N. D. 1988. *Surveillance in Health and Disease.* Oxford: Oxford University Press.

Feinleib, M. 1983. "Data bases, data banks and data dredging: the agony and the ectasy." *J. Chron. Dis.* 37:783–790.

Fox, J. P. 1981. "Record linkage and occupational mortality." In *Recent Advances in Occupational Health.* J. Corbett McDonald, ed. Edinburgh: Livingstone.

Fraser, P., Beral, V., and Chilvers, C. 1978. "Monitoring disease in England and Wales: methods applicable to routine data-collecting systems." *J. Epid. Com. Health* 32: 294–302.

Frost, W. H. 1941. "The familial aggregation of infectious diseases." In *The Papers of Wade Hampton Frost, M.D.,* K. F. Maxcy, ed. New York: The Commonwealth Fund, pp. 543–552.

Gillum, R. F. 1978. "Community surveillance for cardiovascular disease: methods, problems, applications—a review." *J. Chron. Dis.* 31:87–94.

Gordis, L., Lilienfeld, A. M., and Rodriguez, R. 1969. "An evaluation of the Maryland Rheumatic Fever Registry." *Pub. Health Rep.* 84:333–339.

Halperin, W., and Baker, E. L., eds. 1992. *Public Health Surveillance.* New York: Van Nostrand Reinhold.

Harlow, S. D., and Linet, M. S. 1989. "Agreement between questionnaire data and medical records: the evidence for accuracy of recall." *Am. J. Epidemiol.* 129:233–248.

Heaseman, M. A., and Clarke, J. A. 1979. "Medical record linkage in Scotland." *Health Bull.* 37:97–103.

Heston, J. F., Kelly, J.A.B., Meigs, J. W., and Flannery, J. T. 1986. *Forty-five Years of Cancer Incidence in Connecticut.* NCI Monograph No. 70., Washington, D.C.: U.S. Government Printing Office.

Hinds, M. W., Skaggs, J. W., and Bergeisen, G. H. 1985. "Benefit-cost analysis of active surveillance of primary care physicians for hepatitis A." *Am. J. Pub. Health* 75:176–177.

Horn, P. L., Lowell, D. M., LiVolsi, V. A., and Boyle, C. A. 1985. "Reproducibility of the cytologic diagnosis of human papilloma virus infection." *Acta Cytologica* 29: 692–694.

Jabine, T. 1987. "Reporting chronic conditions in the National Health Interview Survey. A review of tendencies from evaluation studies and methodological test." National Center for Health Statistics. *Vital Health Stat.* 2:105.

Jekel, J. F. 1984. "The Rainbow Reviews: publications of the National Center for Health Statistics." *J. Chron. Dis.* 37:681–688.

Kovar, M. G. 1989. "Data Systems of the National Center for Health Statistics." National Center for Health Statistics. *Vital Health Stat.* 1:23.

Krueger, D. E. 1957. "Measurement of prevalence of chronic disease by household interviews and clinical evaluations." *Am. J. Pub. Health* 47:953–960.

Landis, J. R., and Koch, G. G. 1977. "The measurement of observer agreement for categorical data." *Biometrics* 33:159–174.

Langmuir, A. D. 1963. "The surveillance of communicable diseases of national importance." *N. Engl. J. Med.* 268:182–192.

———. 1971. "Evolution of the concept of surveillance in the United States." *Proc. R. Soc. Med.* 64:681–689.

Lerner, P. R. 1974. "Social Security Disability Applicant Statistics, 1970." United States Department of Health, Education, and Welfare, Social Security Administration, Office of Research and Statistics Pub No. (SSA) 75-11911, Washington, D.C.: U.S. Government Printing Office.

Lilienfeld, A. M., Parkhurst, E., Patton, R., and Schlessinger, E. R. 1951. "Accuracy of supplemental medical information on birth certificates." *Pub. Health Rep.* 66:191–198.

Lilienfeld, A. M., Bross, I.D.J., and Sartwell, P. E. 1953. "Observations on an outbreak of infectious hepatitis in Baltimore during 1951." *Amer. J. Publ. Health* 43:1085–1096.

Madow, W. G. 1967. "Interview data on chronic conditions compared with information derived from medical records." National Center for Health Statistics. *Vital Health Stat.* 2:23.

———. 1973. "Net differences in interview data on chronic conditions and information derived from medical records." National Center for Health Statistics. *Vital Health Stat.* 2:57.

Marier, R. 1977. "The reporting of communicable diseases." *Am. J. Epidemiol.* 105: 587–90.

Marquis, K. H., Cannell, C. F., and Laurent, A. 1971. "Reporting health events in household interviews, effects of reinforcement, question length, and reinterviews." National Center for Health Statistics. *Vital Health Stat.* 2:45.

McCall, M. G., and Acheson, E. D. 1968. "Respiratory disease in infancy." *J. Chron. Dis.* 21:349–59.

McDonald, G. W., Fisher, G. F., and Pentz, P. C. 1966. "Diabetes screening activities, July 1958 to June 1963." In *Chronic Diseases and Public Health,* A. M. Lilienfeld and A. J. Gifford, eds. Baltimore: The Johns Hopkins Press, pp. 652–662.

Milham, S. 1963. "Underreporting of incidence of cleft lip and palate." *Amer. J. Dis. Child.* 106:185–188.

Morrison, A. S. 1992. *Screening in Chronic Disease,* 2nd ed. New York: Oxford University Press.

Most, A. S., and Peterson, D. R. 1969. "Myocardial infarction surveillance in a metropolitan community." *JAMA* 208:2433–2438.

Muir, C., Waterhouse, J., Mack, T., Powell, J., Whelan, S., eds. 1987. *Cancer Incidence in Five Continents, Volume V.* Lyon: IARC.

National Center for Health Statistics. 1963. *Origin, Program, and Operation of the U.S. National Health Survey.* PHS Pub. No. 100, Series 1, No. 1, United States Department of Health, Education, and Welfare, Washington, D.C.: U.S. Government Printing Office.

National Center for Health Statistics. 1968. "Design and methodology for a national survey of nursing homes." National Center for Health Statistics. *Vital Health Stat.* 2:7.

Nelson, L. M., Longstreth Jr, W. T., Koepsell, T. D., and van Belle, G. 1990. "Proxy respondents in epidemiologic research." *Epid. Rev.* 12:71–86.

Newcombe, H. B. 1969. "The use of medical record linkage for population and genetic studies." *Methods Inf. Med.* 8:7–11.

———. 1974. "Record linkage for studies of environmental carcinogenesis." In *Proceedings Tenth Canadian Cancer Conference, 1973.* Toronto: University of Toronto Press.

Office of Population Censuses and Surveys. 1973. *General Household Survey: introductory report.* London: HMSO.

———. 1978. "Household mortality from the longitudinal study." *Population Trends, No. 14.* London: HMSO.

Rutstein, D. D., Berenberg, W., Chalmers, T. C., Child, C. G., Fishman, A. P., and Perrin, E. B. 1976. "Measuring the quality of medical care: a clinical method." *N. Engl. J. Med.* 294:582–588.

Rutstein, D. D., Mullan, R. J., Frazier, T. M., Halperin, W. E., Melius, J. M., and Sestito, J. P. 1983. "Sentinel health events (occupational): a basis for physician recognition and public health surveillance." *Am. J. Pub. Health* 73:1054–1062.

Sanders, B. S. 1962. "Have morbidity surveys been oversold?" *Am. J. Pub. Health* 52:1648–1659.

Schaffner, W., Scoot, H. D., Rosenstein, B. J., and Byrne, E. B. 1971. "Innovative communicable disease reporting." *HSMHA Health Reps.* 86:431–436.

Sherman, I. L., and Langmuir, A. D. 1952. "Usefulness of communicable disease reports." *Pub. Health Rep.* 67:1249–1257.

Soda, T. A. 1965. "A nation-wide simple morbidity survey in Japan." In *Trends in the Study of Morbidity and Mortality.* Geneva: World Health Organization, pp. 181–196.

Soda, T. A., and Kosaki, N. 1975. *Twenty Years of the Japanese National Committee on Vital Statistics.* Geneva: World Health Organization.

Spiegelman, M. 1968. *Introduction to Demography.* Rev. ed. Cambridge, Mass.: Harvard University Press.

Strom, B. L., ed. 1989. *Pharmacoepidemiology.* New York: Churchill, Livingstone.

Sydenstricker, E. 1974. "Statistics of morbidity." In *The Challenge of Facts, Selected Public Health Papers of Edgar Sydenstricker,* R. V. Kasius, ed. New York: Milbank Memorial Fund, Prodist, pp. 228–245.

Thacker, S. B., and Berkelman, R. L. 1988. "Public health surveillance in the United States." *Epid. Rev.* 10:164–190.

Thacker, S. B., Redmond, S., and Rothenberg, R. M. 1986. "A controlled trial of disease surveillance strategies." *Am. J. Prev. Med.* 2:345–350.

United States National Health Survey. 1961. *Reporting of Hospitalization in the Health Interview Survey.* Health Statistics Series D, No. 4, U.S. Department of Health, Education and Welfare, Washington, D.C.: Public Health Service.

Vogt, R. L., LaRue, D., Klaucke, D. N., and Jillson, D. A. 1983. "Comparison of an active and passive surveillance system of primary care providers for hepatitis, measles, rubella, and salmonellosis in Vermont." *Am. J. Pub. Health* 73:795–797.

Woolsey, T. D., Lawrence, P. S., and Balamuth, E. 1962. "An evaluation of chronic disease prevalence data from the Health Interview Survey." *Am. J. Pub. Health* 52:1631–1637.

World Health Organization. 1985. *Report of the expanded programme on immunization.* WHO, Geneva (EPI/GEN/85/1).

————. 1988. *Report of the expanded programme on immunization.* WHO, Geneva (EPI/GEN/88/Wp. 4).

Yerushalmy, J. 1947. "Statistical problems in assessing methods of medical diagnosis, with special reference to X-ray techniques." *Pub. Health Rep.* 62:1432–1449.

7

MORBIDITY STUDIES

As with mortality, epidemiologists are interested in the occurrence of morbidity by **time, place and persons.** The reasoning processes used in interpreting morbidity data are similar to those applied to mortality statistics, but such data are not bound by the limitations of death certificates. One can therefore use more personal characteristics for analysis. In addition, epidemiologists often conduct their own morbidity studies, **cross-sectional surveys,** in selected communities and thus obtain information that is particularly relevant to the etiological hypotheses for the specific disease under consideration.

TIME

One aspect of the distribution of an illness in time was considered in the discussion of incubation periods in Chapter 3; basically, these periods represent the time distribution of the onset of disease after exposure to an etiological agent. Much of the discussion of time trends of mortality in Chapter 5 applies equally well to trends in the incidence and prevalence of disease.

An aspect of time distribution that has not been discussed previously is the seasonal trend of disease. Many diseases, particularly the infectious ones, occur more frequently at particular times of the year. In some instances, there are clear-cut explanations for the seasonality; many arthropod-borne diseases, such as Lyme disease, occur more frequently during the summer months because the arthropod vectors of the disease are present then (Figure 7–1) (Ciesielski et al., 1989). The seasonal distribution of asthma attacks is quite different, showing an

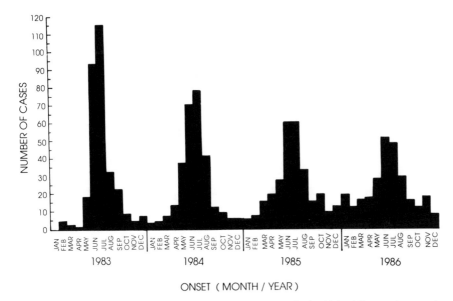

Figure 7–1. Reported number of Lyme disease cases in the United States, by onset month, 1983–1986. *Source:* Ciesielski et al. (1989).

increase in the early fall and reaching its highest levels in the late fall (Figure 7–2). Weiss (1990) examined the seasonality of hospitalization for asthma in the United States between 1982 and 1986 among persons aged less than 35 years, 35 to 64 years, and 65 years and older (Figure 7–3). He observed a distinct peak in asthma hospitalizations among persons 5 to 34 years of age during the fall months, while the pattern for older adults tended to peak in the winter and spring. The pattern for the younger age group probably reflects seasonal changes in the environmental allergen "triggers" of the disease. The patterns among the older adults

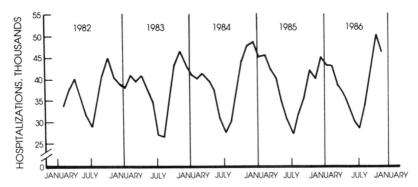

Figure 7–2. Number of hospitalizations for asthma in the United States, 1982–1986, by month. *Source:* Weiss (1990).

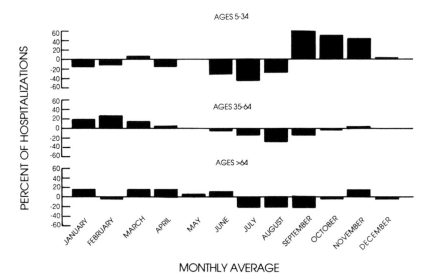

Figure 7–3. Deviation from the average monthly number of hospitalizations for asthma in the United States during 1982–1986, in the stated month, for three different age groups. *Source:* Weiss (1990).

resemble those for bronchitis, influenza, and pneumonia. In older adults, asthma occurrence may therefore be related to co-morbidity with an infectious agent. For instance, a bronchitic infection in an older adult might trigger the asthmatic attack.

The seasonal occurrence of a disease has been used to differentiate between diseases. In his classic study of endemic typhus fever conducted at a time when many investigators thought that endemic typhus in the United States was identical to epidemic typhus fever in Europe, Maxcy (1926) noted that the two diseases differed in their seasonal distribution (Figure 7–4). Together with other epidemiologic evidence (to be discussed below), this observation indicated that these were two distinct diseases with different modes of transmission.

PLACE

The same issues that have been considered in interpreting the occurrence of mortality by place also apply to morbidity. Morbidity data, however, make it possible to analyze disease distribution in smaller geographic areas than do mortality data, as morbidity data are usually derived from surveys in which living respondents can be interviewed. Therefore, one can consider very specific factors that influence morbidity distributions and more specific and definitive etiological hypotheses can be developed.

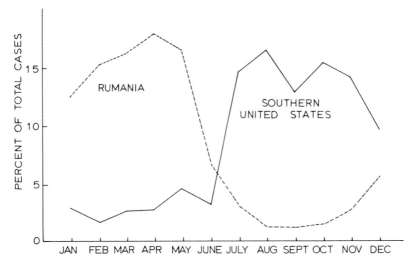

Figure 7–4. Percent distribution of cases of endemic typhus fever by month, Southern United States (Alabama and Savannah, Ga.), 1922–1925 and epidemic typhus fever in Rumania, 1922–1924. *Source:* Maxcy (1926).

A classic example of the use of place in deriving etiological inferences is the above-mentioned study of endemic typhus fever (Maxcy, 1926). At the time of that study, it was known that Old World (epidemic) typhus fever was transmitted from person to person by the louse. From clinical, serological, and experimental evidence, many investigators considered the two diseases to be similar and therefore inferred that endemic typhus was also louse-borne.

Maxcy observed the focal distribution of the disease in certain areas, among them Montgomery, Alabama. Using a ''spot map,'' he analyzed the distribution of cases of disease by place of residence (Figure 7–5) and found no distinct localization of cases. Considering the question of contact, however, he felt that an employed person would be exposed to an even greater number of contacts at his place of occupation than at home and, therefore, he distributed the cases according to place of employment (Figure 7–6). This suggested a focal center of the disease in the heart of the business district. A more detailed analysis of the places of employment indicated a high attack rate among those working at food depots, groceries, feed stores, and restaurants. This led Maxcy to suggest a rodent reservoir of the disease—rats or mice—and transmission by fleas, mites, or louse in terms of the differences in the cases' seasonal distribution (Figure 7–4), their distribution by place of employment (Figures 7–5 and 7–6), and the lack of evidence of communicability from person to person. His inferences were subsequently shown to be correct in an investigation by Dyer that incriminated the rat as the reservoir and the rat flea as the insect vector of *Rickettsia Mooseri (R. Typhi)* (Woodward, 1970).

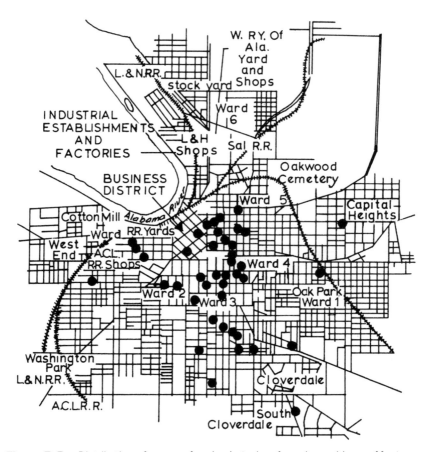

Figure 7–5. Distribution of cases of endemic typhus fever by residence, Montgomery, Alabama, 1922–1925. *Source:* Maxcy (1926).

A more recent example of the use of place in epidemiologic investigations is Gordis's study of rheumatic fever in Baltimore, Maryland. Between 1960–1964 and 1968–1970, he found that the incidence of rheumatic fever among black children in Baltimore, Maryland, had declined by 35.4 percent while the rates for white children had remained essentially unchanged (Figure 7–7) (Gordis, 1973, 1985). One explanation for this observation was the effectiveness of inner-city comprehensive-care programs in Baltimore in providing prompt and efficacious treatment of streptococcal infections. Eligibility for these programs was based on residence in specified census tracts. Gordis compared the annual incidence rate of rheumatic fever among inner-city black children in Baltimore resident in census

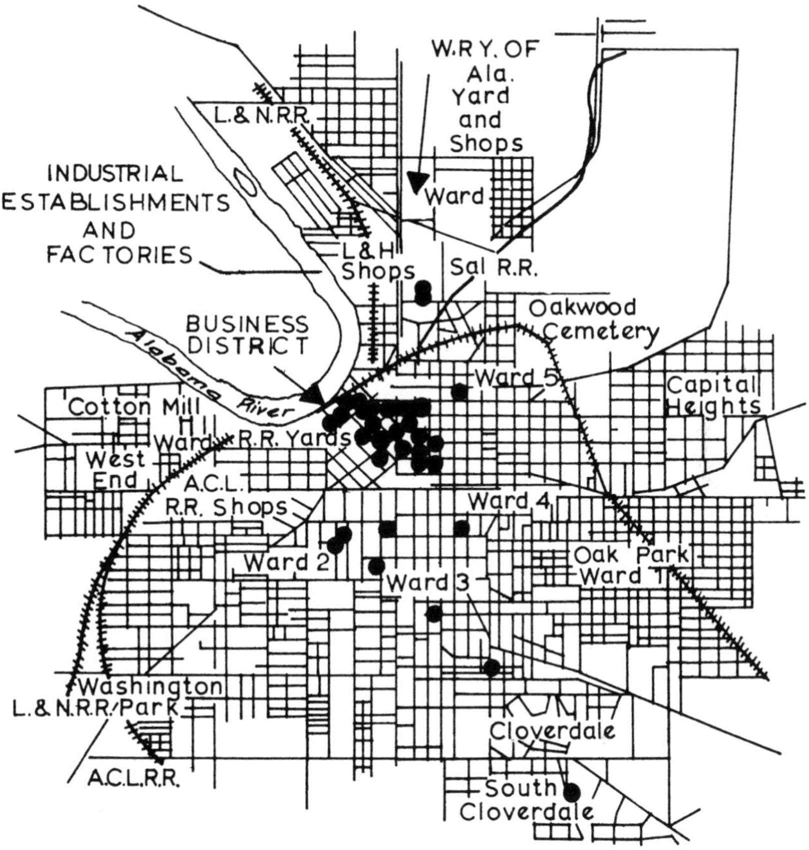

Figure 7–6. Distribution of cases of endemic typhus fever by place of employment or, if unemployed, by place of residence, Montgomery, Alabama, 1922–1925. *Source:* Maxcy (1926).

tracts eligible for treatment in the comprehensive-care programs with the rate of those resident in census tracts not eligible for care (Figure 7–8). The results showed a decline in the incidence of rheumatic fever among children resident in the areas eligible for comprehensive care but not among those who were not eligible for such care. This finding suggested that the programs had altered the natural history of streptococcal infection and thus reduced the occurrence of subsequent rheumatic fever.

The direct influence of place on the occurrence of a disease is illustrated by Lyme disease, caused by a spirochete, *Borrelia burgdorferi*, and spread by

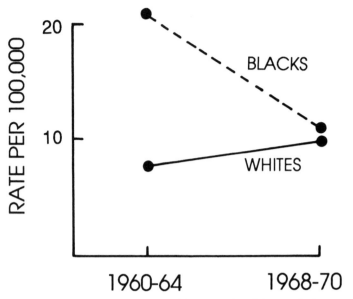

Figure 7–7. Average annual incidence of first attacks of rheumatic fever, ages 5 to 19 years, by race, Baltimore, Maryland, 1960–1970. *Source:* Gordis (1985).

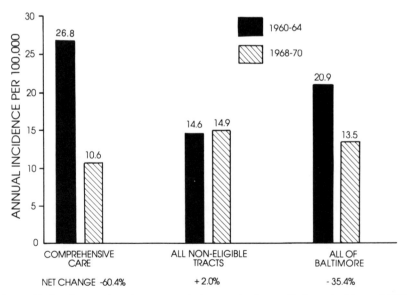

Figure 7–8. Comprehensive care and changes in rheumatic fever incidence 1960–1964 and 1968–1979, Baltimore, black population, ages 5 to 14 years. *Source:* Gordis (1985).

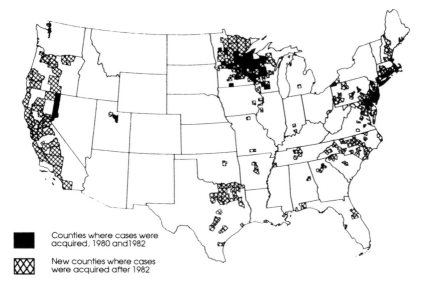

Counties where cases were
acquired, 1980 and 1982

New counties where cases
were acquired after 1982

Figure 7–9. Cases of Lyme disease in the United States, by county of acquisition, 1980–1986 (excluding 1981). *Source:* Ciesielski (1989).

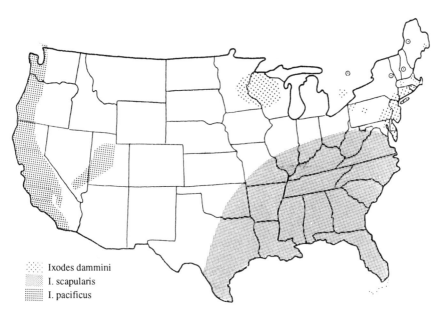

Ixodes dammini
I. scapularis
I. pacificus

Figure 7–10. Geographic distribution in the United States of tick species carrying *B. burgdorferi. Source:* Anderson (1989).

infected Ixodid ticks. Figure 7–9 shows the counties of the United States in which cases of Lyme disease occurred during 1980–1986 (excluding 1981) (Ciesielski et al., 1989). The four regions of the country in which the disease has been reported correspond to the distribution of the three Ixodid tick species that carry the disease (Figure 7–10) (Anderson, 1989). The temporal spread of the disease by the various tick species can be seen in Figure 7–9. No cases developed in counties in which none of the three Ixodid species were present.

These studies illustrate the various ways in which place influences the occurrence of disease. In one instance, endemic typhus, the important place was that of employment, where a disease reservoir was present. In another, place represented an intervention that altered the natural history of streptococcal infection. In the last example, Lyme disease, place represented the presence of the tick species necessary for the continued spread of the etiological agent.

TIME AND SPACE CLUSTERS

A term that has been used increasingly in recent years to describe the distribution of disease in time or place, or both, is "cluster." A clustering of cases in time might indicate that certain etiological factors were introduced into the environment at that time, for example, an infectious agent, a drug, or an environmental pollutant (Centers for Disease Control, 1990; Rothenberg et al., 1990). The food-poisoning outbreak discussed in Chapter 1 was a clustering of cases of gastroenteritis due to exposure to contaminated food. The increase in mortality among asthmatics discussed in Chapter 5 also represented a temporal clustering that resulted from the introduction of a particular "therapeutic" agent. In these instances, it was possible to compute either attack rates or mortality rates when analyzing the data. Clustering of cases in space in Maxcy's spot maps showed the focal distribution of endemic typhus, thus providing the evidence that finally incriminated an animal reservoir and mode of infection.

Space-time clustering data were valuable in unraveling the etiology of infectious diseases, so it is not surprising that interest has now developed in studying the clustering of cases of diseases of unknown etiology to determine whether they may have an infectious origin. For example, there have been many studies of clusters of cases of leukemia and other forms of cancer where an infectious agent is considered to be a possible etiological factor (Caldwell, 1990; Grufferman and Delzell, 1984). These studies have resulted in the development of a variety of complex statistical techniques to determine whether or not these "clusters" could have arisen by chance alone. The advantages and disadvantages of the various statistical techniques utilized is a controversial area of epidemiology (Smith,

1982; Tango, 1984; Shaw et al., 1988; Raubertas, 1988; Centers for Disease Control, 1990).

A major problem in many of these studies is that they deal only with clusters of cases and generally do not take into consideration the varying concentrations of the population in the communities where the cases appear. The occurrence of a cluster should be viewed as only a lead to the possible common exposure of a segment of the population to an etiological agent that may possibly be infectious or toxic. If the search for an infectious or toxic agent is of major interest, these studies should be followed by epidemiologic studies comparing population groups such as families, neighborhoods, and schools whose members have been exposed. Secondary attack rates can then be computed and compared, as has been done most recently for multiple sclerosis (Kurtzke and Hyllested, 1986, 1988; Kurtzke et al., 1988). If the clusters are limited to families, it becomes necessary to consider the possible influence of genetic factors as well as environmental factors that are common to family members.

PERSONS

Epidemiologists are interested in variables that may influence morbidity such as age, gender, ethnicity, and social status. The number of personal characteristics available for study is not as limited as in analyses of mortality data, where the information must often be obtained from death certificates. Routinely collected morbidity statistics share some of the limitations of mortality data, but the variables included in the National Health Survey or in disease registers are generally more extensive than those on death certificates.

An epidemiologist who wishes to determine the incidence or prevalence of a disease entity in a community by means of a morbidity survey can include any factor thought relevant to the investigation, such as demographic, physiological, biochemical, or immunological characteristics and personal living habits. This would permit the analysis of the relationship of these factors to the disease within the surveyed population in terms of individual characteristics (see Chapter 1, p. 12). However, the epidemiologist is also interested in the distribution of the relevant factors in the community as a whole. Consistency in the distribution of a set of these factors with that of morbidity in the population clearly strengthens the evidence upon which an etiological inference is based; this will be discussed in Chapter 12.

The few personal characteristics already reviewed in Chapter 5 in the context of mortality statistics are also pertinent to morbidity studies. These will be discussed together with several additional factors.

Age

Many infectious diseases such as measles and chickenpox are considered child-hood diseases; that is, their highest frequency of occurrence is in the younger age groups. Before the widespread use of measles vaccination in the United States, the incidence rate of measles increased sharply from about one to four years of age, probably as a result of the increasing early socialization of the child and thus increasing exposure to the causative virus (Figure 7–11). This age group also had a low proportion of immune individuals because they had not previously been exposed to the virus. After age four, the incidence rate gradually decreased until it approached zero at about 12–15 years of age. Since an attack of measles conferred life-long immunity, the increasing incidence rate up to age four resulted in a high proportion of immune individuals in the age group from four to about thirteen years and few susceptibles who remained to be infected.

One aspect of age that we have not yet considered is the relationship of maternal age at the time of birth to disorders in the offspring. The relationship of maternal age to infant mortality and prematurity has been known for years, although there have been no widely accepted biological explanations. Perhaps the most consistently observed relationship between maternal age and disease in the offspring is the markedly increased incidence of Trisomy 21 (Down's Syndrome) with increasing maternal age (Figure 7–12) (Harlap, 1974; Hook and Lindjso, 1978).

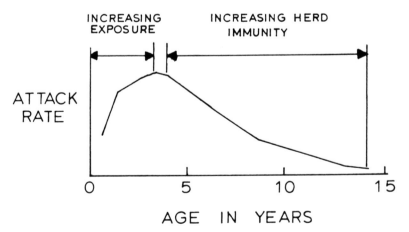

Figure 7–11. Measles age-specific incidence.

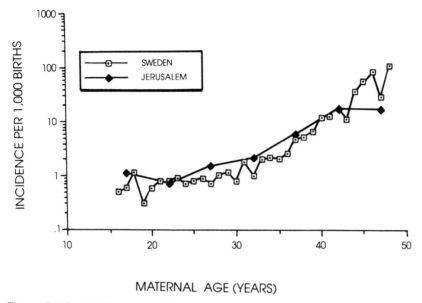

Figure 7–12. Incidence rate of Trisomy 21 (Down's Syndrome) by maternal age in Jerusalem, Israel, 1964–1970, and Sweden, 1968–1970. *Source:* Hook and Linksjo (1978) and Harlap (1974).

Gender

As with mortality, one observes differences in morbidity that are gender-related. Biological and behavioral factors related to gender contribute to differences in the prevalence or incidence of a variety of conditions including heart disease, accident-related disabilities, and autoimmune diseases. The initial observation in the AIDS outbreak that the disease occurred only among men provided one of the clues to the means of disease transmission. Men still have a higher prevalence of HIV infection; the nature of disease transmission, the source of the outbreak, and the behavior of a subgroup of men account for this gender difference.

In the epidemiology of kuru, a neurologic disorder endemic in the New Guinea highlands, it was noted that women were at much greater risk of developing the disease than were men (Gajdusek, 1977). Subsequent investigations revealed that the disease was caused by a "slow" virus transmitted during a cannibalistic ritual in which the brains of the deceased were consumed. Since the women were usually given the task of preparing the body for funeral, they often consumed the uncooked brains. In this instance, the epidemiologic characterization of the disease provided an important insight into the etiology of the condition.

Race and Ethnicity

As discussed in Chapter 5, variables such as race, ethnicity, and religion may be associated with some genetic traits such as sickle-cell anemia or Tay-Sach's disease but can also be associated with a wide range of life-style characteristics, such as diet, smoking, alcohol consumption, and childbearing patterns, all of which can be related to health outcomes. Furthermore, race and ethnicity are often associated with socioeconomic status, which may be related to educational level, access to health care, occupation, and other variables that may affect health.

An example was a small epidemic of tapeworm infestation due to *D. latum* among Jewish housewives in the 1940s. Knowing the ethnic group and its eating habits, the investigators were able to trace the epidemic to contaminated fish; housewives became infected by sampling uncooked gefilte fish as they tasted its seasoning (Desowitz, 1978).

SUMMARY

Demographic studies of morbidity concern the classic epidemiologic triad of time, place, and person. **Time** may be viewed from the perspective of temporal trends, whether of morbidity or mortality. And it can also be viewed in terms of the seasonality of a disease. Some diseases characteristically occur in the fall or winter; others in the spring or summer. Whatever the seasonal pattern is, it carries important epidemiologic information about the etiology and natural history of the disease.

Place also conveys information about the etiology and natural history of a disease. If clusters of the disease exist, they may reflect a common exposure to the etiologic agent (such clusters can also occur by chance). Spot maps, in which a geographical feature of cases of the disease (e.g., residence, place of employment) is placed on a map, can provide insight into the etiology or transmission of the agent for a disease.

The characteristics of those **persons** who have developed a disease (in comparison with those who have not developed it) provide further information about the epidemiologic profile or pattern of the disease. Variation in the risk of disease with age may suggest endogenous and exogenous influences on the development of the condition. Gender, ethnicity, religion, and other personal characteristics may help identify those at high risk for a disease, leading to etiologic hypotheses and screening programs.

STUDY PROBLEMS

1. In the United States, St. Louis encephalitis, eastern equine encephalitis, and western equine encephalitis show similar seasonal incidence patterns, with a peak in the summer and early autumn, and few cases developing at other times of the year. Explain this pattern.
2. In the 1930s and the 1940s, the most common agent of hospital-acquired (nosocomial) infections was the staphlococcus bacteria. In the 1950s, it was the streptococcus bacteria. During the 1960s and 1970s, the most common agents were gram negative bacteria. What reasons might explain this changing etiology of nosocomial infections?
3. What factors might be responsible for the reemergence of tuberculosis in the late 1980s and early 1990s as a major cause of morbidity in the United States?
4. In the United States National Health Interview Survey, information was obtained from a sample of households on whether or not anyone in the household had diabetes. Additional information was also obtained regarding several aspects of diabetes, such as treatment and disability, for the periods July 1964–June 1965 and during 1973. The prevalence rate per 1,000 population obtained at these two times by age group and sex are shown in the following table.

AGE (YEARS)	1964–1965		AGE (YEARS)	1973	
	MALE	FEMALE		MALE	FEMALE
All ages	10.5	13.8	All ages	16.3	24.1
<25	1.2	1.3	<17	1.1	1.6
25–44	6.2	6.2	17–44	6.9	10.8
45–54	15.4	20.0 ⎫	45–64	40.6	44.4
55–64	32.0	41.4 ⎭			
65–74	47.1	60.6 ⎫	65+	60.3	91.3
75+	47.0	50.8 ⎭			

(a) What inferences would you derive from these data?
(b) Would you desire any additional information? If so, what?
(c) List a few types of studies that are suggested by the data.

5. The Third National Cancer Survey was conducted in seven metropolitan areas and two entire states of the United States during the three-year period 1969–1971 to obtain information on the incidence of different forms of cancer according to a variety of population characteristics. For all areas combined, the following average annual age-specific incidence rates (per 100,000 population) for cancer of the esophagus as a primary site were observed in white and black males. Discuss possible reasons for the difference in rates between the two groups.

AGE (YEARS)	WHITES	BLACKS
35–39	0.3	1.8
40–44	0.7	8.8
45–49	2.6	22.6
50–54	6.0	40.3
55–59	12.2	59.5
60–64	18.4	59.0
65–69	22.6	66.1
70–74	24.1	108.2
75–79	34.2	57.7
80–84	37.6	46.7
85+	32.1	43.4

6. On St. Lawrence Island, in the Bering Sea, an epidemic of mumps occurred in 1956. A survey demonstrated the following age-specific incidence rates, which were compared with those observed among families in Baltimore during an epidemic in 1959–60. What are the reasons for the difference in age-specific incidence rates between these two areas?

AGE (YEARS)	INCIDENCE RATE PER 100 EXPOSED SUSCEPTIBLES	
	ST. LAWRENCE ISLAND	BALTIMORE
<1	17	12
1–4	56	60
5–9	86	54
10–19	82	18
20–49	68	19
50+	21	0

REFERENCES

Anderson, J. F. 1989. "Epizootiology of *Borrelia* in *Ixodes* tick vectors and reservoir hosts." *Rev. Inf. Dis.* 11(Suppl 6):S1451–S1459.

Caldwell, G. G. 1990. "Twenty-two years of cancer cluster investigations at the Centers for Disease Control." *Am. J. Epidemiol.* 132(Supplement):S43–S47.

Centers for Disease Control. 1990. "Guidelines for investigating clusters of health events." *MMWR* 39(No. RR-11):1–23.

Ciesielski, C. A., Markowitz, L. E., Horsley, R., Hightower, A. W., Russell, H., and Broome, C. V. 1989. "Lyme disease surveillance in the United States, 1983–1986." *Rev. Inf. Dis.* 11(Suppl 6):S1435–1441.

Desowitz, R. S. 1978. "On New Guinea tapeworms and Jewish grandmothers." *Natural History* 85:22–27.

Gajdusek, D. C. 1977. "Unconventional viruses and the origin and disappearance of kuru." *Science* 197:943–960.

Gordis, L. 1973. "Effectiveness of comprehensive-care programs in preventing rheumatic fever." *New Engl. J. Med.* 289:331–335.

———. 1985. "The virtual disappearance of rheumatic fever in the United States: lessons in the rise and fall of disease." *Circulation* 72:1155–1162.

Grufferman, S., and Delzell, E. 1984. "Epidemiology of Hodgkin's disease." *Epi. Rev.* 6:76–106.

Harlap, S. 1974. "Down's syndrome in West Jerusalem." *Am. J. Epidemiol.* 97:225–232.

Hook, E. B., and Lindjso, A. 1978. "Down's syndrome in live births by single year maternal age interval in a Swedish study: comparisons with results from a New York State study." *Am. J. Hum. Genet.* 30:19–27.

Kurtzke, J. F., and Hyllested, K. 1986. "Multiple sclerosis in the Faroe Islands: II. clinical update, transmission, and the nature of multiple sclerosis." *Neurology* 36:307–328.

———. 1988. "Validity of epidemics of multiple sclerosis in the Faroe Islands." *Neuro-epi.* 7:190–227.

Kurtzke, J. F., Hyllested, K., Arbuckle, J. D., Baerentsen, D. J., Jersild, C., Madden, D. L., Olsen, A., and Sever, J. L. 1988. "Multiple sclerosis in the Faroe Islands: IV. the lack of a relationship between canine distemper and the epidemics of MS." *Acta Neur. Scand.* 78:484–500.

Maxcy, K. F. 1926. "An epidemiological study of endemic typhus (Brill's disease) in the Southeastern United States with special reference to its mode of transmission." *Pub. Health Reps.* 41:2967–2995.

Raubertas, R. F. 1988. "Spatial and temporal analysis of disease occurrence for detection of clustering." *Biometrics* 44:1121–1129.

Rothenberg, R. B., Steinberg, K. K., and Thacker, S. B. 1990. "The public health importance of clusters: a note from the Centers for Disease Control." *Am. J. Epidemiol.* 132(Supplement):S3–S5.

Shaw, G. M., Selvin, S., Swan, S. H., Merrill, D., and Schulman, J. 1988. "An examination of three spatial disease clustering methodologies." *Int. J. Epidemiol.* 17:913–919.

Smith, P. G. 1982. "Spatial and temporal clustering." In *Cancer Epidemiology and Prevention*, D. Schottenfeld and J. F. Fraumeni, eds. Philadelphia: W. B. Saunders.

Tango, T. 1984. "The detection of disease clustering in time." *Biometrics* 40:15–26.

Weiss, K. B. 1990. "Seasonal trends in U.S. asthma hospitalizations and mortality." *JAMA* 263:2323–2328.

Woodward, T. E. 1970. "President's address: Typhus verdict in American history." *Transactions Amer. Clin. Climatol. Assoc.* 82:7–8.

III

EPIDEMIOLOGIC STUDIES

From the demographic studies in a community or population group described in Chapter 4 to 7, the epidemiologist may observe a statistical association between a population characteristic and the occurrence of a disease. Such associations, however, may be subject to an "ecological fallacy," as noted in Chapter 1. Clinical and/or experimental observations may also suggest an association. One attempts to confirm such associations by conducting **epidemiologic studies,** which determine whether these diseases or conditions are more often present in persons with the characteristic of interest than in those without it.

Epidemiologic investigations may be viewed as the application of the scientific method to populations. Just as a biological investigator wishes to observe the effect of a simple modification in the laboratory environment of two identical species, in the epidemiologic study one seeks to compare the effect of an exposure to a single factor on the incidence of disease in two otherwise identical populations.

Epidemiologic studies may be characterized as **experimental** or **observational** (Figure III–1). The major difference between the two is that in an experimental setting, the epidemiologist *controls the conditions* under which the study is to be conducted; in an observational setting, the epidemiologist is *not able* to control these conditions. In experiments, the epidemiologist controls the method of assigning subjects to either the treatment or the comparison groups. A commonly used means of assignment is to randomly allocate similar persons to the treatment or the comparison group; such an experimental study is called a **randomized clinical trial** and is discussed in Chapter 8. Most of the other types of experiments assign treatment to communities as an aggregate and are known as

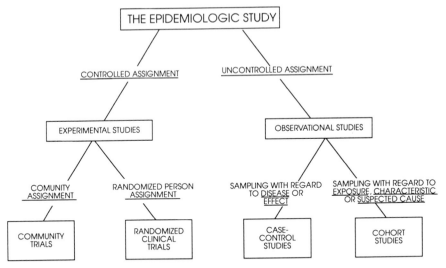

Figure III–1.   The anatomy of the epidemiologic study.

community trials; they are discussed in Chapter 9. Clearly, if there is an alternative between an experimental or an observational study, the former is preferred as the epidemiologist has greater control of the conditions under which the study is carried out. Experiments, however, are not always feasible. For example, consider conducting an experiment on the effects of cigarette smoking; one would have to randomly assign persons either to a group that would be required to smoke or to one that would not be allowed to smoke until the experiment was concluded. Such an experiment would be neither ethical nor practical.

In contrast to experimental epidemiologic studies (in which the epidemiologist assigns the exposure), in observational investigations the epidemiologist observes the associations between exposure and outcome. There are two methods of conducting such investigations: cohort studies and case-control studies. In a **cohort study,** one begins with a group of persons exposed to the factor of interest and a group of persons not exposed. These persons are then followed for the development of various conditions. Such studies are considered in Chapter 10.

Alternatively, in a **case-control study,** one assembles a group of persons with a disease (cases) and a comparison group of persons without the particular disease under investigation (controls); the history of past exposure to the factor of interest is then compared between the cases and the controls. Case-control studies are discussed in Chapter 11.

By its nature an observational study, in which the investigator has no control over exposure assignment, is open to alternative explanations for associations that are excluded in an experimental study. One common alternative explanation is known as **confounding,** in which the association between exposure to a factor and the consequent development of disease is distorted by an additional variable that is itself associated both with the factor and with the disease. An example was given in Chapter 4, in which the confounding effect of age was adjusted for in the comparison of mortality among residents of Alaska and Florida. The control of confounding in observational studies, a major activity of the epidemiologist, is discussed in Chapters 10 and 12 as well as the Appendix.

The synthesis of information provided by epidemiologic studies, together with that from demographic studies and from biology and medicine, is considered in Part IV, ''Using Epidemiologic Data.''

8

EXPERIMENTAL EPIDEMIOLOGY: I. RANDOMIZED CLINICAL TRIALS

The strength of the experimental method lies in the investigator's direct control over the assignment of subjects (either individually or aggregated) to study groups. In observational studies, by contrast, the investigator essentially accepts the conditions as they are and makes observations about the populations to help answer questions about health and disease.

Broadly considered, there are two forms of epidemiologic experiments: (1) randomized clinical trials and (2) community trials or experiments (the latter are also referred to as *field experiments*). In **randomized clinical trials,** the efficacy of a preventive or therapeutic agent or procedure is tested in *individual subjects.* In **community trials,** as the term implies, a *group of persons as a whole* is used to determine the efficacy of a drug, procedure, or intervention. One example of such a community trial is the evaluation of fluoride in preventing dental caries, discussed in Chapter 1.

DESIGN AND CONDUCT OF THE RANDOMIZED CLINICAL TRIAL

To simplify the discussion, we will consider randomized clinical trials in terms of evaluating the efficacy of a drug in the treatment of a disease. However, such trials can also be used to evaluate a prophylactic agent, such as a vaccine; a public health procedure, such as a screening method; or a medical procedure, such as an operation (e.g., coronary artery bypass graft surgery). Specific conditions of the trial may have to be changed depending upon its purpose, but the general methods and principles, for the most part, remain the same.

The randomized clinical trial is an experiment in which individuals are **randomly** assigned to two (or more) groups, known as the "treatment" and the "comparison" groups. The treatment group is given the drug being tested and the comparison group is given the drug in current use; if no such drug exists, then a placebo, an inert substance such as a sugar pill or saline injection, is used. This approach is directly comparable to that of laboratory experiments.

Randomization

In the randomized clinical trial, the treatment and comparison groups should be comparable in all respects except the one being studied, i.e., the drug being tested (Hill, 1951, 1977; Altman, 1991; Fleiss, 1986; Peto et al., 1976, 1977; Meinert, 1986). The epidemiologist can achieve comparability on factors that are known to have an influence on the outcome, such as age, sex, race, or severity of disease, by *matching* for these factors. But one cannot match persons for factors whose influence is not known or cannot be measured. This problem can be resolved by the random assignment of individuals to the treatment and comparison groups. Randomization helps to ensure that the distribution of *all* factors—known and unknown, measurable and not measurable—except for the therapy being studied, is based on chance and not some factor, such as patient preference, that may lead to a bias in assignment. In addition, randomization is the means by which the investigator avoids introducing conscious or subconscious bias into the process of allocating individuals to the treatment or comparison groups. Preventing biased assignment is important as it permits a more definitive interpretation of the trial results.

Types of Randomized Clinical Trials

Within this basic framework there are several types of randomized clinical trials:

1. **Therapeutic trials,** in which a therapeutic agent or procedure is given in an attempt to cure the disease, *relieve* the symptoms, or prolong the survival of those with the disease.
2. **Intervention trials,** in which the investigator *intervenes* before a disease has developed in individuals with characteristics that increase their risk of developing the disease.
3. **Preventive trials,** in which an attempt is made to determine the efficacy of a *preventive* agent or procedure among those without the disease. These trials are also referred to as **prophylactic trials.**

Table 8–1 provides examples of these three kinds of studies. One should note that a fine line exists between the three types of clinical trials; indeed, intervention studies can be viewed as special types of either a therapeutic or a preventive trial.

If, in a randomized clinical trial of the first type, the therapeutic agent successfully cures the disease, relieves its symptoms, or increases survival, then that agent may be used to treat the disease. One such trial was that of early photocoagulation for persons who have developed diabetic retinopathy (Early Treatment Diabetic Retinopathy Study Research Group, 1991). Those who received this treatment had a 29 percent decrease in the incidence of severe visual loss five years after the therapy. Similarly, in the Beta-Blocker Heart Attack Trial (BHAT), those who received propanolol after a heart attack had 28 percent less mortality during the next 27 months than those who did not receive the drug (β-Blocker Heart Attack Trial Research Group, 1982).

The second type of trial, the treatment of risk factors by intervention, is illustrated by evaluations of drugs intended to reduce hypercholesterolemia and thus decrease the risk of developing coronary heart disease. If, in a randomized controlled trial, a drug successfully lowers serum cholesterol levels and this, in turn, reduces the incidence of coronary heart disease, the utility of the drug has been demonstrated. In addition, a strong link has been added to the chain of evidence showing a causal relationship between elevated serum cholesterol levels and coronary heart disease. An example of this approach is the Coronary Primary Prevention Trial (CPPT). In this randomized trial, individuals who received cholestyramine experienced a 19 percent reduction in coronary heart disease risk compared with persons in the placebo group (Lipid Research Clinics Program, 1984). The **cessation experiment** is also included in this category. Such a study differs from the others in that, instead of the addition of a mode of treatment, an attempt is made to evaluate the termination of a living habit considered to be of etiological importance. One such trial is the Oslo Heart Study, in which 1,232 men at high risk of cardiovascular disease were randomly allocated into two

Table 8–1.   Types and Examples of Randomized Clinical Trials

TYPE	EXAMPLE
Therapeutic	AZT treatment for AIDS
	Simple mastectomy for breast cancer
Intervention	AZT treatment of HIV-positive subject without symptoms of AIDS
	Mammography to detect asymptomatic breast cancer
	Cholesterol-lowering drugs to decrease the risk of myocardial infarction
Preventive	Hepatitis B vaccination for hepatitis and hepatocellular carcinoma prevention
	Education in use of condoms to reduce the risk of HIV transmission and infection

groups (Hjerman et al., 1981). One group received nutritional advice on lowering the lipid content of their diets and an educational program on cigarette smoking cessation; the other group received no advice regarding either diet or smoking cessation. After five years, the mean serum cholesterol concentration among those in the intervention group was 13 percent lower than those in the control group; the serum triglyceride concentration was 20 percent lower in the intervention group compared with the control group. Also, average cigarette smoking levels declined by 45 percent more in the intervention group than in the control group. Cessation of a high-cholesterol diet and cigarette smoking (in the intervention group) resulted in a 47 percent decline in myocardial infarction and sudden death risk.

The last type of study, the testing of a preventive agent, is illustrated by the evaluation of a vaccine for a given disease or of some form of chemoprophylaxis, such as aspirin to prevent myocardial infarction or stroke. If a randomized clinical trial shows that the vaccine or chemoprophylactic agent lowers the incidence of the disease, then that vaccine or agent may have value as a preventive measure (Shapiro et al., 1988). An example of such a trial is the Physicians' Health Study, which randomized 22,071 United States physicians to receive either aspirin or a placebo to reduce cardiovascular disease morbidity and mortality (Hennekens and Eberlein, 1985). There was a 39 percent decline in nonfatal myocardial infarction rates in the group that took aspirin compared with the control group (Steering Committee of the Physicians' Health Study Research Group, 1988).

The general principles are essentially the same in conducting clinical trials for infectious and noninfectious diseases, but the spectrum of noninfectious diseases (see Figure 3–9) is more complex. Each stage in the course of a chronic disease usually lasts a number of years, varying with the disease and the individual, and it is often difficult to make the distinctions between the stages. In addition, the etiological agent(s) is often unknown. In many chronic diseases, however, something is usually known about factors that are associated with an increased risk of developing the disease. These "risk factors" include such characteristics as elevation of serum cholesterol (in the case of coronary heart disease) and high blood pressure (in both cerebrovascular disease and coronary heart disease). Thus, in diagramming the natural history of a chronic disease, we can replace "etiological agent" in Figure 3–9 with "risk factor" (Figure 8–1). The stage to which the disease has progressed at the time the trial is started determines the type of trial. The relationship between the risk factor and possible etiological factors for three diseases is shown in Table 8–2.

General Plan of a Clinical Trial

The plan of a clinical trial is formally stated in a **protocol,** which contains the *objectives* and *specific procedures* to be used in the trial. It must be written before

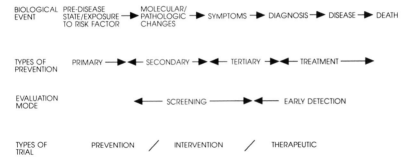

Figure 8–1. Diagrammatic representation of natural history of an infectious or non-infectious disease. *Source:* Meyskens (1988).

the start of the trial and should contain such information as the methods for selecting and then allocating the study groups, details on the performance of any laboratory tests, and the administration of the drug or other therapy. Once the protocol has been written, the epidemiologist compiles a ''manual of operations.'' During the course of the trial, if any questions arise because of a given situation, the manual of operations is referred to as the guide for what the investigator is to do. An outline for a typical protocol is presented in Table 8–3. Bearman's description of how to write such a protocol is an excellent guide (Bearman, 1975). More recently, several textbooks on the subject have appeared (Meinert, 1986; Fleiss, 1986).

Selection of Study Groups

At the beginning of a clinical trial, a decision must be made regarding the characteristics of the population to be studied; that is, what age and sex groups, disease characteristics, etc. are eligible for inclusion in the experiment. For example, in the Hypertension Detection and Follow-Up Project (HDFP), a randomized trial of the efficacy of systematic antihypertensive therapy, the criteria for inclusion in the study population were an age of 30 to 69 years, an average home screening diastolic blood pressure of 95 mmHg or above and a confirmed follow-up average

Table 8–2. Spectrum of Selected Diseases Divided Into Three Categories

	PREDISEASE STATE	
ETIOLOGICAL FACTOR	RISK FACTOR	DISEASE
Diet?	Elevated serum cholesterol ----≫	Coronary heart disease
Virus?	Hepatitis B ------------------≫	Hepatocellular carcinoma
???	Elevated blood pressure -------≫	Stroke

Table 8–3.   General Outline of a Protocol for a Clinical Trial

1. Rationale and background for study
2. Specific objectives of study
3. Concise statement of the study design (masking, randomization schemes, types and duration of treatments, number of patients)
4. Criteria for including and excluding subjects (including subject recruitment)
5. Outline of treatment procedures
6. Definition of all clinical, laboratory, and other methods
7. Methods of assuring the integrity of the data
8. Major and minor outcomes (e.g., death, myocardial infarction)
9. Provisions for observing and recording side effects
10. Procedures for handling problem cases
11. Procedures for obtaining the informed consent of subjects
12. Procedures for periodic review of trial
13. Procedures for analyzing results
14. Procedures for termination of trial
15. Procedures for communicating results of trial to study subjects and other interested persons
16. Appendices: Forms

Source: Adapted from Bearman (1975).

diastolic blood pressure of 90 mmHg or above, absence of terminal illness, and noninstitutional residence (Davis et al., 1986). In brief, the investigator selects a reference or "target" population that may be composed of persons with a certain disease or set of characteristics related to a disease, or persons in specific age groups, geographic areas, or occupations that would suggest their inclusion in the study. The type of reference population selected depends on the purpose of the study as well as the difficulties involved in subject recruitment.

Sample Size

The number of persons (the **sample size**) necessary to detect an effect of a drug or procedure must be computed from various statistical formulae that have been developed (Meinert, 1986; Fleiss, 1986). The importance of having a sufficient number of subjects can be seen in an example.

Suppose that one conducts a randomized trial of the effectiveness of a given drug in treating lung cancer. The epidemiologist hopes to detect a decrease in mortality one year after initiation of the treatment of at least 50 percent compared with the current therapy. There are four possible outcomes of this trial (Table 8–4). If the trial shows that the drug was effective (as defined by the epidemiologist in this example, efficacy would mean that it decreased mortality by at least 50 percent during the year after treatment began) and in reality it is, then the epidemiologist has reached a correct conclusion. The same can be said if the treat-

Table 8–4. The Possible Outcomes of a Randomized Clinical Trial

		ACTUAL EFFECT	
		TREATMENT EFFECTIVE	TREATMENT NOT EFFECTIVE
Conclusion Resulting from Trial	Treatment Effective	Correct Conclusion	Type I Error ("α-error") (False Positive)
	Treatment Not Effective	Type II Error ("β-error") (False Negative)	Correct Conclusion

ment was in reality not effective and the trial shows this (i.e., it decreased mortality by less than 50 percent).

If the trial result is a false positive one (i.e., the trial result indicates that the treatment is effective but in reality it isn't), then a **Type I error** (also known as an "α-error") has occurred. Alternatively, if the trial conclusion is a false negative one, then a **Type II error** (or "β-error") has taken place. The chances (or probability) of having a Type I error or a Type II error are related. If the epidemiologist reduces the chance of a Type I error, the chance of a Type II error increases, and vice versa. The only ways to simultaneously decrease both Type I and Type II errors are to either (1) increase the sample size or (2) increase the size of the minimum effect that the trial will detect, e.g., to use a decrease in mortality of at least 75 percent instead of 50 percent.

One measure frequently used to characterize the adequacy of the sample size to detect an effect is the **power** of the trial. Power is equal to $1 - P(\text{Type II error})$, where $P(\text{Type II})$ is the chance of a Type II error. Often, the minimum power for a trial is set at 80 percent, but other levels of power and Type I errors are also used by investigators, depending on the circumstances surrounding the trial. Freiman and her colleagues (1978) noted that in many trials in which the treatment was found not to be efficacious, the sample size was inadequate to detect a 25 to 50 percent improvement among those treated. The consequences of an inadequate sample size in a randomized clinical trial extend beyond missing an important therapeutic improvement. In one instance, an outbreak of surgical wound infections was attributed to use of an ineffective prophylactic antibiotic; the sample size of the trial suggesting that the antibiotic was efficacious was, in fact, too small to demonstrate such efficacy (Lilienfeld et al., 1986).

Use of Historical Controls

One type of comparison group should be mentioned because of its frequent use in evaluating preventive and therapeutic agents (Sacks et al., 1982; Ederer, 1975b;

Peto et al., 1976). **Historical controls** are selected from patients who have been treated *in the past* in one way so that their outcome can be compared with that of patients treated with a new method. This term is also used to describe a group of patients having a much broader prior therapeutic experience with a standard form of treatment. Clearly, there was no random assignment of patients to treatment and control group. Such a comparison may provide acceptable evidence if previous experience with a disease indicates that the standard method of treatment had resulted in a very high case-fatality rate, such as 95 percent (i.e., an invariable clinical course), while the new treatment has a marked effect, resulting in, say, a 50 percent fatality rate. This was the case with penicillin. Before its introduction, the case-fatality rate from certain infectious diseases, such as bacterial endocarditis, was almost 100 percent, and this was sharply reduced when these diseases were treated with penicillin. In most instances, however, the difference between new and old treatment methods is not so marked, and the clinical course of the untreated disease is not so fatal.

Incidence, case-fatality, and mortality rates for a given disease may vary with time. Relying on historical experience when assessing the effect of a new therapy may therefore result in a misleading inference. In a classic demonstration of this phenomenon, Pocock (1977) noted that reliance on such an approach would result in marked variability and incorrect conclusions regarding the efficacy of cancer chemotherapeutic agents. Another example of the hazards posed by the use of historical controls is provided by the Coronary Drug Project (1970), a randomized trial comparing the efficacy of several drugs for the long-term therapy of coronary heart disease in middle-aged men with previous myocardial infarction. The observed mortality rate in the control group was 4 percent, 33 percent less than the expected rate of 6 percent that had been previously observed in a group of myocardial infarction patients (Coronary Drug Project Research Group, 1975). Comparison of the mortality rate for any of the treatments with the expected rate might mislead an investigator to conclude that the treatments are more efficacious than they truly are.

Allocation

The subjects, once recruited, are randomly assigned to either the treatment or comparison groups. Simple random allocation can be refined by using such methods as "stratification" (Zelen, 1974; Green and Byar, 1978). This technique takes advantage of some of the factors that are known to influence the disease being studied. For instance, participants are often classified by sex and age, usually in five- or ten-year age groups known as "strata," since matching by individual years of age is impractical. When an individual is of the desired sex and within a certain age stratum, the person is randomly assigned to either the treatment or the comparison group from that stratum. It may also be desirable to stratify by severity of disease as severity generally has an effect on the outcome of the disease. Participants classified by severity of disease can *then* be randomly assigned to treatment or comparison groups by methods assuring approximately equal numbers in both groups within each category of severity. The study group receives the new treatment, preventive agent, or whatever type of intervention is under investigation, and the comparison group receives the usual, accepted treatment.

An example of the recruitment and allocation of study subjects into strata is given in Figure 8–2, from the Hypertension Detection and Follow-up Project (Davis et al., 1986). This trial compared the effect of intensive intervention to control hypertension with that of "usual care." The initial screening served to identify eligible hypertensives, to stratify them by diastolic blood pressure into three groups (90–104 mmHg, 105–114 mm Hg, and 115 mmHg or greater), and then to assign them randomly to either the intensive intervention group or the usual care group. The stratification was necessitated by the strong gradiant of mortality associated with increasing diastolic blood pressure. It allowed the inves-

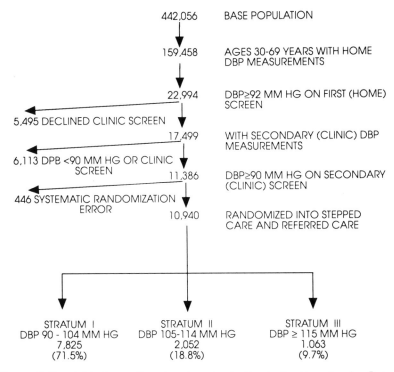

Figure 8–2. Subject recruitment and randomization in the Hypertension Detection and Follow-Up Study. *Source:* Davis et al. (1986).

tigators to examine the effect of intensive intervention not only in those with marked hypertension, i.e., a diastolic blood pressure of 115 mmHg or greater, but also in those with "mild" hypertension, i.e., a diastolic blood pressure of 90–104 mmHg.

Multicenter Comparison Groups

If the study is a multicenter one involving many clinics (which is often necessary to obtain a sufficient number of subjects), a comparison group is needed at each center. Each center represents a separate stratum; one center's comparison group *cannot* serve as a comparison group for the other centers. This is illustrated in Table 8–5, with the results from the two centers in the Swedish Breast Cancer Screening Trial, a randomized clinical trial that attempted to determine the efficacy of low-dose mammography to reduce breast cancer mortality (Tabar et al., 1985). The data in Table 8–5 show the breast cancer death rates among women screened in two counties in Sweden. Although the rates in the comparison groups differ from each other, the proportional decline in the mammography group mortality is the same in both counties (about 33 percent). Without a comparison group at each center, one might have decided that the technique was not effective since the death rate among women having mammography in Kopparberg County was higher than the death rate from breast cancer for comparison subjects in Ostergotland County (131 vs. 124 per 100,000).

Compliance with Treatment

Investigators cannot be certain that a treatment is or is not effective unless they can be assured that the treatment group is actually receiving the treatment; thus, it is necessary to continue to assess compliance with therapy during the trial (Haynes et al., 1978). A common strategy for assessing the compliance of patients in taking their medication, when it is a pill, is to give them more pills than needed for a given time period. They are instructed to return the unused pills, which are then counted. A comparison is made between the number of pills returned and

Table 8–5. Breast Cancer Mortality per 100,000 Women in the Swedish Breast Cancer Screening Study

	KOPPARBERG COUNTY	OSTERGOTLAND COUNTY
Mammography Group	130.6	92.2
Comparison Group	207.0	123.9

Source: Tabar et al. (1985).

the amount that should have been returned if the patient had taken the proper number.

Other ways of assessing the probability of adherence to assigned therapy have been used. In the previously mentioned Veterans Administration antihypertensive study, patients had to pass certain ''reliability'' tests before they could be included in the trial. For example, patients unlikely to be compliant with the treatment, such as homeless persons and alcoholics, were excluded from the trial. A biological method of measuring compliance with therapy was used in the Anturane Reinfarction Trial (Anturane Reinfarction Trial Research Group, 1978). Since Anturane has the pharmacologic effect of lowering serum uric acid levels, the investigators determined the serum uric acid levels in both the treatment and comparison groups to assess compliance. Similarly, in the Aspirin Myocardial Infarction Study (AMIS), the urine of participants was examined for salicylates as an indication of compliance (Aspirin Myocardial Infarction Study Research Group, 1980).

Determination of the Effect

The clinical trial requires that observations be made for each participant concerning the effect of the treatment being evaluated. In some situations, the individual participant is essentially the ''observer'' of the effect, as in the assessment of pain; in other situations a physician must determine if the individual's disease status has been altered or if the disease has been prevented. Unfortunately, knowledge of whether the participant was in the treatment or comparison group can influence the observation or care, resulting in *biased assessment of effect,* either consciously or subconsciously. Of course, if death is the outcome or effect being measured, the potential for bias in assessing outcome is considerably diminished. To remove these sources of bias in the observations, three procedures for making the necessary observations have been developed: single masking, double masking, and triple masking. (Meinert, 1986; Hill, 1951; Ederer, 1975a; Ballentine, 1975; Armitage, 1975). Sometimes, the term ''blinding'' is used in place of ''masking.''

Single masking

In a single-masked study, the participants are not given any indication whether they are in the treatment or comparison group. The object of single masking is to *prevent the participant from introducing bias* into the observations; this is often accomplished by means of a placebo. An example of the need for a placebo can be found in the mammary artery coronary bypass surgery trials of the 1950s for the treatment of angina pectoria; the comparison group underwent a sham procedure in which only the skin was cut (Dimond et al., 1958). In one particular trial, 10 of 13 patients who were operated on showed marked reduction in the degree of angina pectoria; however, all five of the patients who had only a skin incision (the mammary artery was not ligated) also reported marked improvement! This suggested that an individual's perception of pain was influenced by the belief that he had received the operation.

Double masking

Double masking seeks to remove biases that occur as a *result of either the subject or the observer of the subject being influenced by knowledge* that the subject is in the comparison or treatment group. The bias due to the subject's knowledge of his or her assignment can be eliminated by single masking, as already described; eliminating the bias that may result from the observer's knowledge requires that the observer also be masked with respect to the subject's allocation. Thus, in a double-masked study, neither the subject nor the observer (or assessor) of the subject has knowledge of the subject's group allocation. Double masking thereby minimizes not only bias in assessment but also any possible bias in the care of the subjects.

When examination of the subjects is not necessary to measure the outcome and an objective test such as an electrocardiogram or laboratory procedure is available, it is a simple matter to assemble the records and have them interpreted by someone not directly involved in the study. In addition, it is desirable to use mortality as the outcome of a study, if possible, since this leaves little room for subjective judgment. Even so, when specific causes of death are used as outcomes, their determination can be biased by knowing in which group the subject belongs. This potential bias in the determination of the cause of death can be prevented by masking the individuals who are assigning cause-of-death codes to deceased study participants.

Triple masking

Triple-masked studies carry the concept of masking one step further than does a double-masked study; *the subject, the observer of the subject, and the person reviewing the data* are all masked with regard to the group to which a specific individual belongs.

An overview of the various types of masking is schematically presented in Table 8–6.

Problems in Randomized Clinical Trials

Volunteers and nonparticipants

In experimental epidemiologic studies, only subjects who consent to participate will enter the study. This limits the inferences that can be derived from their

Table 8–6. Overview of the Various Types of Masking Used in
Randomized Clinical Trials

	TYPE OF MASKING		
	SINGLE	DOUBLE	TRIPLE
Subject	X	X	X
Observer	—	X	X
Data analyst	—	—	X

X = Masked with respect to subject's allocation.

— = May be aware of subject's allocation.

results since it has been shown that volunteers can differ in significant ways from nonparticipants (Crocetti, 1970; Wilhelmsen et al., 1976).

The design of the National Diet-Heart Study, an intervention trial regarding dietary fat intake, made it possible to compare the characteristics of those who volunteered and those who did not (American Heart Association, 1968; Crocetti, 1970). The volunteers were found to be more frequently nonsmokers, concerned about health, members of community organizations, active in community affairs, employed in professional and skilled positions, and they had received more formal education. A larger proportion of volunteers than nonparticipants were Protestants or Jews and lived in households with children. If any of these characteristics were also related to the outcome being measured, the investigator would have to limit the inferences from the study's results and generalize cautiously.

The problem of differences between volunteers and nonparticipants can be dealt with, to some extent, by following the nonparticipants in the same way as the volunteers to determine their outcome. Sampling the nonparticipants often allows for their characterization. Even if such follow-up is limited to mortality data, comparisons between the volunteer and nonparticipant groups provide valuable information on the extent to which the results may be generalized.

Refusals to continue in the study

In any follow-up study, there will be subjects who drop out of the study at some point. In the National Diet-Heart Study, Crocetti found that the long-term participants were more aware of the relationship of diet to heart disease and more active in community organizations than the short-term participants. Similar findings have been reported by Wilhelmsen et al. (1976) in a primary prevention trial of cardiovascular risk factors (hypertension and cigarette smoking). The occurrence of dropouts could bias the results of a study. As with nonparticipants, this problem can be partially solved by obtaining whatever information is available on the characteristics of the dropouts in addition to determining their outcomes.

It may be advisable to select a random sample of dropouts for intensive follow-up depending on their number and the difficulty of obtaining information about them.

Loss to follow-up

The need to keep the proportion of persons lost to follow-up at a minimum will be discussed in the context of cohort studies (see Chapter 10). Attempts should be made to obtain such minimal information on this group as mortality data. It may be necessary to randomly select a sample on which to focus these efforts.

Intervention studies

In the treatment of risk factors and cessation experiments, there is a special problem that reflects the biological features of some chronic, noninfectious diseases. Does a negative result in a risk-factor intervention study indicate that no causal relationship exists between the risk factors that were experimentally modified and the specific disease? The answer is "no," or "not necessarily," since it is quite conceivable that the underlying pathological process could represent the cumulative effect of exposure to the etiological agent over many years and that this process had already reached an irreversible state in those studied. Thus, either type of study may lead to a negative finding from which a negative inference cannot be drawn. There is no general rule for interpreting negative results of cessation and risk-factor treatment studies of chronic disease. The results of each study must be evaluated in terms of the current knowledge of the particular disease.

Integrity of the Data

A frequently overlooked aspect of the design of a clinical trial is maintaining the integrity of the data; this issue is critical to the success of a multicenter trial and is of general importance in any trial (Meinert, 1986; CIOMS, 1960). The epidemiologist must be certain that the data from the trial are accurately recorded, as well as accurately transferred from one data storage medium to another. All research data forms should have clear instructions.

One way of assuring that the integrity of the data has not been violated is to have a group of epidemiologists or biostatisticians not involved in the trial conduct an audit of the data. This was done in the Anturane Reinfarction Trial discussed above. An independent audit of the completed trial found coding errors in less than one percent of the data, a very acceptable rate.

Analysis of the Results

The epidemiologist should first examine the characteristics of the two groups at baseline to assess their comparability, determining whether randomization resulted in the formation of comparable and evenly balanced groups. The British Physicians' Aspirin Trial, an investigation of aspirin as a prophylactic medication to prevent cardiovascular and cerebrovascular disease, offers a good example of this (see Table 8–7) (Peto et al., 1988). Clearly, the two groups were comparable on a large number of characteristics.

After ascertaining the comparability of the treatment and comparison groups, the investigator must determine whether the treatment was effective. The groups are compared and the size of the differences assessed. Statistical tests of significance are used as a guide (and only as a guide) in these comparisons. The data are examined for internal consistency; the researcher assesses the quality of the data and searches for patterns to help interpret and explain the findings. Many of the statistical methods are very specific in their area of application, and new methods are constantly being devised (Peto et al., 1976, 1977; Meinert, 1986; Fleiss, 1986). A discussion of these techniques is beyond the scope of this book.

Table 8–7.   Selected Baseline Characteristics of British Physicians' Aspirin Trial Study Groups at Entry

	ASPIRIN GROUP	COMPARISON GROUP
Number of Participants	3,429	1,710
Age (Years)		
<60	1,604 (46.8%)	804 (47.0%)
60–69	1,349 (39.3%)	658 (38.5%)
70–79	476 (13.9%)	248 (14.5%)
Smoking		
Never	859 (25.1%)	395 (23.1%)
Ex-smoker	1,512 (44.1%)	776 (45.4%)
Current Smoker, cigarettes only		
<20/day	224 (6.5%)	123 (7.2%)
≥20/day	205 (6.0%)	109 (6.4%)
Other, or mixed, current smoker		
	625 (18.2%)	307 (18.0%)
Systolic blood pressure (mmHg)		
<130	816 (23.8%)	473 (27.7%)
130–149	1,235 (36.0%)	584 (34.2%)
>149	612 (17.8%)	288 (16.8%)
Not known	766 (22.3%)	365 (21.3%)

Source: Adapted from Peto et al. (1988).

When analyzing results, it is worthwhile to compare the information obtained early in a study on the dropouts and persons lost to follow-up with that obtained on those who remained in the study, and thus determine whether there are any differences between these groups. To avoid bias, the investigator usually should assume the most conservative outcome (i.e., the outcome that is least favorable for the treatment under evaluation) for those patients who have withdrawn from the study or have been lost to follow-up. A broad estimate of the effect of these groups on the overall findings can be made by calculating the two extremes of a range: one based on assuming the most conservative outcome and the other based on assuming the best possible outcome. Of course, this determination depends on the outcome used in a specific study.

A schematic outline of a clinical trial is given in Figure 8–3. Simply stated, the investigator specifies all aspects of the trial before it starts. One then follows that protocol rigidly. Perhaps the best advice for the conduct of a randomzed experiment is that given by Cornfield (1959): "Be careful."

ETHICAL CONSIDERATIONS

Clinical trials are similar in many ways to the observational studies discussed in Chapters 10 and 11. Because of the random assignment of subjects to the treatment and comparison groups, however, certain ethical questions arise. These ethical issues are of increasing concern to investigators, institutions, and sponsoring agencies. A detailed consideration of these issues is beyond the scope of this book. The reader is referred to Hill's (1977) and Chalmers's (1975) discussions of this issue. Hill has aptly stated the dilemma facing the investigator:

> The question at issue, then, is whether it is proper to withhold from any patient a treatment that might, perhaps, give him benefit. The value of the treatment is, clearly, not proven; if it were, there would be no need for a trial. But, on the other hand, there must be some basis for it—whether it be from evidence obtained in test tubes, animals or even in a few patients. There must be some basis to justify a trial at all.

Before a trial can be carried out, the consent of the subjects to participate must be obtained; it is important that the subjects be informed that they may be assigned to *either* the treatment or comparison groups. The risks of having the treatment must be explained; the possible benefits of the treatment must also be explained. If the subjects, provided with this information, still decide to participate in the study, then they are said to have given their **informed consent.** Such consent should be obtained in writing in accordance with regulations of govern-

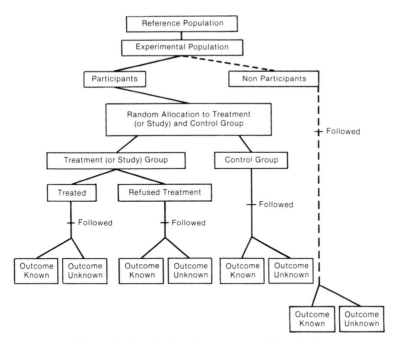

Figure 8–3. Outline of randomized clinical trial.

mental agencies (in the United States) or of the institution where the trial is to be conducted.

The investigator may, nonetheless, be troubled by the idea of withholding a possibly beneficial treatment from someone who is ill or at the risk of developing a disease. Green's statement is one of the better responses to this problem (Hill, 1977):

> Where the value of a treatment, old and new, is doubtful, there may be a higher moral obligation to test it critically than to continue to prescribe it year-in-year-out with the support merely of custom or wishful thinking.

Hill has provided some general criteria for the ethical conduct of clinical trials (Table 8–8). The investigator must also consider whether it is ethical if *no trial* is conducted.

The demand by persons with AIDS (through organizations representing their interests) that potential therapies be released and licensed for use before thorough scientific testing has led to a reexamination of current U.S. Food and Drug Administration (FDA) governmental regulations. The tension between the desire for early release and the requirement for adequate testing can lead to considerable

Table 8–8.   Ethical Considerations in a Randomized Clinical Trial

---

1. Is the proposed treatment safe for (unlikely to bring harm to) the patient?
2. For the sake of a controlled trial, can a treatment ethically be withheld from any patient in the doctor's care?
3. What patients may be brought into a controlled trial and allocated randomly to any of the different treatments?
4. Is it ethical to use a placebo or dummy treatment?
5. Is it proper for the trial to be in any way masked?

Source: Adapted from Hill (1977).

controversy and conflict, but the scientific "rules of evidence" are bypassed at great peril.

META-ANALYSIS

The completion of many randomized clinical trials of common agents in the past two decades has led to the use of "meta-analysis," in which data from similar studies are pooled in a statistically rigorous manner. The purposes of meta-analysis are four-fold: "(1) to improve the statistical power for primary outcomes for subgroups, (2) to resolve uncertainty when reports disagree, (3) to improve estimates of effect size, and (4) to answer questions not posed at the start of the individual trials" (Sacks et al., 1987). Underlying these aims is the assumption that one has access to all of the relevant data from all randomized clinical trials involving a given agent. Conversely, meta-analysis obscures differences among trials. As Meinert (1989) has noted, there is a tendency in meta-analysis to "knowingly or unwittingly" combine the results of different trials while ignoring the potentially important differences among them.

Dickersin and Berlin (1992) have described the historical development of meta-analysis. The term itself apparently was first used by Glass in 1976 in the context of educational research. Since then, a number of meta-analytic reviews have been published, including a recent one of long-term antiarrythmic therapy after a myocardial infarction (Hine et al., 1989). In this meta-analysis, data from the ten available studies were assembled (Figure 8–4). Although one of the studies had a statistically significant finding indicating an effect for therapy, the others did not. The aggregate effect was nil. The investigators concluded that such therapy is not efficacious and thus is not indicated after a myocardial infarction.

Several registries of randomized trials have been established that assist inves-

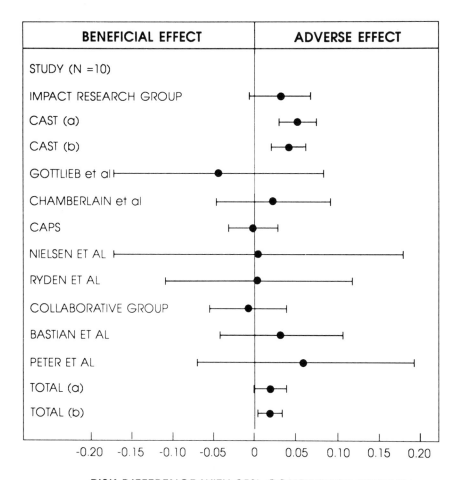

RISK DIFFERENCE WITH 95% CONFIDENCE INTERVAL

Figure 8–4. Mean case-fatality rate differences (and associated 95 percent confidence intervals) in ten randomized clinical trials of antiarrythmic therapy following a myocardial infarction, listed in descending order by quality. *Source:* Hine et al. (1989).

tigators in assembling all of the relevant data for a meta-analysis (Easterbrook, 1992; Dickersin and Berlin, 1992; Boissel, 1986; Simes, 1986; Meinert, 1988). In certain fields, e.g., perinatal medicine, such databases have been operating for some time (Chalmers, 1988). In others, e.g., neurological disorders, such registries need development. For reasons of cost, it is likely that meta-analyses will proliferate in place of large definitive trials; the needed databases should be developed to meet this demand.

For a detailed description of the statistical techniques used in a meta-analysis, the reader is referred to many recent reviews and books (Wolf, 1986; Sacks, et al., 1987; Abramson, 1990; Spector and Thompson, 1991; Louis et al., 1985; Glass et al., 1981; Eddy et al., 1992; DerSimonian and Laird, 1986).

SUMMARY

A randomized clinical trial is an experiment in which all participants are assigned to either the treatment group or the comparison group. These assignments are randomized. The process of randomization, if carried out properly, will provide comparable groups for most factors so that differences in outcomes at the end of the trial can be attributed to the intervention being tested.

There are three types of trials: therapeutic trials (in which the treatment of a disease is evaluated), intervention trials (in which an intervention in persons at elevated risk of developing a disease before the disease develops is evaluated), and preventive trials (in which the efficacy of a preventive agent is evaluated).

In a randomized clinical trial, the study is conducted according to a protocol, which describes in detail the design and rationale for the study. The study population is usually recruited until a predetermined sample size has been met. The sample size is selected to ensure that the study has adequate ''statistical power,'' i.e., so that if the treatment being studied is effective, its efficacy will not be mistakenly missed in the trial. Once the subjects have been recruited, they are randomly assigned to either the treatment or the comparison group. During the course of the trial, a major concern is the compliance of the study population with the study protocol; methods are available to assess the degree of compliance present in a trial. Assessment of an effect from the intervention being tested can be biased if either the subject or the assessor knows the person's group allocation. Masking is used to avoid this bias. It is important to minimize the number of subjects who either drop out or are lost to follow-up in a trial. If possible, the investigator should follow these persons to determine whether their withdrawal from the study introduced an important bias.

The nature of a randomized clinical trial necessitates concern with the ethical basis for its conduct. Often, one is concerned about withholding a possibly beneficial treatment from a patient in order to complete the study. However, one must also be concerned about interrupting a study before the treatment has been demonstrated to be efficacious.

Recently, a new analytic method for pooling the results of randomized clinical trials has been developed: meta-analysis. In this approach, all of the results of randomized trials for a certain issue are assembled and pooled in a statistically rigorous way.

STUDY PROBLEMS

1. Define radomization. List three major objectives in a randomized clinical trial.
2. What types of research on a new agent should be done before using it in a randomized clinical trial?
3. What are the limitations of the randomized clinical trial?
4. A triple-masked multi-center randomized clinical trial of a newly discovered therapeutic drug was conducted recently. Ten centers, all in the same state, participated in the trial; in each center, subjects were randomly assigned to either the experimental or control groups. All observations were sent to a central coordinating center where they were analyzed. The trial indicated that the drug was clearly efficacious (using standard statistical techniques).
   (a) List the various tabulations of the data that would be needed for a proper analysis of the drug's efficacy.
   (b) What inferences can be derived from such a trial?
   (c) List the various problems that could occur during such a trial. How might they be handled?
   (d) What questions should physicians ask themselves about the trial before using the drug in their practices?
5. List several situations in which a randomized clinical trial could be considered unethical. What other methods could be used in these situations? Discuss the limitations of each method.
6. What are the disadvantages of conducting a randomized clinical trial with a small sample size for a new agent when the benefit is small?
7. Can a randomized clinical trial provide useful information about side effects of a new treatment? Suppose that the adverse effects are rare.
8. Surgeons introducing new procedures often use a case series as proof of efficacy. What is the problem with this approach?
9. If one used an α-error value of 0.05 in a randomized clinical trial in which 60 statistical tests were performed, how many of those tests would one expect to be statistically significant even if there were no real difference? How does one deal with the problems posed by this result?

REFERENCES

Abramson, J. H. 1990. ''Meta-analysis: a review of pros and cons.'' *Pub. Health Rev.* 18: 1–47.
Altman, D. G. 1991. ''Randomisation.'' *Br. Med. J.* 302:1481–1482.

American Heart Association. 1968. *The National Diet-Heart Study: Final Report.* American Heart Assoc. Monogr. No. 18, New York: The American Heart Association, Inc.

Anturane Reinfarction Trial Research Group. 1978. "Sulfinpyrazone in the prevention of cardiac death after myocardial infarction." *New Engl. J. Med.* 298:289–295.

Armitage, P. 1975. *Sequential Medical Trials,* 2nd edition. New York: Halsted Press.

Aspirin Myocardial Infarction Study Research Group. 1980. "A randomized, controlled trial of aspirin in persons recovered from myocardial infarction." *J. Am. Med. Assn.* 243:661–669.

Ballentine, E. J. 1975. "Objective measurements and the double masked procedure." *Amer. J. Ophthalmol.* 79:763–767.

Bearman, J. E. 1975. "Writing the protocol for a clinical trial." *Amer. J. Ophthalmol.* 79: 775–778.

B-Blocker Heart Attack Trial Research Group. 1982. "A randomized trial of propranolol in patients with acute myocardial infarction." *J. Am. Med. Assn.* 247:1707–1714.

Boissel, J. 1986. "Registry of multicenter clinical trials: seventh report—1985." *Thromb. Haemost.* 55:282–291.

Chalmers, I. 1988. *Oxford Database of Perinatal Trials.* Oxford, England; Oxford University Press.

Chalmers, T. C. 1975. "Ethical aspects of clinical trials." *Amer. J. Ophthalmol.* 79:753–758.

Cornfield, J. 1959. "Principles of research." *Amer. J. Mental Defic.* 64:240–252.

CIOMS. 1960. *Conference on Controlled Clinical Trials.* Hill, A. B., Chairman. Springfield, Ill.: Charles C Thomas.

Coronary Drug Project Research Group. 1970. "Initial findings leading to modifications of its research protocol." *J. Am. Med. Assn.* 214:1303–1313.

Coronary Drug Project Research Group. 1975. "Clofibrate and niacin in coronary heart disease." *J. Am. Med. Assn.* 231:360–381.

Crocetti, A. F. 1970. "An interview study of volunteers and nonvolunteers in a medical research project." Thesis, Dr.P.H., School of Hygiene and Public Health, The Johns Hopkins University.

Davis, B. R., Ford, C. E., Remington, R. D., Stamler, R., and Hawkins, C. M. 1986. "The Hypertension Detection and Follow-up Program design, methods, and baseline characteristics and blood pressure response of the study population." *Prog. Card. Dis.* 29(3 Suppl 1):11–28.

DerSimonian, R., and Laird, N. 1986. "Meta-analysis in clinical trials." *Controlled Clin. Trials* 7:177–188.

Dickersin, K., and Berlin, J. A. 1992. "Meta-analysis: state-of-the-science." *Epid. Rev.* 14:154–176.

Dimond, E. G., Kittle, C. F., and Crocket, J. E. 1958. "Evaluation of internal mammary artery ligation and sham procedure in angina pectoris (abstract)." *Circulation* 18:712.

Early Treatment Diabetic Retinopathy Study Research Group. 1991. "Early Photocoagulation for diabetic retinopathy." *Ophthalmology* 98:766–785.

Easterbrook, P. J. 1992. "Directory of registries of clinical trials." *Stat. Med.* 11:345–423.

Eddy, D. M., Hasselblad, V., and Shacter, R. D. 1992. *Meta-analysis by the Confidence Profile Method: The Statistical Synthesis of Evidence.* Boston: Academic Press.

Ederer, F. 1975a. "Patient bias, investigator bias, and the double-masked procedure in clinical trials." *Am. J. Med.* 58:295–299.

———. 1975b. "Why do we need controls? Why do we need to randomize?" *Am. J. Ophthalmol.* 79:758–762.

Fleiss, J. L. 1986. *The Design and Analysis of Clinical Experiments.* New York: J. Wiley and Sons.

Freiman, J. A., Chalmers, T. C., Smith Jr., H., and Kuebler, R. R. 1978. "The importance of beta, the Type II Error and sample size in the design and interpretation of the randomized control trial." *New Engl. J. Med.* 299:690–694.

Glass, G. V., McGaw, B., and Smith, M. L. 1981. *Meta-analysis in Social Research.* Beverly Hills, Calif.: Sage Publications.

Glass, G. V. 1976. "Primary, secondary, and meta-analysis of research." *Educ. Res.* 5:3–8.

Green, S. B., and Byar, D. P. 1978. "The effect of stratified randomization on size and power of statistical tests in clinical trials." *J. Chron. Dis.* 31:445–454.

Haynes, R. B., Taylor, D. W., and Sackett, D. L., etc. 1978. *Compliance in Health Care.* Baltimore: The Johns Hopkins University Press.

Hennekens, C. H., and Eberlein, K. 1985. "A randomized trial of aspirin and beta-carotene among U.S. physicians." *Prev. Med.* 14:165–168.

Hill, A. B. 1951. "The clinical trial." *Brit. Med. Bull.* 7:278–282.

———. 1977. *A Short Textbook of Medical Statistics,* 10th ed. Philadelphia: J. B. Lippincott Co.

Hine, L. K., Laird, N. M., Hewitt, P., and Chalmers, T. C. 1989. "Meta-analysis of empirical long-term anti-arrythmic therapy after myocardial infarction." *J. Am. Med. Assn.* 262:3037–3040.

Hjermann, I., Velve Byre, K., Holme, I., and Leren, P. 1981. "Effect of diet and smoking intervention on the incidence of coronary heart disease. Report from the Oslo Study Group of a randomised trial in healthy men." *Lancet* 3:1303–1310.

Lilienfeld, D. E., Vlahov, D., Tenney, J. H., McLaughlin, J. S. 1986. "On antibiotic prophylaxis in cardiac surgery: a risk factor for wound infection." *Ann. Thorac. Surg.* 42:670–674.

Lipid Research Clinics Program. 1984. "The Lipid Research Clinics Coronary Primary Prevention Trial results: II. The reduction in the incidence of coronary heart disease due to cholesterol lowering." *J. Am. Med. Assn.* 251:365–374.

Louis, T. A., Fineberg, H. V., and Mosteller, F. 1985. "Findings for public health from meta-analyses." *Ann. Rev. Public Health* 6:1–20.

Meinert, C. L. 1986. *Clinical Trials.* New York: Oxford University Press.

———. 1988. "Toward prospective registration of clinical trials (editorial)." *Controlled Clin. Trials.* 9:1–5.

———. 1989. "Meta-analysis: Science or religion?" *Controlled Clin. Trials.* 10(45): 257S–263S.

Meyskens Jr, F. L. 1988. "Thinking about Cancer Causality and Chemoprevention." *J. Nat. Cancer Inst.* 80:1278–1281.

Peto, R., Pike, M. C., Armitage, P., Breslow, N. E., Cox, D. R., Howard, S. V., Mantel, N., McPherson, K., Peto, J., and Smith, P. G. 1976. "Design and analysis of randomized clinical trials requiring prolonged observation of each patient: I. Introduction and Design." *Brit. J. Cancer* 34:585–612.

———. 1977. "Design and analysis of randomized clinical trials requiring prolonged observation of each patient: II. Analysis and examples." *Brit. J. Cancer* 35:1–39.

Peto, R., Gray, R., Collins, R., Wheatley, K., Hennekens, C. H., Jamrozik, K., Warlow,

C., Hafner, B., Thompson, E., Norton, S., Gilliland, J., and Doll, R. 1988. "Randomised trial of prophylactic daily aspirin in British male doctors." *Br. Med. J.* 296:313–316.

Pocock S. J. 1977. Letter to the Editor. *Br. Med. J.* 1:1661.

Sacks, H. S., Chalmers, T. C., Smith Jr., H. 1982. "Randomized versus historical controls for clinical trials." *Am. J. Med.* 72:233–240.

Sacks, H. S., Berrier, J., Reitman, D., Ancone-Berk, V. A., and Chalmers, T. C. 1987. "Meta-analysis of randomized controlled trials." *New Engl. J. Med.* 316:450–455.

Shapiro, S., Venet, W., Strax, P., and Venet, L. 1988. *Periodic Screening for Breast Cancer: the Health Insurance Plan Project and Its Sequelae, 1963–1986.* Baltimore: The Johns Hopkins University Press.

Simes, R. J. 1986. "Publication bias: the case for an international registry of clinical trials." *J. Clin. Oncol.* 4:1529–1541.

Spector, T. D., and Thompson, S. G. 1991. "The potential and limitations of meta-analysis." *J. Epid. Com. Health* 45:89–92.

Steering Committee of the Physicians' Health Study Research Group. 1988. "Preliminary report: findings from the aspirin component of the ongoing Physicians' Health Study." *New Engl. J. Med.* 318:262–264.

Tabar, L., Fagerberg, C.J.G., Gad, A., Baldetorp, L., Holmberg, L. H., Grontoft, O., Ljungquist, U., Lundstrom, B., Manson, J. C., Eklund, G., Day, N. E., and Pettersson, F. 1985. "Reduction in mortality from breast cancer after mass screening with mammography." *Lancet* 1:829–833.

Wilhelmsen, L., Ljundberg, S., Wedel, H., and Werko, L. 1976. "A comparison between participants and non-participants in a primary preventive trial." *J. Chron. Dis.* 29:331–339.

Wolf, F. M. 1986. *Meta-analysis: Quantitative Methods for Research Synthesis.* Beverly Hills, Calif.: Sage Publications.

Zelen, M. 1974. "The randomization and stratification of patients to clinical trials." *J. Chron. Dis.* 27:365–375.

9

EXPERIMENTAL EPIDEMIOLOGY:
II. COMMUNITY TRIALS

Experimental epidemiology derives its strength from the investigator's ability to control the conditions under which a study is conducted. One of the principal means of control in a clinical trial is *randomly* allocating individual subjects to the exposed and unexposed groups, as discussed in Chapter 8. Randomized clinical trials are particularly useful when one can identify a high-risk population for which an intervention is available. However, there are situations in experimental epidemiology that do not lend themselves to a randomized clinical trial (Kottke et al., 1985; Puska et al., 1985; Sherwin, 1978).

Experiments that involve communities as a whole are known as "community trials." Such studies have also been called "lifestyle intervention trials," "field trials," and "community-based public health trials" (Fredrickson, 1968; Hulley, 1978; Farquhar, 1978). In a community trial, the group as a whole is collectively studied, while in a randomized clinical trial it is the individual within a group (the experimental or control group) that is studied. If the risk factors for a disease are so prevalent that one cannot easily identify a high-risk group within a population (for which intervention programs could be designed), then an intervention in the community may be needed (Kottke et al., 1985). For example, in the United States, elevated serum cholesterol and cigarette smoking (risk factors for cardiovascular and cerebrovascular disease) are common in the population. Identification of a high-risk group would require extensive screening of people, a process that would be expensive and would require much cooperation from them. Instead, interventions in the general population of the United States to reduce the prevalence of these risk factors (assessed by cross-sectional surveys of the population) may be indicated (Blackburn, 1983). By reducing the prevalence of the risk

179

population, one seeks to lower the incidence of the disease in the
nce the incubation period for a noninfectious disease can be years,
te outcome often assessed in a community trial is reduction in the
isk factors of interest.

mmunity trial, the epidemiologist selects two communities that are
similar in as many respects as possible. Community assent for participation in the
trial is obtained from various political and other community leaders. A survey is
conducted in each community to measure the incidence or prevalence of the
disease of interest and the prevalence of the suspected risk factors for which an
intervention has been developed. Possible interventions include behavior modification (e.g., health education) or consumption of a preventive agent (e.g., fluoride). The intervention is then carried out in one of the communities (the intervention community); the other community (the comparison community or control
community) does not receive it. Then the intervention stops. A survey is again
conducted in each community to measure the incidence of the disease of interest
and the prevalence of the suspected risk factors. The net difference in the incidence of the disease and in the prevalence of the suspected risk factors between
the intervention community and the comparison community is thereby associated
with the intervention.

An example of a community trial is the introduction of fluorides into the
water supply in order to determine whether this would decrease the frequency of
dental caries (see Chapter 1) (Ast and Schlesinger, 1956). Another illustration of
the method is Goldberger's demonstration in 1914–1916 of the dietary etiology
of pellegra (Golderger et al., 1923; Goldberger, 1964). In both of these instances,
however, the interventions were not allocated randomly. Recently, random
assignment of the intervention in community trials has become more
common.

An example of a randomized community trial is the WHO Collaborative
Trial in the Multifactorial Prevention of Coronary Heart Disease (World Health
Organization European Collaborative Group, 1980, 1983). In this study, workers
in 80 factories in four countries (Belgium, Italy, Poland, and the United Kingdom)
were screened between 1971 and 1977 for cigarette smoking, blood pressure,
weight, and serum cholesterol level. The 80 factories were arranged into 40 pairs
of plants of approximately comparable size, location, and type of industry. Within
each pair, one factory was randomly assigned to receive the intervention, which
consisted of a health education program for smoking cessation, cholesterol-low-
ering dietary advice, exercise, weight reduction, and control of hypertension. The
use of randomized assignment of the factories reduced the possible bias in the
assignment of the intervention that might otherwise be present in the study (Gail
et al., 1992; Cornfield, 1978; Buck and Conner, 1982). The results of this trial
were that the more overall risk-factor prevalence was reduced, the greater was

the net decline in cardiovascular disease incidence and mortality. Strong cultural differences in the degree to which risk-factor prevalence could be reduced by a standardized educational intervention were also identified.

CONDUCT OF A COMMUNITY TRIAL

Community trials have six stages (Table 9–1). Each of these stages relies upon the successful completion of the previous steps.

Development of a Protocol

As in a randomized controlled trial, the development of a formal protocol that states the rationale, procedures, and organization of the community trial is the essential first step. The protocol should also include a detailed description of the methods that will be used in periodic assessment of the progress of the study, as well as the methods of analyzing the results of the trial. In addition, the protocol must provide for such contingencies as adverse reactions to the intervention.

Community Selection and Recruitment

The second stage concerns the selection of the communities (intervention and control) that will be involved in the trial. The number and size of the communities that will be needed for the trial can be determined by using standard statistical formulae (Cornfield, 1978; Buck and Donner, 1982; Donner et al., 1981; Donner, 1987). As in a randomized clinical trial, the investigator must assure that the trial has sufficient power to detect the desired intervention effect. Since community-based interventions are expensive, the number of communities to be studied is often quite small. In the Minnesota Heart-Health Program, for example, a community trial of health education to reduce cardiovascular disease risk-factor prevalence (and ultimately cardiovascular disease occurrence), only six communities were studied (Jacobs et al., 1986). The consequence of a small number of

Table 9–1.   Stages in a Community Trial

1. Development of a protocol
2. Community selection and recruitment
3. Establishment of a baseline and community surveillance
4. Intervention selection and assignment
5. Oversight and data monitoring
6. Evaluation

communities in such trials may be the loss of statistical power to detect a difference between the intervention community (or communities) and the control community (or communities).

Ideally, the selected communities are stable, with little migration, and have self-contained medical care systems (Kessler and Levin, 1972). Five criteria are commonly used in the selection of specific communities: unusual prevalence of the disease, unusual prevalence of suspected risk factors, administrative convenience, favorable community relations, and availability of background demographic information on the communities. Since the administrative convenience with which a study can be managed and favorable community relations are the keys to a successful trial, it is these factors that are most important in the selection of the communities to be studied.

The communities should be similar in as many respects as possible. Their size (populations) should be comparable, as should their economies, the ethnicities of their populations, and so on. If any important factor is dissimilar between the two communities, it is possible that any differences in outcome between the communities could be attributed to that factor and not to the intervention. In the Minnesota Heart Health Program, for example, three different community sizes were selected for study: Two communities were "matched" towns, two were "matched" cities, and two were "matched" suburbs (Jacobs et al., 1986).

After the communities have been selected, they must be recruited to participate in the trial. Such recruitment includes obtaining the assent of local and regional elected officials, community leaders, and the local medical communities (Elder et al., 1986). Sherwin (1978) has noted that it is impossible to obtain informed consent from every member of a community involved in a community trial as the investigator would in a randomized clinical trial. However, aside from the practical issue of the difficulty of conducting surveys in communities in which local leaders have told the investigator that they do not want their localities involved in the study, it would also be unethical to proceed with the trial in those communities without consent from their leadership. Once these persons have agreed to the communities' participation, it is important for the investigator to inform the community members themselves that they will be participating in a study, e.g., through notices in the local newspaper and stories on the local television newscasts.

Establishment of a Baseline and Community Surveillance

The establishment of a baseline or starting point for the outcome(s) of interest in the investigation is the next step in the development of a community trial. The outcome may be relatively easy to assess, such as changes in mortality rates (Puska et al., 1985; Jacobs et al., 1986). Mortality changes can be followed by using death certificates in the participating communities. Incidence of disease can also be used as an outcome; however, many of the problems of ascertainment discussed in Chapter 7 must then be considered (Fortmann et al., 1986; Puska, 1991; Gillum, 1978). An intermediate outcome might also be used, such as changes in risk factors for the disease (e.g., dietary saturated fat consumption or prevalence of cigarette smoking).

Once the outcomes of interest have been selected, the investigator must determine the baseline for those outcomes in each of the communities. The method used for determining the baseline should be the same one that will be used at the end of the investigation to assess the effect of the intervention. It may also be desirable to determine the changes in outcome during the trial. Hence, the surveillance systems used, whether they be vital statistics systems, hospital-based case ascertainment, or community surveys, must be relatively low-cost and sensitive to the outcomes of interest (Puska, 1991).

Community surveillance consists of six steps: development of a protocol, community outreach, establishing diagnostic criteria, ascertainment of cases, validation, and data management (Gillum, 1978). Once the system has been planned in a protocol, the investigator must solicit community support for the trial. Endorsements from the communities' political, social, and medical leaders will facilitate the construction of the needed systems; they may also allow access to systems that communities have already established on their own. The definition of the outcomes must then be specified; for example, what diagnostic criteria apply to a myocardial infarction or to a stroke? The means by which the outcome is ascertained are then selected; a method for validating the ascertainment is also selected. Finally, the data collected during surveillance must be properly processed.

Intervention Selection and Assignment

Once the baseline has been established, the next step is to specify the type of intervention that will be used for the communities in the study. In community trials, the intervention is often education (Farquhar et al., 1977; Farquhar, 1978; Puska et al., 1985). For instance, if the hypothesis to be tested in a community trial is that use of condoms reduces the risk of AIDS, then an educational program might be used to increase the rate of condom use in the intervention community.

The assignment of the intervention to be used in the trial is simple: in a nonrandomized trial, the investigator simply assigns the intervention to one of the communities; in a randomized trial, a coin might be flipped to decide which community receives the intervention. For example, in the Community Intervention Trial for Smoking Cessation (COMMIT) study, a randomized community trial of smoking cessation, eleven pairs of communities were randomly assigned by roulette to either an intensive smoking cessation program (the intervention) or to no program (the comparison) (COMMIT, 1991; Gail et al., 1992). It is always possible that an investigator might unknowingly favor one community over the other one—which is the reason that randomization should be used.

Oversight and Data Monitoring

During the course of a community trial, data are collected and analyzed to determine whether the intervention is having any injurious effect; if such an effect were found, then the trial would have to be stopped. Such data collection and analysis permits surveillance (see Chapter 6, p. 104) of the outcomes that will

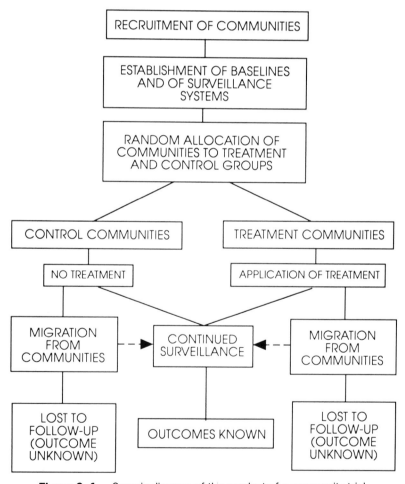

Figure 9–1.   Generic diagram of the conduct of a community trial.

be used to assess the effectiveness of the intervention (Gillum, 1978; Puska, 1991). A committee of experts not otherwise associated with the trial may meet regularly to decide whether the trial should continue, from an ethical perspective.

Evaluation

At the conclusion of the trial, the data are analyzed to determine if the intervention was effective. In the first stage of the analysis, no adjustment is made for any potential confounding factors. Since communities as an aggregate, and not as individuals, are compared, however, it is important also to analyze the data with such adjustments.

A major consideration in the evaluation of a trial is the statistical power to validly conclude from the trial that an intervention is effective. The concept of power in a community trial is the same as in a randomized clinical trial (see Chapter 8, p. 161). In the Minnesota Heart-Health Program, for example, the population being studied, about 430,000 persons, is sufficiently large to allow for the detection of a differential 14-percent decline in cardiovascular disease mortality with an Type I error of 5 percent and a power of 85 percent (Jacobs et al., 1986).

A diagram summarizing the conduct of a community trial is shown in Figure 9–1.

NONRANDOMIZED COMMUNITY TRIALS

Two nonrandomized community trials, both started in 1972, provide interesting examples of this type of experimental design. The North Karelia Project developed in response to a community's desire to reduce its high cardiovascular disease rates. It focused on community health education, training of health care providers, increased availability of healthier foods, and the development of community-based health behavior support networks. In contrast, the Stanford Five-City Project focused on community-based health education efforts as the means to reduce cardiovascular morbidity.

The North Karelia Project

The North Karelia Project exemplifies the concepts of a community trial described above. This community trial was launched after the rural Finnish province of North Karelia recognized that it had the highest frequency of cardiovascular disease in the world (Figure 9–2) (Puska et al., 1985). Representatives of North

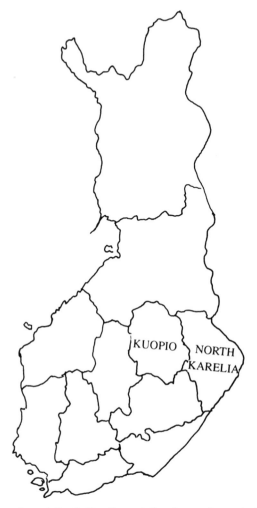

Figure 9–2. Location of North Karelia and Kuopio provinces in Finland. *Source:* Adapted from Salonen et al. (1983).

Karelia petitioned the Finnish government to undertake activities to reduce the occurrence of cardiovascular diseases. Local authorities, in collaboration with scientists and the World Health Organization, developed a protocol for a community trial. The interventions focused on reducing three major risk factors for cardiovascular disease (cigarette smoking, serum cholesterol level, and hypertension) that were known to be quite prevalent within the community as a whole and on improving medical care for those having myocardial infarctions or strokes.

A comparison province, Kuopio, with a population similar to that in North Karelia, was selected (Figure 9–2). Surveys were conducted in both provinces to provide baseline data for these three risk factors. Concurrently, myocardial infarc-

Table 9–2. Prevalence per 100 Population of Smoking among Residents of North
Karelia and Kuopio Communities in 1972, 1977, 1982, and 1987, by Gender

| YEAR | MEN | | WOMEN | |
	NORTH KARELIA	KUOPIO	NORTH KARELIA	KUOPIO
1972	52	50	10	11
1977	44	45	10	12
1982	36	42	15	15
1987	36	41	16	15

Source: Vartiainen et al. (1991).

tion and stroke registries were established in both areas. An intervention program
was then undertaken in North Karelia, including health education among influ-
ential citizens, training for health care providers, community health education,
screening for hypertension, and development of needed health care facilities. The
program was evaluated in 1977, 1982, and 1987 (Vartiainen et al., 1991). After
the first evaluation, efforts were begun to reduce the prevalence of cardiovascular
disease risk factors throughout Finland (Puska et al., 1985). Hence, any comparisons between North Karelia and Kuopio after 1977 must take into account the
national programs that affected both comparison communities.

The results of the third evaluation of the North Karelia Project are shown in
Tables 9–2, 9–3, and 9–4. Notable declines in the three major cardiovascular risk
factors in North Karelia can be seen; however, there are also decreases for the
comparison community, albeit smaller than for North Karelia. For most of the
risk factors examined, the declines were greatest between 1972 and 1982. For
the 1982–1987 period, the changes were slight. Ischemic heart disease mortality
data for North Karelia and the rest of Finland (including Kuopio) underscore the
impact of these declines in risk factors (Table 9–5) (Tuomilehto et al., 1989).
Although ischemic heart disease mortality in North Karelia declined for both men
and women from the early 1970s through the early 1980s, the death rates have

Table 9–3. Mean Serum Cholesterol Concentrations (mg/dL) among Residents of
North Karelia and Kuopio in 1972, 1977, 1982, and 1987, by Gender

| YEAR | MEN | | WOMEN | |
	NORTH KARELIA	KUOPIO	NORTH KARELIA	KUOPIO
1972	274	265	270	264
1977	258	261	254	251
1982	244	242	236	232
1987	242	240	231	227

Source: Vartiainen et al. (1991).

Table 9–4. Mean Diastolic Blood Pressure (mmHg) among Residents of North Karelia and Kuopio in 1972, 1977, 1982, and 1987, by Gender

YEAR	MEN		WOMEN	
	NORTH KARELIA	KUOPIO	NORTH KARELIA	KUOPIO
1972	92.0	93.3	92.4	91.3
1977	88.6	92.6	86.3	88.4
1982	86.7	88.9	84.5	84.8
1987	88.1	89.1	83.2	83.9

Source: Vartiainen et al. (1991).

remained constant during the mid-1980s. This pattern contrasts with that for the rest of Finland, which experienced most of its decline in ischemic heart disease mortality in the late 1970s through the mid-1980s. These changes have been attributed to declines in the prevalence of cardiovascular disease risk factors (Salonen et al., 1989).

The Stanford Five-City Project

Another recent example of a nonrandomized community trial is the Stanford Five-City Project, an attempt to determine whether community health education can decrease the rate of cardiovascular disease (Farquhar et al., 1985; Farquhar et al., 1990). In 1972, the first phase of this trial (the Stanford Three-Community Study) was started in three California communities; it was an attempt to modify the same

Table 9–5. Average Annual Age-Adjusted Ischemic Heart Disease Death Rate per 100,000 Persons in North Karelia and the Rest of Finland from 1969 to 1986, by Gender

PERIOD	MEN		WOMEN	
	NORTH KARELIA	REST OF FINLAND	NORTH KARELIA	REST OF FINLAND
1969–1971	715	491	132	90
1972–1974	637	470	96	87
1975–1977	592	469	89	80
1978–1980	538	417	82	71
1981–1982	501	383	75	63
1983	541	343	56	58
1984	509	343	81	57
1985	526	342	75	58
1986	439	317	93	54

Source: Tuomilehto et al. (1989).

three risk factors (cigarette smoking, elevated serum cholesterol levels, and high blood pressure) by community education (Farquhar et al., 1977). In two of the communities, extensive mass-media campaigns were conducted over a period of two years. In one of these, face-to-face counseling was also provided for a small subgroup of high-risk individuals. The third community served as a comparison.

In each community, people were interviewed and examined before the educational campaign began. One or two years later their knowledge and behavior with respect to diet and smoking were assessed. Physiological indicators of risk—blood pressure, relative weight, and plasma cholesterol—were also measured. The baseline values of the risk factors were remarkably uniform in these communities. After two years of campaigning, the mass media and the combination of mass media plus face-to-face instruction had significant positive effects on all factors except relative weight. The comparison of the treated and control communities yielded an estimated decrease in risk of developing cardiovascular disease of approximately 25 percent (Maccoby et al., 1977). These results were sufficiently encouraging that in 1980 the investigators extended the trial to five communities.

The Stanford Five-City Project involves two intervention communities and three control communities. The education campaign began in 1980 and continued for over five years. The first results of the trial (through 1985) showed small but distinct decreases within the intervention communities in the prevalence of all cardiovascular disease risk factors examined, except for body-mass index (Figure 9–3). Future analyses will deal with both cardiovascular disease and stroke mortality.

RANDOMIZED COMMUNITY TRIALS

Both the North Karelia Project and the Stanford Five-City Project developed in response to local concerns about high cardiovascular disease mortality rates. The use of randomization to assign the intervention to either North Karelia or Kuopio would not have been practical or ethical. The Stanford Five-City Project was an extension of a previous trial, the Stanford Three-Community Study, for which random assignment would also have been problematic, since two of the three communities shared a common television station that was to be used for the intervention. Recent community trials, however, have been started with randomized assignment of the intervention. As in randomized clinical trials, the use of randomized assignment helps to ensure that the distribution of all factors—known and unknown, measurable and not measurable—except for the intervention being studied, is based on chance and not some factor, such as investigator preference, that may lead to a bias in assignment. The Aceh Study, a randomized community

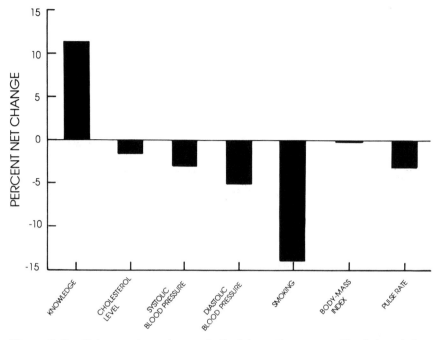

Figure 9–3. Net percentage changes in the intervention communities in knowledge and risk factors for persons 25 to 74 years old in the Stanford Five-City Project. *Source:* Farquhar et al. (1990).

trial of vitamin A supplementation and childhood mortality, illustrates this type of epidemiologic study.

The Aceh Study developed from epidemiologic observations suggesting that children with ophthalmologic indications of mild vitamin A deficiency had elevated death rates as a result of that deficiency (Sommer et al., 1986). Sommer and his colleagues sought to determine whether administration of vitamin A to children with such deficiency would reduce the associated mortality. The residents of an area of Indonesia, the Aceh Province, where xerophthalmia is endemic, were selected as the population to be studied.

Within the province, 2,048 villages in which there was no current or planned vitamin supplementation program were available for the study. From those villages, 450 were systematically selected for inclusion; these villages were then randomly assigned to either intervention (n = 229) or control (n = 221) groups. Some of the communities (18) were found to have started vitamin A supplementation programs before the baseline surveys began; adjacent villages (from among the 2,048) were substituted for them. The study was designed to be large enough to observe a 20-percent decline in mortality in the intervention communities with a Type I error of 5 percent and a power of 80 percent. A baseline survey of all 450 villages was undertaken. All children 0–5 years old were examined for active xerophthalmia; those with the disease were referred for intervention and were excluded from the trial.

The community intervention consisted of a single capsule of 200,000 IU vitamin A and 40 IU vitamin E. These capsules were given to children 1–5 years old by volunteers in the intervention communities about 1–3 months after the baseline survey. Capsules were also distributed six months later in both intervention and control communities during a follow-up examination.

In the trial, 29,236 children were enumerated at baseline; follow-up information was available on 89.0 percent of the treated children and 88.4 percent of the control children. During the follow-up period of six months, 53 children in the intervention villages and 75 children in the control villages died, a reduction in mortality of 34 percent (Figure 9–4). In the intervention villages, xerophthalmia prevalence declined by 85 percent. The investigators concluded that vitamin A supplementation in areas in which vitamin A deficiency is common would likely reduce mortality associated with the deficiency.

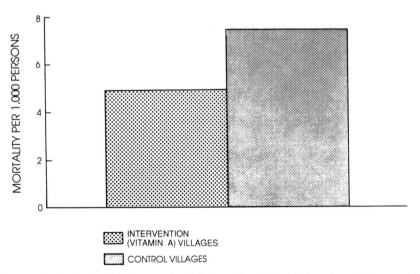

Figure 9–4.   Reduction in mortality in intervention (vitamin A) and control groups in the Aceh Study. *Source:* Adapted from Sommer et al. (1986).

LOSS TO FOLLOW-UP

Major concerns in any community trial are that some of the study population (either intervention or control) will be lost to follow-up and that the composition of the study population will change during the course of the trial (Buck and Donner, 1982). Over time, there is movement of persons both into and out of the community. Those who leave the community may be different from those who stay with regard to the factors being studied. The loss of persons from either group can create problems in interpreting the results of the trial. Persons who move into the community after the intervention has been administered, for instance, would not have been exposed to it, yet their health experience would be incorporated with that of the community during the evaluation stage of the trial (Gillum et al., 1980). Also, if there are more persons lost to follow-up in the intervention group than in the control group, the effectiveness of the intervention may be obscured (Farquhar et al., 1990).

COMMUNITY TRIALS VERSUS RANDOMIZED CLINICAL TRIALS

The difference between randomized clinical trials and community trials (randomized or not) is that in the former, the unit of intervention assignment is the individual and in the latter, a community. To help decide which design is more appropriate, four criteria are useful (Blackburn, 1984; Farquhar, 1978; Kottke et al., 1985):

1. *Complexity of the interventions.* If the disease and the intervention are more complex than can be addressed in a randomized clinical trial, a community trial may be more appropriate. For example, smoking cessation as a means of preventing cardiovascular disease and cancer depends in part on minimizing the stimulus to smoke in the smoker's environment. In a randomized clinical trial setting it is often difficult to modify the smoker's environment in this way, while in a community trial it may be less difficult.

2. *Type of factors targeted for intervention.* In randomized clinical trials, intervention for life-style factors, such as use of condoms for AIDS prevention, is often more difficult than for factors amenable to medical intervention, such as hypertension (Syme, 1978). In such situations, a community trial may be more practical.

3. *High prevalence of disease.* If the disease is common in the population, then a community trial may reach a larger group in the population than

would a randomized clinical trial. Hence, the public health impact of the intervention would be more cost-effective. Xerophthalmia in Indonesia and HIV infection among homosexual men in the United States are examples of such high-prevalence conditions.

4. *Health policy formulation.* If a local or regional health care system is inadequate to provide the needed intervention, then a community trial may be necessary to provide the scientific basis for public health policy.

The choice between a randomized clinical trial and a community trial essentially depends on the size of the population to be studied. The larger that population is, the more desirable a community trial becomes (Kottke et al., 1985). This is a matter of cost. For instance, hypercholesterolemia is prevalent in many communities in the United States. Screening and intervention for all persons with elevated serum cholesterol levels in these communities would consume many health care resources. Suppose that an educational program had been developed that purported to lower dietary cholesterol intake. Use of such a program, if effective, would likely consume fewer resources than screening and treating the entire population of those communities. Yet only a community trial could demonstrate its efficacy.

SUMMARY

A community trial is an experimental epidemiologic study design in which entire communities are assigned to either intervention or control groups. This approach is useful when the outcome of interest is so common that it is difficult to identify a high-risk group. It is an alternative to a randomized clinical trial.

The first step in the conduct of a community trial is the development of a protocol in which all of the procedures, definitions, and justifications for the conduct of the trial are stated. The next step is the recruitment of the communities that will be studied. Baselines for the factors targeted for intervention and the outcomes of interest are then established. Surveillance procedures to monitor changes in the factors and the outcomes are also implemented at this time. The intervention is then implemented. Data monitoring continues throughout the conduct of the trial. At the trial's conclusion, the data are analyzed to determine if the intervention had the desired effect. Until recently, intervention assignment in a community trial was not randomized. This was partly the result of the small numbers of communities studied. Recent trials with larger sample sizes, however, have used randomized assignment to reduce the possibility of bias in the results of a study.

STUDY PROBLEMS

1. What is the major difference between randomized clinical trials and community trials? Between natural experiments and human community trials?
2. List the different reasons for conducting community trials.
3. What are the limitations, if any, on the inferences that can be derived from the Stanford Five-City Project regarding the effects of community education in the control of cardiovascular diseases?
4. In previous chapters, the problem of ecological fallacy was discussed. You will recall that it arose from deriving inferences from observations of groups, such as communities, or geographical or political units, rather than of individuals as in a clinical trial or an observational study. Are community trials subject to the ecological fallacy? Explain.
5. In Chapter 8 the use of historical controls in clinical trials was discussed. If historical controls are used in community trials, what factors must be taken into consideration in interpreting the results of such a study?
6. It is generally accepted that the design of a randomized clinical trial is more important than the analysis of its results. Why? Is this also true of a community trial? Explain.
7. List some situations in which it would be preferable to conduct a community trial rather than a randomized clinical trial.
8. The housefly feeds on typhoid bacilli–infected excreta in the sickroom or privy and is able to carry such excreta from the sick to the healthy. In a city with a stable population, the privies were often open and accessible to the housefly. In a period of a few months toward the end

MONTH	TYPHOID CASES OCCURRING YEAR BEFORE FLYPROOFING	TYPHOID CASES OCCURRING YEAR AFTER FLYPROOFING
January	8	9
February	0	5
March	4	7
April	6	4
May	41	11
June	41	18
July	109	10
August	82	5
September	14	7
October	15	8
November	7	2
December	2	4
Total	329	90

of the year, the privies were all made flyproof. The number of cases listed on page 194 of typhoid fever occurred in the city the year before and the year after the privies were made flyproof, by month.

(a) What inferences could you derive from these data?

(b) Are there any additional data you would like to have before deriving any inferences? If so, list the kinds of data.

REFERENCES

Ast, D. B., and Schlesinger, E. R. 1956. "The conclusion of a ten-year study of water fluoridation." *Amer. J. Pub. Health* 46:265–271.

Blackburn, H. 1983. "Research and demonstration projects in community cardiovascular disease prevention." *J. Pub. Health Pol.* 4:398–421.

———. 1984. "Commentary: observation versus experiment." *Stat. Med.* 3:401–403.

Buck, C., and Donner, A. 1982. "The design of controlled experiments in the evaluation of non-therapeutic interventions." *J. Chron. Dis.* 35:531–538.

COMMIT Research Group. 1991. "Community Intervention Trial for Smoking Cessation (COMMIT): summary of design and intervention." *J. Nat. Cancer Inst.* 83:1620–1628.

Cornfield, J. 1978. "Randomization by group: A formal analysis." *Am. J. Epidemiol.* 108:100–102.

Donner, A., Birkett, N., and Buck, C. 1981. "Randomization by cluster: sample size requirements and analysis." *Am. J. Epidemiol.* 114:906–914.

Donner, A. 1987. "Statistical methodology for paired cluster designs." *Am. J. Epidemiol.* 126:972–979.

Elder, J. P., McGraw, S. A., Abrams, D. B., Ferreira, A., Lasater, T. M., Lonpre, H., Peterson, G. S., Schwertfeger, R., and Carleton, R. A. 1986. "Organizational and community approaches to communitywide prevention of heart disease: the first two years of the Pawtucket Heart Health Program." *Prev. Med.* 15:107–117.

Farquhar, J. W., Wood, P. D., Breitrose, H., Haskell, W. L., Meyer, A. J., Maccoby, N., Alexander, J. K., Brown Jr., B. W., McAlister, A. L., Nash, J. D., and Stern, M. P. 1977. "Community education for cardiovascular health." *Lancet* 1:1192–1195.

Farquhar, J. W. 1978. "The community-based model of life style intervention trials." *Am. J. Epidemiol.* 108:103–111.

Farquhar, J. W., Fortmann, S. P., Maccoby, N., Haskell, W. L., Williams, P. T., Flora, J. A., Taylor, C. B., Brown Jr., B. W., Solomon, D. S., and Hulley, S. B. 1985. "The Stanford Five-City Project: design and methods." *Am. J. Epidemiol.* 122:323–334.

Farquhar, J. W., Fortmann, S. P., Flora, J. A., Taylor, C. B., Haskell, W. L., Williams, P. T., Maccoby, N., and Wood, P. D. 1990. "Effects of communitywide education on cardiovascular disease risk factors. The Stanford Five-City Project." *J. Am. Med. Assn.* 264:359–365.

Fortmann, S. P., Haskell, W. L., Williams, P. T., Varady, A. N., Hulley, S. B., and Farquhar, J. W. 1986. "Community surveillance of cardiovascular diseases in the Stanford Five-City Project. Methods and initial experience." *Am. J. Epidemiol.* 123:656–669.

Fredrickson, D. S. 1968. "The field trial: some thoughts on the indispensible ordeal." *Bull. N.Y. Acad. Med.* 44:985–993.

Gail, M. H., Byar, D. P., Pechacek, T. F., and Corle, D. K. 1992. "Aspects of statistical design for the Community Intervention Trial for Smoking Cessation (COMMIT)." *Controlled Clin. Trials* 13:6–21.

Gillum, R. F. 1978. "Community surveillance for cardiovascular disease: methods, problems, applications—a review." *J. Chron. Dis.* 31:87–94.

Gillum, R. F., Williams, P. T., and Sondik, E. 1980. "Some considerations for the planning of the total community prevention trials—when is sample size adequate?" *Community Health* 5:270–278.

Goldberger, J., Waring, C. H., and Tanner, W. F. 1923. "Pellagra prevention by diet among institutional inmates." *Pub. Health Reps.* 38:2361–2368.

Goldberger, J. 1964. *Goldberger on Pellagra.* M. Terris, ed. Baton Rouge: Louisiana State University Press.

Hulley, S. B. 1978. "Symposium on CHD prevention trials: design issues in testing life style intervention." *Am. J. epidemiol.* 108:85–86.

Jacobs Jr., D. R., Luepker, R. V., Mittelmark, M. B., Folsom, A. R., Pirie, P. L., Mascioli, S. R., Hannan, P. J., Pechacek, T. F., Bracht, N. F., Carlaw, R. W., Kline, F. G., and Blackburn, H. 1986. "Communitywide prevention strategies: evaluation design of the Minnesota Heart Health Program." *J. Chron. Dis.* 39:775–788.

Kessler, I. I., and Levin, M. L., eds. 1972. *The Community as an Epidemiological Laboratory.* Baltimore: Johns Hopkins University Press.

Kottke, T. E., Puska, P., Salonen, J. T., Tuomilehto, J., and Nissinen, A. 1985. "Projected effects of high-risk versus population-based prevention strategies in coronary heart disease." *Am. J. Epidemiol.* 121:697–704.

Maccoby, N., Farquhar, J. W., Wood, P. D., and Alexander, J. 1977. "Reducing the risk of cardiovascular disease: effects of a community-based campaign on knowledge and risk." *J. Community Health* 3:100–114.

Puska, P., Nissinen, A., Tuomilehto, J., Salonen, J. T., Koskela, K., McAlister, A., Kottke, T. E., Maccoby, N., and Farquhar, J. W. 1985. "The community-based strategy to prevent coronary heart disease: conclusions from the ten years of the North Karelia Project." *Ann. Rev. Public Health* 6:147–193.

Puska, P. 1991. "Intervention and experimental studies." In *Oxford Textbook of Public Health,* 2nd ed. Holland, W. W., Detels, R., Knox, G., eds.). Oxford: Oxford University Press.

Salonen, J. T., Puska, P., Kottke, T. E., Tuomilehto, J., and Nissinen, A. 1983. "Decline in mortality from coronary heart disease in Finland from 1969 to 1979." *BMJ* 286: 1857–1860.

Salonen, J. T., Tuomilehto, J., Nissinen, A., Kaplan, G. A., Puska, P. 1989. "Contribution of risk factor changes to the decline in coronary incidence during the North Karelia Project: a within-community approach." *Int. J. Epid.* 18:595–601.

Sherwin, R. 1978. "Controlled trials of the diet-heart hypothesis: some comments on the experimental unit." *Am. J. Epidemiol.* 108:92–102.

Sommer, A., Tarwotjo, E., Djunaedi, E., West Jr., K. P., Loeden, A. A., Tilden, R., and Mele, L. 1986. "The Aceh Study Group. Impact of vitamin A supplementation on childhood mortality. A randomised controlled community trial." *Lancet* 1:1169–1173.

Syme, S. L. 1978. "Life style intervention in clinic-based trials." *Am. J. Epidemiol.* 108: 87–91.

Tuomilehto, J., Puska, P., Korhonen, K., Mustaniemi, H., Vartiainen, E., Nissinen, A., Kuulasmaa, K., Niemensivu, H., and Salonen, J. T. 1989. "Trends and determinants of ischemic heart disease mortality in Finland: with special reference to a possible leveling off in the early 1980s." *Int. J. Epid.* 18(Suppl 1):S109–S117.

Vartiainen, R., Korhonen, H. J., Pietinen, P., Tuomilehto, J., Kartovaara, L., Nissinen, A., and Puska, P. 1991. "Fifteen-year trends in coronary risk factors in Finland, with special reference to North Karelia." *Int. J. Epid.* 20:651–662.

World Health Organization European Collaborative Group. 1980. "Multifactorial trial in the prevention of coronary heart disease: 1. recruitment and initial findings." *Eur. Heart J.* 1:73–80.

———. 1982. "Multifactorial trial in the prevention of coronary heart disease: 3. incidence and mortality results." *Eur. Heart J.* 4:141–147.

10

OBSERVATIONAL STUDIES:
I. COHORT STUDIES

In the experimental method, an investigator studies the effect of a change in the genetic composition or environment of a cell, an organ, or an organism and makes a comparison with a similar cell, organ, or organism that has not been subjected to that change. This ideal is the basis of both experimental and observational epidemiologic studies. In an experimental epidemiologic study, the investigator assigns the treatment; however, in the observational study, the investigator can only *observe* the outcomes associated with the individual exposures experienced by participants in the study. The investigator does not control the assignment of that exposure experience.

The data collected in an observational study can be tabulated in the form of a fourfold table, as shown in Table 10–1. If two similar groups can be identified that differ only by being exposed to a given environmental factor, e.g., oral contraceptives, or by possessing a particular characteristic, e.g., a specific blood group, the epidemiologist can follow these two groups and observe the incidence of disease in each. This type of investigation is known as a "cohort" study and is the subject of this chapter. In many situations, however, it is impractical for the epidemiologist to identify groups of individuals based upon their exposure histories or characteristics. One can more readily identify those individuals who have ("cases") or do not have ("controls") the disease of interest; the individuals' histories of past exposure to the factor or characteristic of interest can then be obtained and compared. This type of investigation is known as a "case-control" study, and will be discussed in Chapter 11.

The general concept of a cohort study is relatively simple, although such studies can be conducted in several ways. A sample of the population is selected and information is obtained to determine which persons either have a particular

Table 10–1.   The Distinction between Cohort and Case-Control Studies

	CASE–CONTROL STUDY ↓	
ETIOLOGICAL CHARACTERISTIC OR EXPOSURE	DISEASED GROUP (CASES)	NONDISEASED GROUP (CONTROLS)
COHORT STUDY → Present (exposed) Absent (not exposed)		

characteristic (such as a behavior or physiological trait) that is suspected of being related to the development of the disease being investigated, or have been exposed to a possible etiological agent. These individuals are then followed for a period of time to observe who develops and/or dies from that disease or physiological condition (such as decline in a pulmonary function test). The necessary data for assessing the development of the disease can be obtained either directly (by periodic examinations of everyone in the sample) or indirectly (by reviewing physician and hospital records, disease registration forms, and death certificates). Incidence or death rates for the disease are then calculated, and the rates are compared for those with the characteristic of interest and those without it. If the rates are different (either absolutely or relatively), an association can be said to exist between the characteristic and the disease. It is important to obtain information on other general characteristics of the study groups, such as age, gender, ethnicity, and occupation, in addition to the specific characteristic of interest, in order to account for the influence of any factors that are known to be related to the disease. Statistical methods are available for such analyses (Breslow and Day, 1987; Kelsey et al., 1986; Kahn and Sempos, 1989; Fleiss, 1981).

This type of study has been described by a variety of terms: "prospective," "incidence," "longitudinal," "forward-looking," and "follow-up," but "cohort study" will be used in this book. A distinction should be noted between cohort studies, described in this chapter, and cohort analyses, discussed in Chapter 5. In cohort studies individuals are followed or traced, whereas in cohort analyses there is no actual follow-up of persons; the follow-up is *artificially constructed* by the analysis of mortality (or morbidity) in successive age groups over a series of time periods (see p. 94).

MEASURING ASSOCIATION IN COHORT STUDIES

The data collected in a cohort study consist of information about the exposure status of the individual and whether, after that exposure occurred, the individual developed a given disease. These data may be tabulated into a 2 × 2 table (Table

Table 10–2.   Framework of a Cohort Study

ETIOLOGICAL CHARACTERISTIC OR EXPOSURE	DEVELOPED DISEASE	DID NOT DEVELOP DISEASE	TOTAL
Present (exposed)	a	b	a+b
Absent (not exposed)	c	d	c+d

10–2). The incidence rate among those persons exposed to the factor being investigated is a/(a + b), while the rate for those not so exposed is c/(c + d). The epidemiologist is interested, then, in determining whether the incidence rate for those exposed is greater than the rate for individuals not exposed, i.e., is a/(a + b) greater than c/(c + d)? If it is, then an association is said to exist between the factor and the subsequent development of disease. The question then asked by the epidemiologist is: How strong is the association?

Relative Risk

The **relative risk** ("RR") is used to measure the strength of an association in an observational study (Cornfield, 1951):

$$\text{Relative Risk (RR)} = \frac{\text{Incidence rate of disease in exposed group}}{\text{Incidence rate of disease in unexposed group}}$$

The variance, confidence limits, and statistical tests for the relative risk may be found in the Appendix (p. 317). In a cohort study, if the incidence of myocardial infarction among cigarette smokers was 3 per 1,000 and that for nonsmokers was 1 per 1,000, then the relative risk of myocardial infarction for smokers compared to nonsmokers would be:

$$\text{RR} = \frac{(3/1,000)}{(1/1,000)} = 3.0$$

This value of the relative risk means that a cigarette smoker is three times as likely to develop a myocardial infarction as is a nonsmoker.

The magnitude of the relative risk reflects the strength of the association; i.e., the greater the relative risk, the stronger the association. A relative risk of 3.0 or more indicates a strong association; for cigarette smoking and lung cancer, for instance, it is greater than 10.0, signifying a very strong relation (United States Surgeon General, 1982). In contrast, the relative risk for a family history of breast cancer (sister or mother) and female breast cancer is about 2.0, indicating a moderate association (Kelsey, 1979). A relative risk between 1.0 and 1.5 indicates a weak association.

Relative risks may also be less than 1.0 in value, suggesting a protective effect from exposure to a factor. For example, in a cohort study in Mali of meningococcal vaccine efficacy conducted during an epidemic of meningococcal meningitis, Binken and Bond (1982) found that the incidence rate of the disease among those vaccinated was 0.7 per 10,000 persons and among those not vaccinated 4.7 per 10,000 persons over the 5-week period following the vaccination campaign. Hence, the relative risk of meningitis for those vaccinated compared to those not vaccinated was 0.15, meaning that the risk of developing meningitis for someone who was vaccinated is only 15 percent of that for someone who was not vaccinated. This relative risk suggests a strong association between vaccination and protection from developing the disease.

Inferences about the association between a disease and exposure to a factor are considerably strengthened if information is available to support a gradient in the relationship between the degree of exposure (or ''dose'') to the factor and the disease. Relative risks can be calculated for each dose of the factor. The general approach is to treat the data as a series of 2×2 tables, comparing those exposed at various levels of the factor with those not exposed at all. An example of this type of analysis is the study by Vessey and his colleagues (1989) of the relationship between oral contraceptive use and ovarian cancer.

In the early 1970s, the possibility of a relation between oral contraceptive use and gynecologic cancer occurrence was suggested. During the period 1968–1974, 17,032 white married women, aged 25 to 39 years, were recruited at the Oxford Family Planning Association clinics in England and Scotland (Vessey et al., 1976). Of those enrolled, 6,838 were parous women who used oral contraceptives and 3,154 were parous women who used an intrauterine device (IUD). Some of these women were followed for up to 20 years (from 1968) and deaths were recorded by specific cause. The risk of mortality from ovarian cancer for different duration levels of oral contraceptive use are shown in Table 10–3 compared with those who had no exposure, i.e., women who used an IUD. The relative risks of death from ovarian cancer for oral contraceptive users relative to nonusers were:

RR (less than 48 months of oral contraceptive use) = 12.1/9.2 = 1.32

RR (48–95 months of oral contraceptive use)   = 1.8/9.2 = 0.20

RR (more than 96 months of oral contraceptive use) = 1.5/9.2 = 0.16

Table 10–3. Mortality Rates per 100,000 Women-Years and Relative
Risk of Ovarian Cancer by Duration of Use of Oral Contraceptives

TOTAL DURATION OF USE	OVARIAN CANCER MORTALITY RATE	RELATIVE RISK[a] OF OVARIAN CANCER
Never[b]	9.2	1.00
≤ 47 months	12.1	1.32
48–95 months	1.8	0.20
96+ months	1.5	0.16

[a]Compared to "Never" users
[b]Intra-uterine device users
Source: Vessey et al. (1989).

This pattern of declining relative risk of ovarian cancer with increased duration
of oral contraceptive use suggests that these pharmaceuticals might protect against
this disease. A statistical significance test to determine whether such relative risks
are different from 1.0 was developed by Cochran (1954), and a method for calculating an overall (pooled) relative risk for all categories was developed by
Mantel and Haenszel (1959) (see Appendix, p. 320). If several studies of the same
epidemiologic problem have been carried out at different times and in different
places, it may be useful to scrutinize the estimates and then determine whether
they are similar (Breslow and Day, 1987; Greenland, 1987; Kahn and Sempos,
1989).

Attributable Fraction

A measure of association that is influenced by the frequency of a characteristic
in a population is the **attributable fraction** (also known as the "attributable
risk"). Levin (1953) originally defined it in terms of lung cancer and smoking as
the "maximum proportion of lung cancer attributable to cigarette smoking."
Attributable fraction can also be defined as the maximum proportion of a disease
in a population that can be attributed to a characteristic or etiologic factor. Another
way of using this concept is to think of it as the proportional decrease in the
incidence of a disease if the entire population were no longer exposed to the
suspected etiological agent. Although we are discussing attributable fraction in
the context of cohort studies, this measure of association is also useful in the
interpretation of case-control investigations (see Chapter 11).

As an example of the calculation of the attributable fraction, suppose that
the incidence of lung cancer in the overall population is 120 cases per 100,000
persons; among nonsmokers in that population, it is 30 cases per 100,000 persons;

and among smokers, it is 330 cases per 100,000 persons. The relative risk of lung cancer among smokers compared to nonsmokers would then be 11.0 (330 per 100,000 / 30 per 100,000). Also assume that 30 percent of the population smokes. If the 30 percent of the population that smokes were to stop, then the incidence of lung cancer in that group would be reduced from 330 cases per 100,000 persons to 30 cases per 100,000 persons. The attributable fraction of lung cancer for cigarette smoking would then be:

$$
\begin{aligned}
\text{Attributable Fraction (AF)} &= \frac{0.3 \ (330 \ \text{per} \ 100,000 \ - \ 30 \ \text{per} \ 100,000)}{120 \ \text{per} \ 100,000} \\
&= \frac{0.3 \ (300 \ \text{per} \ 100,000)}{120 \ \text{per} \ 100,000} \\
&= \frac{90 \ \text{per} \ 100,000}{120 \ \text{per} \ 100,000} \\
&= 75\%
\end{aligned}
$$

An alternative way to calculate the attributable fraction is:

$$
\text{Attributable Fraction (AF)} = \frac{P \ (RR \ - \ 1)}{P \ (RR \ - \ 1) \ + \ 1} \times 100\%
$$

where RR = the relative risk and P = proportion of the total population that has the characteristic; the derivation of this formula can be found in the Appendix (p. 319). In the lung cancer example, P is 30 percent and RR is 11.0. The attributable fraction would therefore be:

$$
AF = \frac{0.3 \ (11.0 \ - \ 1)}{0.3 \ (11.0 \ - \ 1) \ + \ 1} = \frac{3.0}{3.0 \ + \ 1} = \frac{3.0}{4.0} = 75\%
$$

Standard error and confidence limits have been derived for the attributable fraction by Walter (1975, 1976) (see Appendix).

The effect of various values of the relative risk (RR) and various proportions of those with a characteristic in the population (P) on the values of the attributable fraction is shown in Table 10–4. When the frequency of a characteristic in a population is low (e.g., 10 percent) and the relative risk for that characteristic in a given disease is also low (e.g., 2), only a small proportion (9 percent) of the cases of disease can be attributed to that characteristic (Adams et al., 1989). However, with a high relative risk (e.g., 10) and a high proportion of the population having the characteristic (e.g., 90 percent), a much larger percentage (89

Table 10–4.   Attributable Fractions* as a Proportion for Selected Values of Relative
Risk and Population Proportion with the Characteristic

| P = PROPORTION OF POPULATION | RR = RELATIVE RISK | | | |
WITH CHARACTERISTIC (%)	2	4	10	12
10	.09	.23	.47	.52
30	.23	.47	.73	.77
50	.33	.60	.82	.84
70	.41	.67	.86	.89
90	.47	.73	.89	.91
95	.49	.74	.90	.92

*Attributable fraction $= \dfrac{P\,(RR\,-\,1)}{P\,(RR\,-\,1)\,+\,1}$

percent) of cases can be attributed to it. In these calculations, it is assumed that
other etiological factors are equally distributed among those with and without the
characteristic.

The measurement of attributable fraction is particularly useful in planning
disease control programs (Walter, 1975, 1976; Stellman and Garfinkel, 1989). It
enables health administrators to estimate the extent to which a particular disease
is due to a specific factor and to predict the effectiveness of a control program in
reducing the disease by eliminating exposure to the factor. For example, epidemiologic studies have suggested that throughout the world, the hepatitis B virus
is the etiologic agent for 75 percent to 90 percent of primary hepatocellular cancer
(Beasley, 1988). A global hepatitis B vaccination campaign could therefore
greatly reduce the occurrence of this cancer.

Computations of attributable fraction are also helpful in developing strategies for epidemiologic research, particularly if there are multiple factors. In the
United States, for example, it is estimated that in certain age groups, 80 to 85
percent of lung cancer can be attributed to cigarette smoking. Other etiological
factors apparently play a relatively minor role, and the investigator interested in
ascertaining these factors may decide to limit further studies to nonsmoking lung
cancer patients. In general, if close to 100 percent of a disease is attributable to
one or more factors, a search for additional etiological factors may not be prof-
itable unless one is interested in studying other characteristics that influence those
already exposed to a high-risk factor.

Exposure Assessment

A crucial aspect of the design of cohort studies concerns the categorization of
subjects into ''exposed'' and ''unexposed'' groups that can be compared with

respect to disease incidence. If subjects cannot be correctly categorized, a cohort study is not feasible. An example of this inability to correctly classify exposure arose when epidemiologists at the Centers for Disease Control attempted to plan a cohort study of Vietnam veterans in regard to their exposure to Agent Orange, a defoliant that contained the toxic contaminant dioxin (Lilienfeld and Gallo, 1989; Centers for Disease Control Veterans Health Study, 1988). It was hoped that by learning about troop locations each day and comparing them to areas where the defoliant was sprayed the same day, an exposure score could be computed for each subject. However, when this score was compared with serum dioxin levels in a sample of such persons, it was clear that the exposure score would not be valid. Thus, the correct classification of exposure was problematic. The cancellation of the cohort study led to great protest by veterans' organizations who felt that their possible health risks were being ignored. However, conducting a cohort study with this high potential for misclassification might have led to results that underestimated the health risks of exposure to Agent Orange, if such risks actually exist.

Exposure assessment is important in all cohort studies, not only in those of occupational exposures. For example, the possible role of cardiovascular risk factors, such as hypertension and hypercholesterolemia, in pediatric atherosclerosis and adult cardiovascular disease is currently being studied in a cohort study of several thousand children in Bogalusa, Louisiana (Berenson and McMahon, 1980; Berenson, 1986). The exposure to these factors during childhood can be assessed directly, rather than trying to do so later in life.

TYPES OF COHORT STUDIES

Cohort studies can be classified as follows:

1. Concurrent studies
   (a) General population sample
   (b) Select groups of the population
       (i) Special groups—professional, veteran, etc.
       (ii) Exposed groups—occupational, etc.
2. Nonconcurrent studies
   (a) Population census taken in the past—usually special and unofficial
   (b) Select groups of the population
       (i) Special groups—professional, veteran, etc.
       (ii) Exposed groups—occupational, etc.

Concurrent and nonconcurrent cohort studies are contrasted in Figure 10–1. In a **concurrent study,** those with and without the characteristic or exposure are

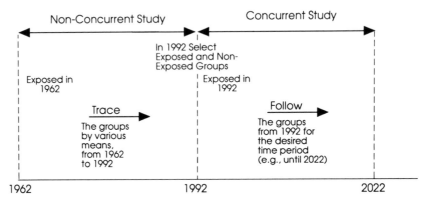

Figure 10–1. Diagrammatic representation of concurrent and nonconcurrent cohort studies.

selected at the start of the study (1992 in Figure 10–1) and *followed* over a number of years by a variety of methods. In a **nonconcurrent study,** the investigator goes back in time (to 1962 in Figure 10–1), selects his or her study groups, and *traces* them over time, usually to the present, by a variety of methods. These two types of cohort studies must be distinguished because they involve different methodological problems.

A simple example of a nonconcurrent cohort study would be an investigation of the safety of silicone breast implants. The epidemiologist might locate a group of plastic surgeons, each of whom used only one brand of silicone breast implant. The patient records of these surgeons would be reviewed for patients who had an implant placed two or three decades ago. Alternatively, if the epidemiologist identified a group of community hospitals in which silicone breast implant procedures were conducted, the medical records of the hospitals could be reviewed to provide information on the patients and the brand of implant used for each procedure. Regardless of the means by which the patients were identified, they would be followed up to the present time by contacting either the patient or the patient's family. For each brand of implant, the morbidity and mortality experience of the patient group would then be compared with that of the general population.

Concurrent Studies

In concurrent studies, the investigator begins with a group of individuals and follows them for a number of years. This was the approach used in the American Cancer Society's Cancer Prevention Study I (CPS I) of the health effects of cigarette smoking (Hammond, 1966; Garfinkel, 1985). The design of this study was similar to that of an earlier, smaller study (Hammond and Horn, 1958). For this investigation, 68,116 volunteers were recruited between October 1, 1959 and February 15, 1960. Each volunteer was asked to enroll families in which at least one person was 45 years of age or older. All persons in each household were asked to complete forms detailing their smoking histories, family history, medical history, occupational history, and various health habits. Follow-up was conducted every year (through the volunteers), and every two years subjects were asked to complete a follow-up questionnaire. Death certificates were obtained for each reported death. About 1,045,000 completed forms were received from persons residing in 1,121 counties in 25 states. Through September 30, 1962, 97.4 percent of the participants were successfully traced; 971,362 were reported to be alive, 46,212 had died, and 27,513 could not be traced. Age- and cause-specific and age-standardized mortality rates by history of tobacco use were computed from the collected data. Since tobacco use differed so markedly between men and women, the data were analyzed separately by gender. Figures 10–2 and 10–3 illustrate some of the findings for men in this classic study.

Figure 10–2 shows an increasing risk of mortality from bronchogenic (or lung) cancer with increasing number of cigarettes smoked and lower mortality rates among ex-smokers than among current smokers. Figure 10–3 shows that the mortality rates among ex-smokers decrease as the period of time since they had stopped increases, except for those who had stopped smoking within a year of entry into the study. This exception may reflect the fact that some of the men gave up smoking because they had already been diagnosed as having lung cancer. Such findings (the outcomes associated with cessation of exposure) are important

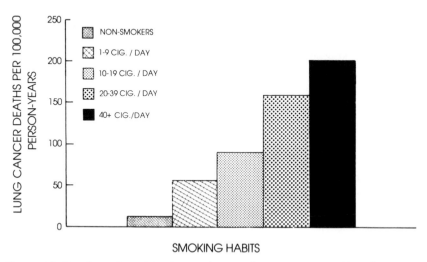

Figure 10–2. Age-adjusted death rates from malignant neoplasm of lung for men by amount of cigarette smoking at beginning of cohort study in 1959–1960. *Source:* Hammond (1966).

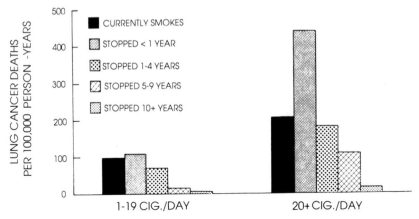

Figure 10–3. Age-adjusted death rates from malignant neoplasm of lung among men who had never smoked, who had stopped smoking, and who were still smoking at beginning of cohort study in 1959–60. *Source:* Hammond (1966).

in deriving etiological inferences from cohort studies (a subject that will be discussed in detail in Chapter 12). The groups in the CPS I study were not probability samples of the general population, which would have been preferable, but a probability sample of the required size would have been impossible to obtain. A similar study, known as the Cancer Prevention Study II, was started by the American Cancer Society in the late 1970s in order to examine more recent exposures of persons who may have been too young to participate in the CPS I study. Data collected in this ongoing investigation are now being analyzed.

A similar approach was used by Hirayama (1981a, b) in his pioneering study of passive smoking and lung cancer. He had collected information on the smoking habits of spouses of 91,540 nonsmoking wives and 20,289 nonsmoking husbands in six prefectures in Japan in 1965. The mortality of these men and women was assessed from death certificates during the 14 years of follow-up. Nonsmoking spouses of smokers had an elevated risk of lung cancer compared with that for nonsmoking couples (Figure 10–4). For nonsmoking men whose wives smoked 20 or more cigarettes daily, the risk was more than twice that of nonsmoking men married to nonsmoking women.

In some situations a cohort study can be conducted in a population selected from a well-defined geographical, political, or administrative area. This is particularly feasible when the disease or cause of death is fairly frequent in the population and does not require recruitment of a large number of persons for the study. The Framingham Heart Study is a good example of this type of cohort study (Dawber, 1980). It was initiated in 1948 by the United States Public Health Service to study the relationship of a variety of factors to the subsequent development

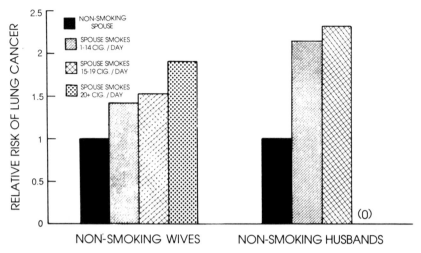

Figure 10–4. Age-adjusted relative risk of lung cancer among nonsmoking husbands and wives, by the smoking habits of their spouses. *Source:* Adapted from Hirayama (1981a).

of heart disease. The town of Framingham, Massachusetts, was chosen for its population stability, cooperation with previous community studies, presence of a local community hospital, and proximity to a large medical center. The initial population sample was a group of persons 30 to 62 years old that, when followed over a period of twenty years, would result in enough new cases or deaths from cardiovascular disease to ensure statistically reliable findings. The town's population in this age group was approximately 10,000. A sample of 6,507 men and women was selected. About 98 percent of the 4,469 respondents were free of coronary heart disease at the initial examination (Feinleib, 1985). Another 740 volunteers were also included in the cohort as part of a community outreach effort to ensure the continued participation in the study by each cohort member. After the first examination, each person was reexamined at two-year intervals for a thirty-year period. Information was obtained on several factors that could be related to heart disease, such as serum cholesterol level, blood pressure, weight, and history of cigarette smoking. Table 10–5 presents the incidence rates of coronary heart disease (CHD) among men and women during the first thirty years of follow-up by initial systolic blood pressure, gender, and age (Stokes et al., 1989). There is an increasing risk of CHD with increasing initial systolic blood pressure in the 35- to 64-year-old age group, a gradient of CHD disease which is slightly steeper in the older male age group and slightly less steep for the women.

The Framingham Heart Study also illustrates a strength of the cohort study:

Table 10–5. Average Annual Incidence per 1,000 Persons of Coronary Heart Diseae in Framingham, Massachusetts, 30-Year Follow-Up, by Systolic Blood Pressure and Gender

SYSTOLIC BLOOD	AGE 35–64		AGE 65–94	
PRESSURE (mmHg)	MEN	WOMEN	MEN	WOMEN
<120	7	3	11	10
120–139	11	4	19	13
140–159	16	7	27	16
160–179	23	9	34	35
>180	22	15	49	31

Source: Stokes et al. (1989).

investigating a variety of outcomes associated with a given exposure. For example, in addition to investigating the association between systolic blood pressure and CHD, for example, the Framingham investigators explored the relation between systolic blood pressure and stroke; a strong relationship between increased systolic blood pressure and elevated stroke risk was found.

The Framingham Heart Study became a prototype for similar studies in Tecumseh, Michigan, and other areas (Keys, 1970; McGee and Gordon, 1976; Napier et al., 1970). However, the difficulties in selecting general population samples for such studies tend to make investigators utilize a special group that for one reason or another can be followed more easily; certain professional groups, people enrolled in medical care programs, veterans, and others. In Doll and Hill's (1964) classic cohort study of cigarette smoking and lung cancer, for instance, a questionnaire was sent to all physicians on the British Medical Register who were living in the United Kingdom (see Chap. 1, p. 9). Follow-up was simplified because the subjects were physicians and therefore maintained contact with several professional organizations. Information from death certificates that listed "physician" as occupation was obtained from the Registrar General's Office. Lists were also obtained from the General Medical Council or the British Medical Association for deaths that had occurred abroad or in the military service.

A more recent example of the use of a unique population is the Oral Contraception Study of the Royal College of General Practitioners (1974) in England (Kay, 1984). Between May 1968 and July 1969, 23,000 oral contraceptive users and an equal number of nonusers, matched only for age and marital status, were recruited by physicians from among their patients. The oral contraceptive users selected were the first two women in each calendar month for whom the physicians wrote a prescription for an oral contraceptive. A nonuser was selected by the following procedure: starting with the user's record, returned to its correct place in the doctor's file, each subsequent record was examined in alphabetical order until the next record was found for a woman whose year of birth was within three years either side of that of the user and who had never used an oral contraceptive. Both the user and the nonuser had to be either married or known to be "living as married." These 46,000 women were followed with regard to their morbidity and mortality experience. In 1974, 1977, 1978, 1981, and 1988, progress reports were issued, showing associations between oral contraceptive use and (1) deep venous thrombosis, (2) acute myocardial infarction, and (3) subarachnoid hemorrhage (Table 10–6).

A similar approach was used by Hennekens and his colleagues (1979) in the Nurses' Health Study. These investigators sent questionnaires on possible risk factors (e.g., oral contraceptive use, smoking habits) to 121,700 nurses in 1976. Follow-up questionnaires were sent every two years thereafter to update risk factor information and to ascertain newly diagnosed conditions. Such data allow the epidemiologist to determine the effect of changes in risk factors on subsequent health events.

Concurrent cohort studies are not limited to noninfectious diseases. An example of the application of this method to infectious diseases is the study by Beasley et al. (1981, 1988) implicating the hepatitis B virus in the etiology of primary hepatocellular cancer. These investigators recruited 21,227 male Taiwanese government civil servants between November 1975 and June 1978, and 1,480 from a cohort study of risk factors for cardiovascular disease. Of these 22,707 men, 3,454 were hepatitis B surface antigen (HBsAg) positive, indicating past infection with the hepatitis B virus. By the end of 1986, 161 participants had developed primary hepatocellular cancer. The HBsAg positive group had a significantly higher rate of the disease than did the HbsAg negative group (Table 10–7). The relative risk of death from primary hepatocellular carcinoma among those who were HBsAg positive compared with that for those who were negative

Table 10–6.   Age-Adjusted Relative Risks of Oral Contraceptive Users Compared to Nonusers

DISEASE (ICD–9 CATEGORY)	RELATIVE RISK (ORAL CONTRACEPTIVE USER TO NONUSER)
Nonrheumatic heart disease and hypertension (400–429)	5.6
Ischemic heart disease (410–414)	3.9
Subarachnoid hemorrhage (430)	4.0
Cerebrovascular accident (431–433)	2.1
Deep thrombosis of the leg, pulmonary embolism (450–453)	(*)

Source: Adapted from Layde et al. (1981).

*Rate for nonusers was 0.0; no relative risk could be calculated.

Table 10–7.   Relation between HBsAg Antibody Status on Entrance to Study and Subsequent Development of Primary Hepatocellular Carcinoma through December 31, 1986

HBSAg STATUS	NUMBER	CASES OF PRIMARY HEPATOCELLULAR CARCINOMA	AVERAGE ANNUAL[1] INCIDENCE RATE OF PRIMARY HEPATOCELLULAR CARCINOMA PER 100,000 POPULATION
Positive	3,454	152	494.5
Negative	19,253	9	5.3

Relative risk of death from primary hepatocellular carcinoma among those who are HBsAg positive compared with those who are negative is (494.5/100,000)/(5.3/100,000) = 98.4.

[1]For 8.9 years of follow-up.

Source: Beasley (1988).

was 98.4, indicating a very strong association between HBsAg status and primary hepatocellular carcinoma.

The concurrent cohort study is particularly useful when the investigator does not know what the specific agent is when the study begins. In early 1984, for example, before the human immunodeficiency virus (HIV–1) had been identified as the etiologic agent for the acquired immunodeficiency syndrome (AIDS), the Multicenter AIDS Cohort Study (MACS) was begun to investigate the etiology and natural history of the disease (Kaslow et al., 1987). In Baltimore, Chicago, Los Angeles, and Pittsburgh, 4,955 homosexual men were recruited between April, 1984 and March, 1985. Each recruit provided blood, urine, feces, saliva, and semen specimens, which were stored for future analyses. The study population is reexamined every six months to determine if the participants have antibodies to the HIV–1 virus and, if so, what AIDS manifestations, if any, have developed. As hypotheses concerning the various manifestations of AIDS are developed, these specimen banks will be used to test those hypotheses.

In the concurrent cohort studies discussed so far, the study population was divided into those with and those without one or more possible etiological factors. The groups were sometimes classified according to different degrees of exposure or to levels of a characteristic such as the presence of the hepatitis B surface antigen. The incidence and mortality rates of these subgroups were then compared. The study groups were selected because they offered particular advantages for follow-up and information about a specific factor was obtainable from them. In a different type of concurrent study, a specific group that has been exposed to a possible etiological factor is selected and followed to determine the effects of this exposure as compared with the experience of a population not exposed to that substance. This method has been especially useful in studies of the effects of exposure to substances in occupational environments. The elucidation of the relation between occupational exposure to asbestos and lung cancer provides an example of this strategy.

In 1955, Doll reported that the relative risk of lung cancer in a group of asbestos factory workers compared to the general population was 10. In 1963, Selikoff and his co-workers began a cohort study of 370 members of the International Association of Health and Frost Insulators and Asbestos Workers (IAH-FIAW) (Selikoff et al., 1968). Follow-up of this cohort continued until 1967, when the investigation ended. The study findings suggested that there was an interaction between asbestos exposure and cigarette smoking in the development of respiratory cancer. These investigators initiated a study in 1967 of all U.S. and Canadian members of the IAHFIAW (Selikoff, 1979). The union provided the investigators with a membership list for 1966. Each member was mailed a questionnaire in which he was questioned about his smoking habits and the use of a mask while working. Some 17,800 men were followed from January 1, 1967 until December 31, 1976; 2,271 men died during the nine-year period. A control group, which had not been exposed to asbestos, was selected from the roster of 1,045,000 persons enrolled by the American Cancer Society in 1959 for the CPS I study described earlier. The control group, selected to be similar to the exposed group except for the exposure to asbestos, consisted of ''men, not a farmer, no more than a high school education, a history of occupational exposure to dust, fumes, vapors, gases, chemicals, or radiation, and alive as of January 1, 1967.'' This group numbered 73,763 such persons. Follow-up of the nonexposed individuals was conducted in September, 1972. Official mortality statistics were used to extrapolate the observed mortality through 1976.

One of the major findings of this study is the positive interaction between both cigarette smoking and asbestos in markedly elevating the risk of lung cancer (Table 10–8). This type of relation is indicated by the fact that the death rate for

Table 10–8.   Age-Adjusted Lung Cancer Death Rates per 100,000 Man-Years, by Cigarette Smoking Status and Occupational Exposure to Asbestos Dust

	NONSMOKERS	CIGARETTE SMOKERS
Not exposed to asbestos dust	11.3	122.6
	(1.0)*	(10.9)
Exposed to asbestos dust	58.4	601.6
	(5.2)	(53.2)

*Figure in parentheses is relative risk of lung cancer mortality compared with that for nonsmoking persons not exposed to asbestos dust.

Source: Hammond et al. (1979).

the combination of cigarette smoking and asbestos exposure was five times that of arette smokers without asbestos exposure and ten times that of nonsmoking persons with asbestos exposure. One might expect the relative risk for smoking workers to be about 15 if no positive interaction were present; however, it was 53, indicating such an interaction.

Nonconcurrent Studies

In nonconcurrent cohort studies, the period of observation starts from some date in the past, as illustrated in Figure 10–1; aside from the observation period, however, all other aspects of a nonconcurrent cohort study are the same as for a concurrent cohort investigation. These studies cannot be conducted with samples of the general population unless the investigator has access to a census of a community, usually unofficial, which was conducted in the past. Samples of the population covered by the census can then be selected and traced from the time of the census (Comstock, Abbey, and Lundin, 1970).

Nonconcurrent studies usually involve specially exposed groups or industrial populations because past census information is often unavailable and employment, medical, or other types of records usually are available. This is illustrated by the study of the relation between polycythemia vera (PV) and leukemia, which had been clinically observed since 1905 (Modan and Lilienfeld, 1965). The increased medical use of radiation treatment for PV and the observations of the leukemogenic effect of ionizing radiation in various studies raised the question as to whether the development of leukemia in patients with PV was part of the disease's natural history or a result of treatment with X-ray and/or P^{32}, a radioactive isotope. A study was undertaken to estimate the risk of developing leukemia among patients with PV and to determine whether it was increased as a result of P^{32} and/or X-ray treatment. Medical records of patients with PV who had been seen during 1947–1955 in seven medical centers were obtained at the same time as those of two comparison groups: (a) patients with polycythemia secondary to lung disease and (b) patients with questionable polycythemia. These groups were then classified by method of treatment into four categories: (1) no radiation treatment, (2) X-ray alone, (3) P^{32} only, and (4) a combination of X-ray and P^{32}. The patients were traced through December 31, 1961. Leukemia occurred predominantly in patients who had received some form of radiation, either X-ray, P^{32}, or a combination of the two (Figure 10–5). This finding has since been confirmed in a randomized clinical trial (Berk et al., 1981).

Nonconcurrent cohort studies of industrial exposures to possible etiological agents of disease can only be carried out by using company records of past and present employees that include information on the date that they begin their employment, age at hiring, the date of departure, and whether they are living or

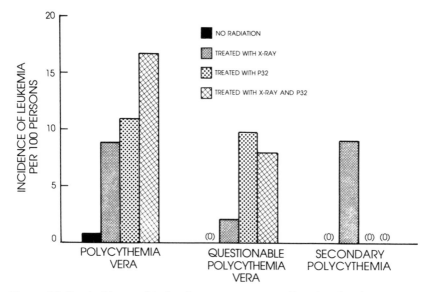

Figure 10–5. Incidence of leukemia among persons with polycythemia vera, questionable polycythemia vera, and secondary polycythemia vera. *Source:* Modan and Lilienfeld (1965).

dead. The mortality experience can be determined and compared with that of another industry, or with the mortality rate of the state where the industry is located, or of the country as a whole. This approach was used by Rinsky and his colleagues (1987) in a study of the relationship between exposure to benzene and leukemia mortality.

The study population consisted of all 1,165 nonsalaried white men employed in a rubber hydrochloride department of any of three plants in Ohio engaged in the manufacture of this natural rubber film for at least one day between January 1, 1940 and December 31, 1965. The cohort was assembled by using company personnel records. The cohort was traced through December 31, 1981, using vital status data from the Social Security Administration, the Ohio Bureau of Motor Vehicles, and a commercial tracing service. Death certificates were obtained for all deceased members. At the same time, an industrial hygienist used company records of benzene exposure to estimate the cumulative occupational exposure to benzene of each person in the cohort. At the time these exposure estimates were developed, the industrial hygienist did not know which of the cohort members had died from leukemia or from other causes.

The observed mortality from leukemia (nine deaths) was then compared with that expected if the cohort had had the same mortality experience as the United States population during the same time period. The results, shown in Figure 10–6, indicated a striking relationship between cumulative occupational exposure to benzene and leukemia mortality.

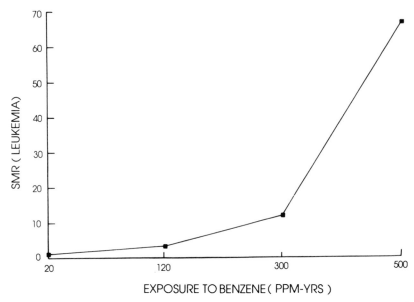

Figure 10–6. Standardized mortality ratio for 1,165 white men with at least one day of exposure to benzene from January 1, 1940 through December 31, 1965, according to cumulative exposure (parts of benzene per million particles × years of exposure). *Source:* Adapted from Rinsky et al. (1987).

STUDY PROCEDURES

A major source of difficulty in carrying out cohort studies is maintaining follow-up of the selected groups of persons. This is least troublesome in concurrent cohort studies for obvious reasons. At the very start of such studies, methods can be adopted for keeping in contact with the population on an annual basis, including periodic home visits, telephone calls, and mailed questionnaires, or even all three. The names and addresses of several friends and relatives can be obtained at the beginning of a study so that they may be contacted if the person moves out of the community. (Geographic mobility of people, particularly in the United States, can pose a problem.) To minimize the difficulties posed by tracing a cohort, cohort studies are often conducted in a health maintenance organization, in which the study population can be relatively easily followed. Another approach is to use a health or disability (for morbidity) or life (for mortality) insurer's clientele, as there is an economic incentive for the study population to inform the insurance company of the outcomes of interest. For deaths in the United States that have occurred since 1979, the National Death Index (administered by the National Center for Health Statistics) will inform investigators of the year and place of death for a given person (User's Manual, National Death Index, 1981).

In many countries, national or regional registries for cancer and other diseases can be used to follow up subjects in a cohort study.

Despite the best efforts, a certain number of individuals will likely be lost to follow-up. Even for this group, information on mortality status can often be obtained from state vital statistics bureaus. Their mortality experience can then be compared with that of the individuals not "lost to follow-up" to determine if there are any differences between the two groups. In addition, the successfully traced group can be compared to the "lost" group with respect to several known characteristics. To the extent that they show similar frequencies of a variety of characteristics of interest in the study, one's confidence is increased that no bias has been introduced into the findings by the lost group.

In a nonconcurrent cohort study, when one goes back perhaps twenty or thirty years to select a study group, the problem of tracing becomes more difficult. Every available source of information about subjects in the study should be used. Table 10–9 presents the various means used by Modan (1966) in determining the survivorship status of patients in his study of polycythemia vera and leukemia. In all cohort studies, it is desirable to trace as high a percentage of the study group as possible. Questions are frequently raised about the possibility of bias in the results if the degree of follow-up is less than 95 percent. This issue has been considered in several studies. Modan and Lilienfeld (1965) found that a very good estimate of the total mortality rate was obtained from the first 77 percent of the patients traced, although the group that was reached first had a somewhat higher leukemia mortality rate than those traced later. In a study of the outcome of neurosis, on the other hand, Sims (1973) found considerable differences

Table 10–9. Distribution of Sources of Information on Patient's Survivorship Status in the Study of Polycythemia Vera and Leukemia

SOURCE OF INFORMATION	NUMBER OF PATIENTS	PERCENT
Patient	158	12.9
Local physician	201	16.4
Relative	103	8.4
Hospital	540	44.2
Neighbors	49	4.0
Postmaster	18	1.5
Town-County clerk	20	1.6
Health department	89	7.3
Other	24	2.0
Untraced	20	1.6
Total	1,222	100.0

Source: Modan (1966).

between the patients who were easily contacted and those who were traced with more effort. Only three deaths had occurred among the first 110 patients traced (59 percent of the study group), but eighteen additional deaths were discovered in the sixty-six patients (36 percent of the study group) who were found by more intensive tracing. Rimm and his colleagues (1990) have noted that even the type of mail service used during follow-up can affect response rates. Thus, it appears that the pattern varies in different studies and, perhaps, with different diseases, so that a general rule cannot be established about the degree of follow-up necessary to ensure unbiased conclusions. The safest course is to attempt to achieve as complete a follow-up as possible.

ANALYSIS OF RESULTS

General Strategy

It has already been made clear that the results of cohort studies are preferably analyzed in terms of relative risks, which provide a relatively simple expression of the relation between mortality rates from different diseases in the groups being compared. This is particularly true if the follow-up observations are made in the same period for all the study groups.

Many cohort studies, however, whether concurrent or nonconcurrent, involve lengthy and varying periods of observations. Persons are lost to follow-up or die at different times during the course of the study, and consequently they are under observation for different time periods. In some studies, persons are enlisted or enter the study at different times and, if the follow-up is terminated at a specific time, they will have been observed for different lengths of time. Two related methods are available for analyzing the results of such studies:

1. The calculation of person-years or months of observation as the denominator for the computation of incidence or mortality rate.
2. Actuarial, life table, or survivorship analysis (also known as cumulative incidence or mortality analysis).

Person-years of observation are often used as denominators in the computation of rates in cohort studies, as in the Royal College of General Practitioner's Oral Contraceptives Study. They are particularly useful when several factors, such as age, sex, and varying periods of observation (which result from persons entering and leaving the study at different ages and times), make the computation of an actuarial life table difficult or impossible. This analytic approach takes into consideration both the number of persons who were followed and the duration of

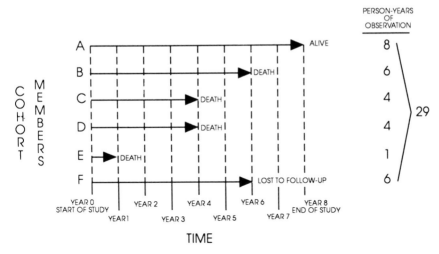

Figure 10–7. Diagrammatic illustration of contribution of person-years observed in a hypothetical eight-year cohort study of six persons (A,B,C,D,E, and F).

observation. In Figure 10–7, six persons are followed during an eight-year con-current cohort study. Four of these persons (B, C, D, and E) die during the course of the follow-up. One person (A) is alive at the end of the study, and one person (F) is lost to follow-up after six years. The total number of person-years of obser-vation (during which the cohort members were at risk of dying) is 29 years. The death rate in this study is therefore 4 deaths/29 person-years of observation (13.8 per 100 person-years of observation).

The use of person-years of observation makes it possible to express in one figure the time period when a varying number of persons is exposed to the risk of an event such as death or the development of disease. In addition, the age distribution of the groups under observation changes as a study progresses, as do the mortality and morbidity rates over time (Matanoski et al., 1975). The use of person-years is limited by the assumption that the risk of occurrence of an event per unit time is constant during the period of observation for the individual and that that risk is the same among similar persons in the cohort (Sheps, 1966; Breslow and Day, 1987). The overall effect of these limitations is modest and usually acceptable in most cohort studies.

Many regard using life tables (also known as survivorship methods) as the preferred method of analyzing data from cohort studies (see Appendix) (Chiang, 1961; Kahn and Sempos, 1989; Breslow and Day, 1987). They provide direct estimates of the probability of developing or dying from a disease for a given time period, and relative risks can be computed as the ratio of these probabilities. Life table methods can be used when the assumptions for person-years cannot be satisfied.

Latency

Regardless of the technique used to estimate the relative risk of developing a disease, one must also examine the possible effect of different latency or incubation periods. For instance, if a malignancy does not develop for at least a decade after the exposure to the suspected carcinogen began, then persons in the cohort would not be at risk for developing the disease until at least a decade had passed since their first exposure. Only after that decade had passed would those persons begin to accrue person-years of observation or be included in a life table (in the first interval); likewise, only if the disease developed after that first decade would that event be included in the analysis.

Adjustment for Age and Other Factors

The relative risks that are calculated by using either person-years or life table methods are unadjusted for age or other possible **confounding** factors. A confounding factor is one that is related both to the disease of interest and to another factor that is itself associated with the disease. For example, suppose that an epidemiologist conducted a cohort study of cigarette smoking and lung cancer. Many factors related to cigarette smoking (e.g., age, gender, and race) are independently associated with lung cancer. Hence, to measure the true relative risk between lung cancer and cigarette smoking, the epidemiologist would need to adjust the observed relative risk for these and other possible confounding factors. If adjustment for these factors does not change the relative risk, then little or no confounding is said to be present.

The epidemiologist may use two different approaches to adjust (or "control") for possible confounding factors:

1. Stratify the data by the possible confounding factors into multiple 2 × 2 tables to calculate the stratum-specific relative risk. An adjusted relative risk may then be calculated with Mantel-Haenszel techniques.
2. Use statistical techniques to mathematically model the risk of developing the disease, adjusted for the effects of the possible confounding factors. Examples include the logistic, the log-linear, and the proportional hazards models.

Where the entire study groups was exposed, however, it is necessary to use an external comparison or control group. If none is available, the mortality (or, if such data are available, the morbidity) experience of the exposed group is usually compared with that of the entire population living in the same geographical area as the exposed group, with statistical adjustments for age, sex, and calendar time of exposure and follow-up. For mortality, the number of deaths in the exposed group is compared with the expected number, based on the appropriate death rates for that geographical area. This comparison is then expressed as a Standardized Mortality Ratio (SMR) (see Chapter 4). This approach is frequently used in epidemiologic studies of occupational exposures (Monson, 1990). The previously described benzene-leukemia study by Rinsky et al. (1987) provides an example of this type of data analysis (see p. 215).

SUMMARY

In a cohort study, the investigator assembles a group of persons exposed to a possible etiologic factor and another, comparable group not exposed to that factor. These two groups are followed for the development of diseases. The investigator then calculates the incidence rate for a given condition in the exposed and unexposed groups, and a relative risk of developing the disease is calculated from those incidence rates. The stronger the association, the larger the relative risk; relative risks of 3.0 to 4.0 or more are usually indicative of strong associations between the factor and the disease. The proportion of disease in a population that is associated with that factor (assuming an etiologic relation) is the attributable fraction. The larger the attributable fraction of a disease for a given factor, the more difficult it becomes to study other possible agents of that disease.

There are two types of cohort studies: concurrent and nonconcurrent. In a concurrent study, the investigator assembles the exposed and nonexposed groups at the same time that the study is being conducted; these groups are then followed concurrently with the conduct of the study. In a nonconcurrent study the investigator reconstructs the groups in their entirety at some time in the past. This may be done with any set of records that provides information on all members of the population regarding their exposure at the same time in the past. Both groups are then followed to the present for the development of disease.

The process of following up the cohort of persons exposed and not exposed poses the greatest challenge to the epidemiologist in this study design. Inadequate follow-up can result in biased data and either spurious associations or missed relationships. It is also possible that the follow-up conducted in the early phases of a study may provide information on a portion of the cohort that is not reflective of the entire group. Analysis of the data at such a stage might result in different inferences than if one waited until both groups had been followed up completely.

Two methods are available for the analysis of cohort studies: (1) the calculation of incidence rates among those exposed and those not exposed using person-years of observation, and (2) the calculation of life-tables to provide interval-specific incidence rates of disease among those exposed and those not exposed.

The use of person-years assumes that the risk of developing the disease is the same in each time period of follow-up and also that the risk of developing disease for each member of the cohort is the same. The incidence rates for those exposed and those not exposed are then compared by calculating the relative risk of disease, a measure of the strength of the association between the exposure and the disease. The magnitude of the relative risk may be affected by the presence of confounding factors, which may be related to the exposure, to the disease, or both. The effects of confounding may be adjusted for by stratification (calculating stratum-specific relative risks) or by constructing a statistical model of the data. If the entire cohort was exposed to the factor (e.g., an occupational study), an SMR-based analysis may be used to control for possible confounding factors, such as age and gender.

STUDY PROBLEMS

1. It has often been stated that the Standardized Mortality Ratio (SMR) and the relative risk are equivalent. Are they? Why might such a statement be made?
2. How useful is the attributable fraction to the epidemiologist?
3. A certain virus V is suspected of being the cause of infectious disease D. Design a cohort study to elucidate the relationship between V and D. How does the design change if V is a "slow virus" or if D is currently viewed as a noninfectious disease?
4. Internationally, several medical billing data bases are being developed by health maintenance organizations (HMOs) and national health care systems. How can these systems be used to conduct both concurrent and nonconcurrent cohort studies?
5. A few surgeons seek your advice (as the local epidemiologist) concerning a study they would like to conduct to determine the effect of tonsillectomy on subsequent mortality. What might you recommend?

REFERENCES

Adams, M. J., Khoury, M. J., and James, L. M. 1989. "The use of attributable fraction in the design and interpretation of epidemiologic studies." *J. Clin. Epid.* 42:659–662.

Beasley, R. P., Hwang, L.-Y., Lin, C.-C., and Chien, C.-S. 1981. "Hepatocellular carcinoma and hepatitis B virus." *Lancet* 2:1129–1133.

Beasley, R. P. 1988. "Hepatitis B virus. The major etiology of hepatocellular carcinoma." *Cancer* 61:1942–1956.

Berenson, G. S. 1986. "Bogalusa Heart Study." In *Causation of Cardiovascular Risk Factors in Children: Perspectives on Cardiovascular Risk in Early Life.* G. S. Berenson, ed. New York: Raven Press.

Berenson, G. S., and McMahon, G. A., eds. 1980. *Cardiovascular Risk Factors in Children: The Early Natural History of Atherosclerosis and Essential Hypertension.* New York: Oxford University Press.

Berk, P. D., Goldberg, J. D., Silverstein, M. N., Weinfeld, A., Donovan, P. B., Ellis, J. T., Landau, S. A., Laszlo, J., Njean, Y., Pisciotta, A. V., and Wasserman, L. R. 1981. "Increased incidence of acute leukemia in polycythemia vera associated with chlorambucil therapy." *New Engl. J. Med.* 304:441–447.

Binken, N., and Bond, J. 1982. "Epidemic of meningococcal meningitis in Bamako, Mali: epidemiological features and analysis of vaccine efficacy." *Lancet* 2:315–317.

Breslow, N. E., and Day, N. E. 1987. *Statistical Methods in Cancer Research, Vol. 2. The Design and Analysis of Cohort Studies.* Lyon: International Agency for Research on Cancer.

Centers for Disease Control Veterans Health Study. 1988. "Serum 2,3,7,8-tetrachlorodibenzo-p-dioxin levels in U.S. Army Vietnam-era veterans." *JAMA* 260:1249–1254.

Chiang, C. L. 1961. "A stochastic study of the life table and its applications. III. The follow-up study with the consideration of competing risks." *Biometrics* 17:57–78.

Cochran, W. G. 1954. "Some methods of strengthening the common χ^2 tests." *Biometrics* 10:417–451.

Comstock, G. W., Abbey, H., and Lundin, F. E., Jr. 1970. "The nonofficial census as a basic tool for epidemiologic observations in Washington County, Maryland." In *The Community as an Epidemiologic Laboratory: A Casebook of Community Studies.* I. I. Kessler and M. L. Levin, eds. Baltimore, Md.: The Johns Hopkins Press, pp. 73–99.

Cornfield, J. 1951. "A method of estimating comparative rates from clinical data. Applications to cancer of the lung, breast, and cervix." *J. Nat. Cancer Inst.* 11:1269–1275.

Dawber, T. R. 1980. *The Framingham Study: the Epidemiology of Atherosclerotic Disease.* Cambridge, Mass.: Harvard University Press.

Doll, R., and Hill, A. B. 1964. "Mortality in relation to smoking: Ten years' observation of British doctors." *BMJ* 1:1399–1410; 1460–1467.

Doll, R. 1955. "Mortality from lung cancer in asbestos workers." *Br. J. Ind. Med.* 12:81–86.

Feinleib, M. 1985. "The Framingham Study: sample selection, follow-up, and methods of analysis." In *Selection, Follow-up, and Analysis in Prospective Studies: A Workshop.* Garfinkel, L., Ochs, O., Mushinski, M., eds. NCI Monograph No. 67. Washington, D.C.: U.S. Government Printing Office.

Fleiss, J. 1981. *Statistical Methods for Rates and Proportions,* 2nd ed. New York: J. Wiley and Sons.

Garfinkel, L. 1985. "Selection, follow-up, and analysis in the American Cancer Society Prospective Studies." In *Selection, Follow-up, and Analysis in Prospective Studies: A Workshop.* Garfinkel, L., Ochs, O., Mushinski, M., eds. NCI Monograph No. 67. Washington, D.C.: U.S. Government Printing Office.

Greenland, S. 1987. "Quantitative methods in the review of epidemiologic literature." *Epi. Rev.* 9:1–30.

Hammond, E. C. 1966. "Smoking in relation to the death rates of one million men and women.'' In *Epidemiological Studies of Cancer and Other Chronic Diseases.* NCI Monograph 19, pp. 127–204.

Hammond, E. C., and Horn, D. 1958. ''Smoking and death rates—Report on forty-four months of follow-up of 187,783 men. Part I. Total mortality. Part II. Death rates by cause.'' *JAMA* 166:1159–1172; 1294–1308.

Hammond, E. C., Selikoff, I. J., Seidman, H. 1979. ''Asbestos exposure, cigarette smoking, and death rates.'' *Ann. N.Y. Acad. Sci.* 330:473–490.

Hennekens, C. H., Speizer, F. E., Rosner, B., Bain, C. J., Belanger, C., and Peto, R. 1979. ''Use of permanent hair dyes and cancer among registered nurses.'' *Lancet* 1:1390–1393.

Hirayama, T. 1981a. ''Non-smoking wives of heavy smokers have a higher risk of lung cancer: a study from Japan.'' *BMJ* 282:183–185.

———. 1981b. ''Non-smoking wives of heavy smokers have a higher risk of lung cancer'' (letter). *BMJ* 283:1466.

Kahn, H. A., and Sempos, C. T. 1989. *Statistical Methods in Epidemiology.* New York: Oxford University Press.

Kaslow, R. A., Ostrow, D. G., Detels, R., Phair, J. P., Polk, B. F., Rinaldo Jr., C. R. 1987. ''The Multicenter AIDS Cohort Study: rationale, organization, and selected characteristics of the participants.'' *Am. J. Epidemiol.* 126:310–318.

Kay, C. R. 1984. ''The Royal College of General Practitioners' Oral Contraception Study: some recent observations.'' *Clinic. Obs. Gyn.* 11:759–781.

Kelsey, J. L. 1979. ''A review of the epidemiology of human breast cancer.'' *Epi. Rev.* 1: 74–109.

Kelsey, J. L., Thompson, W. D., and Evans, A. S. 1986. *Methods in Observational Epidemiology.* New York: Oxford University Press.

Keys, A., ed. 1970. *Coronary Heart Disease in Seven Countries.* Amer. Heart Assoc. Monog. No. 29. New York: The American Heart Association.

Layde, P. M., Beral, V., and Kay, C. R. 1981. ''Further analyses of mortality in oral contraceptive users. Royal College of General Practitioners' Oral Contraception Study.'' *Lancet* 1:541–546.

Levin, M. L. 1953. ''The occurrence of lung cancer in man.'' *Acta Unio In Contra Cancrum* 9:531–541.

Lilienfeld, D.E., and Gallo, M. 1989. ''2,4–D, 2, 4, 5–T, and 2, 3, 7, 8–TCDD: an overview.'' *Epi. Rev.* 11:28–58.

Mantel, N., and Haenszel, W. 1959. ''Statistical aspects of the analysis of data from retrospective studies of disease.'' *J. Nat. Cancer Inst.* 22:719–748.

Matanoski, G. M., Selter, R., Sartwell, P. E., Diamond, E. L., and Elliott, E. A. 1975. ''The current mortality rates of radiologists and other physician specialists: deaths from all causes and from cancer.'' *Am. J. Epidemiol.* 101:188–198.

McGee, D., and Gordon, T. 1976. *The Framingham Study: The Results of the Framingham Study Applied to Four Other U.S.-Based Epidemiologic Studies of Cardiovascular Disease.* Washington, D.C.: U.S. Government Printing Office.

Modan, B. 1966. ''Some methodological aspects of a retrospective follow-up study.'' *Am. J. Epidemiol.* 82:297–304.

Modan, B., and Lilienfeld, A. M. 1965. ''Polycythemia vera and leukemia—the role of radiation treatment.'' *Medicine* 44:305–344.

Monson, R. 1990. *Occupational Epidemiology,* 2nd edition. Boca Raton, Florida: CRC Press.

Napier, J. A., Johnson, B. C., and Epstein, F. H. 1970. "The Tecumseh, Michigan Community Health Study." In *The Community as an Epidemiologic Laboratory: A Casebook of Community Studies.* I. I. Kessler and M. L. Levin, eds. Baltimore, Md: The Johns Hopkins University Press, pp. 25–46.

Rimm, E. B., Stampfer, M. J., Colditz, G. A., Giovannucci, E., and Willett, W. C. 1990. "Effectiveness of various mailing strategies among nonrespondents in a prospective cohort study." *Am. J. Epidemiol.* 131:1068–1071.

Rinsky, R. A., Smith, A. B., Filloon, T. G., Young, R. J., Okun, A. H., and Landrigan, P. J. 1987. "Benzene and leukemia: An epidemiologic risk assessment." *New Engl. J. Med.* 316:1044–1050.

Selikoff, I. J., Hammond, E. C., and Churg, J. 1968. "Asbestos exposure, smoking, and neoplasia." *JAMA* 204:106–112.

———, ———, and Seidman, H. 1979. "Mortality experience of insulation workers in the United States, 1943–1976." *Ann. N.Y. Acad. Sci.* 330:91–116.

Sheps, M. C. 1966. "On the person-years concept in epidemiology and demography." *Milbank Mem. Fund Q.* 44:69–91.

Sims, A.C.P. 1973. "Importance of a high tracing-rate in long-term medical follow-up studies." *Lancet* 2:433–435.

Stellman, S. D., and Garfinkel, L. 1989. "Proportions of cancer deaths attributable to cigarette smoking in women." *Women Health* 15(2):1–29.

Stokes III, J., Kannel, W. B., Wolf, P. A., D'Agostino, R. B., and Cupples, L. A. 1989. "Blood pressure as a risk factor for cardiovascular disease." *Hypertension* 13 (Supplement 1):I13–I18.

User's Manual: The National Death Index. 1981. U.S. Department of Health and Human Services Publication (PHS)81-1148. Hyattsville, Maryland: National Center for Health Statistics.

United States Surgeon General. 1982. *The Health Consequences of Smoking. Cancer.* Washington, D.C.: U.S. Government Printing Office.

Vessey, M. P., Doll, R., Peto, R., Johnson, B., and Wiggins, P. 1976. "A long-term follow-up study of women using different methods of contraception. An interim report." *J. Biosocial Sci.* 8:373–427.

Vessey, M. P., Villard-Mackintosh, L., McPherson, K., and Yeates, D. 1989. "Mortality among oral contraceptive users: 20-year follow-up of women in a cohort study." *Brit. Med. J.* 299:1487–1491.

Walter, S. D. 1975. "The distribution of Levin's measure of attributable risk." *Biometrika* 62:371–374.

———. 1976. "The estimation and interpretation of attributable risk in health research." *Biometrics* 32:829–849.

11

OBSERVATIONAL STUDIES:
II. CASE-CONTROL STUDIES

In case-control studies, comparisons are made between a group of persons that have the disease under investigation and a group that do not. Usually those with the disease are called ''cases'' and those without the disease are called ''controls.'' Indeed, case-control studies may be viewed as an extension of the case series that a health professional might assemble from his or her practice but with an important addition—the *control group allows for a comparison* to be made with regard to exposure history. Since the exposure history is assessed for some period in the past, case-control studies are also called ''retrospective studies.''

Whether the characteristic or factor of interest is (or was) present in the two groups is usually determined by interview, review of records, or biological assay. The proportion of cases exposed to the agent or possessing the characteristic (or factor) of etiological interest is compared to the corresponding proportion in the control group. If a higher frequency of individuals with the characteristic is found among the cases than among the controls, an association between the disease and the characteristic may be inferred.

When interested in determining whether prior exposure to an environmental factor is etiologically important, the epidemiologist will attempt to obtain a history of such exposure by interviewing the cases and controls. In practice, information on both current and past characteristics is usually obtained. One must constantly be aware that the derivation of inferences depends upon the temporal sequence between the characteristic and the disease.

The data for a case-control study are generally tabulated in the form of a four-fold table, as shown in Table 11–1. Such a table allows for the comparison

Table 11–1. Framework of a Case-Control Study

	NUMBER OF INDIVIDUALS		
	WITH DISEASE	WITHOUT DISEASE	
CHARACTERISTIC	(CASES)	(CONTROLS)	TOTAL
With	a	b	a + b
Without	c	d	c + d
Total	a + c	b + d	a + b + c + d = N

of the prevalence of exposure among the cases, $a/(a + c)$, with that for the controls, $b/(b + d)$.

In a case-control study the odds ratio is an estimate of relative risk calculated as the cross-product of the entries in Table 11–1, ad/bc (see Appendix). Two assumptions are necessary in making this estimate: (a) the frequency of the disease in the population must be small, and (b) the study cases should be representative of the cases in the population and the controls representative of the noncases in the population. This cross-product estimate can be made with either actual numbers or percentages (Cornfield, 1951). The relative risk (or odds ratio) stays the same whatever the frequency of the exposure in a population. For example, whether smoking is highly prevalent or not, for a mother who smokes, the odds ratio describes her increased risk of delivering a low-birth-weight baby.

A study by Hurwitz and his colleagues (1987) of the relationship between the use of various medications and Reye's syndrome shows how the case-control approach can be used to investigate an etiological hypothesis and how the data can be analyzed with a four-fold table. Reye's syndrome is a rare, acute, and often fatal encephalopathy marked by brain swelling, low blood sugar, and fatty infiltration of the liver. Observations from case-series studies, case reports, and smaller case-control studies had implicated aspirin (salicylate) ingestion during viral illness as a possible cause of this disease of children. Cases deemed eligible for the Hurwitz study had to have received a diagnosis of Reye's syndrome from a physician, reported an antecedent respiratory or gastrointestinal illness or chicken pox within the three weeks before hospitalization, and experienced stage II or deeper encephalopathy. The control group consisted of children who did not have Reye's syndrome but did have chicken pox or a respiratory or gastrointestinal illness within a period of a few weeks before selection for the study. In this study there were four types of controls: emergency room patients (ER controls), inpatients (hospital controls), school children at the same school as the patient (school controls), and children located by the use of random-digit telephone dialing (community controls). The controls were matched to the cases on three patient characteristics: age, race, and the presence of an antecedent illness. The key data from the study are shown in Table 11–2. The percentage of salicylate users among

Table 11–2.   Number of Hospitalized Reye's Patients and Number of Pooled Controls with a History of Salicylate Use in Three-Week Period

	CASES OF REYE'S SYNDROME	CONTROLS (POOLED)
Used salicylates	26	53
Did *not* use salicylates	1	87
Total	27	140

Source: Hurwitz et al., 1987.

the cases was 96.3% (26/27) as compared to 37.9% (53/140) among the controls, and the odds ratio (the estimate of relative risk) was calculated as follows:

$$\frac{ad}{bc} = \frac{26 \times 87}{53 \times 1} = \frac{2262}{53} = 42.7$$

The variance, standard error, confidence limits, and significance test for the odds ratio can be computed by the procedures presented in the Appendix.

Children with viral illnesses (chicken pox, upper respiratory, or gastrointestinal) who used salicylates during the illness were 42.7 times more likely to develop Reye's syndrome than were children with the same viral illness who did not use salicylates. Thus, aspirin use during viral illness appeared to be strongly associated with the development of Reye's syndrome, increasing the risk over forty-fold.

While these data provide an estimate of risk, they do not allow one to estimate the incidence of Reye's syndrome in the population of children at risk. To estimate the incidence one would need to know the number of all cases of Reye's syndrome among children (for the numerator) and the number of children who experienced respiratory or gastrointestinal illnesses or chicken pox (the denominator). Most case-control studies do not allow one to estimate incidence because denominator data are not available and numerator data may be incomplete.

THE SELECTION OF CASES AND CONTROLS

Various methods have been used to select cases and controls for case-control studies (Table 11–3) Sometimes investigators select cases from one source and controls from a variety of sources, permitting comparisons with different control groups as in the Reye's syndrome study (see Table 11–4). Consistency of results among studies using different types of control groups increases the validity of inferences that may be derived from the findings.

How many controls should be obtained for each case? Appropriate controls are often scarce or limited. In comparing workers at a factory who were or were not exposed to a substance, for instance, one would be limited to the finite set of workers who worked at the factory. In other situations, appropriate controls are readily available, as when studying normal birth outcomes compared to undesirable birth outcomes. Even when controls are abundant, it may be costly and time-consuming to enroll and interview controls; one would want to include only as many as are needed. In studies of rare diseases the number of cases may be so small that the study has insufficient power to detect meaningful differences in exposure. An increased number of controls—up to four per case—may give the study more power (Gail et al., 1976). When the number of cases is large and the power is greater than 0.9 with only one control per case, additional controls cannot add very much to the power.

In selecting cases one may often use all cases occurring in a defined time

Table 11–3. Some Sources of Cases and Controls in Case-Control Studies*

CASES	CONTROLS
All cases diagnosed in the community (in hospitals, other medical facilities including physicians' offices)	Probability sample of general population in a community obtained by various methods including random-digit dialing
All cases diagnosed in a sample of the general population	Noncases in a sample of the general population or subgroup of a sample of general population (e.g., random-digit dialing)
All cases diagnosed in all hospitals in the community	Sample of patients in all hospitals in the community who do not have the diseases being studied
All cases diagnosed in a single hospital	Sample of patients in same hospital where cases were selected
All cases diagnosed in one or more hospitals	Sample of individuals who are residents in same block or neighborhood of cases
Cases selected by any of the above methods	Spouses, siblings, or associates (schoolmates or workmates) of cases Accident victims

*Various combinations of sources are possible.

Table 11–4. Comparison of Salicylate Exposure among Reye's Patients and Four Types of Controls

| | | CONTROLS | | | |
	CASES	EMERGENCY ROOM	INPATIENT	SCHOOL	COMMUNITY
Exposed to aspirin (%)	96	40	27	44	34
Total N	27	30	22	45	43
Odds ratios	—	39	66	33	44

Source: Hurwitz et al., 1987.

period or geographic area. The researcher then has an idea about the age, race, and gender of the cases, as well as other characteristics. To ensure comparability of cases and controls one may **restrict** the controls to the same age range, race, and gender (or other characteristic) as the cases, or one may **group match** (also known as **frequency match**). For example, the cases can be stratified into different ten-year age groups. The control group can then be similarly stratified. Comparisons can then be made at each factor level between cases and controls with the usual statistical significance tests (Cochran, 1954; Mantel and Haenszel, 1959).

As an alternative to group matching, individual cases and controls can be **pair-matched** for various characteristics so that each case has a pairmate. Ideally, these pairmates should be chosen to be alike on all characteristics except for the particular one under investigation. In practice, if many characteristics are chosen for matching, or if many levels are chosen for each characteristic, it becomes difficult to find matching controls for each of the cases. In epidemiologic studies, there are usually a small number of cases and a large number of potential controls to select (or sample) from. Each case is then classified by characteristics that are not of primary interest, and a search is made for a control with the same set of characteristics. If the factors are not too numerous and there is a large reservoir of persons from which the controls can be chosen, case-control pair matching may be readily carried out. However, if several characteristics or levels are considered and there are not many more potential controls than cases, matching can be difficult. It is quite likely that for some cases, no control will be found; indeed, it may be necessary to either eliminate some of the characteristics from consideration or reduce the number of levels for some of them. With age matching, for example, it is often unlikely that pairs can be formed using one-year age intervals, but five- or ten-year age groups may make matching feasible.

The number of characteristics or levels for which matching is desirable and practical is actually rather small. It is usually sensible to match cases and controls only for characteristics such as age and gender whose association with the disease under study is already known or has been observed in available mortality statistics, morbidity surveys, or other sources. In addition, when cases and controls are matched on any selected characteristic, the influence of that characteristic on the disease can no longer be studied. Hence, caution should be exercised in determining the number of variables selected for matching, even when feasible. If the effect of a characteristic is in doubt, the preferable strategy is not to match but to adjust for these characteristics in the statistical analysis.

POTENTIAL SOURCES OF BIAS

Selection Bias

A method commonly used in conducting case-control studies is to select the cases of the disease under study from one or more hospitals. The control groups usually consist of patients admitted to the same hospital, with diseases other than the one under study. This is a popular method for the initial studies that explore a suspected relation because the data can generally be obtained quickly, easily, and inexpensively. But several assumptions and sources of bias must be considered in analyzing the findings from such studies.

Selection bias is one of the major methodological problems encountered when hospital patients are used in case-control studies. W. A. Guy (see Chapter 2) was the first to suggest that a spurious association between diseases or between a characteristic and a disease could arise because of the different probabilities of admission to a hospital for those with the disease, without the disease, and with the characteristic of interest (Guy, 1856). This possibility was then demonstrated mathematically by Berkson (1946).

The influence of these differences on the study group in the hospital can be illustrated with a hypothetical example.

Let X = Etiological factor or characteristic

A = Disease group designated as cases

B = Disease group designated as controls

Assume that there is no real association between disease A and X in the group population, as indicated in Table 11–5; that is, the percentage of those with A who have X and the percentage of those with B who have X is equal. Assume also that there are different rates or probabilities of admission to the hospital for persons with X, A, and B, each of which acts independently, as follows: X = 50

Table 11–5. Frequency of Characteristic X in Disease
Groups A and B in the General Population

	NUMBER OF INDIVIDUALS IN DISEASE GROUPS	
	A	B
CHARACTERISTIC	(CASES)	(CONTROLS)
With X	200	200
Without X	800	800
Total	1,000	1,000
Percent of total with X	20	20

percent; A = 10 percent; B = 70 percent. Now consider the actual numbers of
people in these groups who are admitted to the hospital:

(a) *For those with A and X:*
    10 percent of the 200 in this category are admitted because
    they have A   = 20
    50 percent of the remaining 180 in this category are admitted
    because they have X   = 90

    Total admitted   = $\overline{110}$
(b) *For those with A and without X:*
    10 percent of the 800 in this category are admitted because
    they have A   = 80
(c) *For those with B and X:*
    70 percent of the 200 in this category are admitted because
    they have B   = 140
    50 percent of the remaining 60 in this category with B are
    admitted because they have X   = 30

    Total admitted   = $\overline{170}$
(d) *For those with B and without X:*
    70 percent of the 800 in this category are admitted because
    they have B   = 560

These numbers are then inserted into the four cells of Table 11–5, allowing
a comparison of disease A (cases) and disease B (controls) with respect to those
who do and do not have the characteristic in our hypothetically constructed hospital population, as shown in Table 11–6. The result is that 58 percent of those
with disease A have X as compared to 23 percent of those with disease B. This
indicates that an association exists between A and X, even though this association

Table 11–6. A Hypothetical Hospital Population
Based on Differential Rates of Hospital Admission

	NUMBER OF INDIVIDUALS IN DISEASE GROUPS	
	A	B
CHARACTERISTIC	(CASES)	(CONTROLS)
With X	110	170
Without X	80	560
Total	190	730
Percent of total with X	58	23

is not present in the general population (the source of the hospital population). This spurious association results from the different rates of admission to the hospital for people with the different diseases and X. However, spurious associations such as this will not arise if either (Kraus, 1954):

1. X does not affect hospitalization, that is, no person is hospitalized simply because of X; or
2. the rate of admission to the hospital for those persons with A is equal to those with B.

One can never be absolutely certain that the first condition is met in any given study. For example, if X represents eye color, it might be assumed that this would not influence the probability of hospitalization. It is possible, however, that persons with a particular eye color belong to an ethnic group whose members are mainly of a specific social class, which, in turn, may influence the probability of their hospitalization. The likelihood of a spurious association is greater if the factor under investigation (i.e., X) is another disease rather than a characteristic or an attribute. The second condition is, of course, the exception rather than the rule since persons with different diseases usually have different probabilities of hospitalization. In any event, one cannot assume that these differences do not exist unless it is demonstrated that there are no differences in the hospitalization rates for individuals regardless of the disease.

In hospital studies, the same factors that may produce a spurious association, also termed "Berksonian" or "selection" bias, can have the reverse effect. The differences in hospital admission rates may conceal an association in a study and fail to detect one that actually exists in the population.

Selection bias is not limited to the analysis of hospital patients. It may be present in any situation or type of population where persons with different diseases or characteristics enter a study group at different rates or probabilities. For example, in studying an autopsy series from a specified hospital population where the autopsy rates differ for the diseases and characteristics being studied in the manner described above, the inferred associations will be biased and may result in a spurious association or mask a real association (McMahan, 1962; Mainland, 1953; Waife et al., 1952).

Selection biases, however, do not necessarily invalidate study findings. This issue should be resolved on its own merits for any particular investigation, and the following means are available to increase the likelihood that an observed association is real:

1. The strength of the association can be evaluated to see if it could result from the type of selection bias described above. A strong association is less likely to result from selection bias than a weak one.

2. Depending on the disease and the personal characteristic (such as serum cholesterol level) or the possible etiological factor (such as cigarette smoking), it may be possible to classify the characteristic or factor into a gradient from low to high levels. If the degree of association between the disease and the characteristic or factor consistently increases or decreases with increasing levels of the characteristic or factor, this ''dose-response relationship'' reduces the likelihood that the association is a result of selection bias. For selection bias to occur, it would be necessary to hypothesize the very unlikely occurrence of a similar gradient of rates of entry into the study group or of hospitalization in a study of hospitalized patients for the characteristic and the disease. This can be illustrated with some data from a recent study of oral contraceptive use and breast cancer among women 45 years old and younger in England (McPherson, et al., 1987). Information was obtained on past oral contraceptive use by women with breast cancer in six London hospitals and two Oxford hospitals during 1980–1984. The same information was obtained from a similarly aged control group (female

Table 11–7.   Duration of Oral Contraceptive Use before
First Term Pregnancy among Female Breast Cancer
Patients and Hospital Controls 45 Years Old and Younger

DURATION OF ORAL CONTRACEPTIVE USE	CASES (%)	CONTROLS (%)
No Use	235 (67%)	273 (78%)
≤ 1 Year	27 (8%)	26 (7%)
1–4 Years	43 (12%)	29 (8%)
> 4 Years	46 (13%)	23 (7%)
Total	351 (100%)	351 (7%)

Source: McPherson et al., 1987.

patients in these hospitals admitted for conditions not related to contraceptive use) during this time period. Table 11–7 presents the results of a comparison of breast cancer patients and controls according to the duration of oral contraceptive use before the first pregnancy. Not only is there a higher proportion of oral contraceptive users among the breast cancer patients than the controls, but the breast cancer patients tended to use oral contraceptives for a longer time period than the control patients. A gradient showing an increase in oral contraceptive use among the cases compared with the controls is evident. Another illustration is provided by Antunes and his colleagues (1979), who examined the possible relationship between estrogen use and endometrial cancer with a case-control research design. Their findings are shown in Figure 11–1. A gradient of duration of postmenopausal estrogen use and endometrial cancer is evident.

3. As a precaution against the influence of selection biases, one may draw controls from a variety of sources. Should the frequency of the study characteristic be similar in each control group and differ from the case group, selection bias would not be a likely explanation for the observed association. The study of Reye's syndrome used controls from an emergency room, in patients, school children, and the community and found consistent results for each group (Table 11–4). In their classic study of lung cancer and smoking Doll and Hill (1952) demonstrated the importance of multiple control groups. They obtained infor-

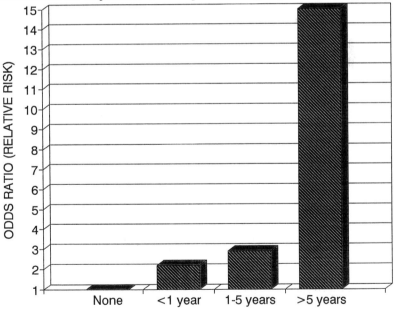

Figure 11–1. Odds ratios for endometrial cancer cases and controls according to duration of use of postmenopausal estrogen. *Source:* Adapted from Antunes, et al. (1979).

mation on the smoking habits of a sample of the general population from a social survey that was conducted in Great Britain during 1951. The smoking habits of patients in their control group were compared with those of persons in the social survey who were residents of Greater London, after adjusting for the age differences between the two groups. Table 11–8 shows the distribution of smoking habits among males in these two groups. The smaller proportion of nonsmokers and the higher proportion of heavy smokers among the controls than in the general population may result from the fact that patients in the control group had diseases that were also related to smoking habits. Thus, the degree of relationship between smoking and lung cancer shown in Table 11–8 was actually underestimated by the use of hospital controls in that investigation.

Representativeness

When cases are drawn from death certificate data bases or centralized registries, it is possible to select a representative sample of cases. This applies to case-control studies of various causes of death or of cancer or other registered illnesses. When cases are drawn from a limited, well-defined population it is also fairly easy to identify all cases. Thus, a case-control study of diarrhea in a day-care center can be designed to interview the parents of every child in the day-care center, or even to examine every child.

Many times it is not easy to identify all the cases of a disease. Even if one canvasses physicians, laboratories, and hospitals to find cases of an illness, there may be people with the illness who are not being treated or who are unaware of their condition. An example might be early miscarriage; a proportion of miscarriages may occur in women who are not aware that they are pregnant (and thus not aware that they miscarried), or women who have not yet been to a physician

Table 11–8. Comparison between Smoking Habits of Male Patients without Cancer of the Lung (Control Group) and of Those Interviewed in the Social Survey: London, 1951

		PERCENT SMOKING DAILY AVERAGE OF CIGARETTES				
SUBJECT	PERCENTAGE OF NONSMOKERS	1–4	5–14	15–24	25+	NUMBER INTERVIEWED
Patient with diseases other than lung cancer	7.0	4.2	43.3	32.1	13.4	1,390
General population sample (Social Survey)	12.1	7.0	44.2	28.1	8.5	199

Source: Doll and Hill (1952).

to begin prenatal care. There is probably no easy way to ensure obtaining a representative sample of women having early miscarriages. Cases of miscarriage drawn from a population of female physicians, for example, would probably select higher educated, higher social class women who are more likely to seek prenatal care earlier in pregnancy. In a study of life style and miscarriages this might introduce a bias, especially if the controls were selected from the general population.

Bias in Obtaining Information

Another bias that may distort the findings from case-control studies develops from the interviewer's awareness of the identity of cases and controls. This knowledge may influence the structure of the questions and the interviewer's manner, which in turn may influence the response. Whenever possible, interviews should be conducted without prior knowledge of the identify of cases and controls, although administrative constraints often prevent such "blind" interviews. In special circumstances, hospital patients may be interviewed at the time of admission so that information of epidemiologic interest is obtained before the patient is seen by a physician and thus before a diagnosis is made establishing the identity of cases and controls. This requires a comprehensive, general-purpose interview routinely administered to all patients admitted. Several epidemiologic studies have utilized a unique set of data from the Roswell Park Memorial Institute, where such a procedure is used (Bross, 1968; Bross and Tidings, 1973; Levin et al., 1950; Levin et al., 1955; Lilienfeld, 1956; Solomon et al., 1968; Winkelstein et al., 1958). Comparing their results with those of studies that depend on more conventional sources of controls provides a means for evaluating possible interviewer bias. A similar approach is used by the Slone Epidemiology Unit which routinely obtains drug histories from patients entering hospitals in the Boston region and other cities.

Patients interviewed as diagnosed cases in studies occasionally have had their diagnoses changed later. If data obtained from the erroneously diagnosed group resemble data from the control rather than the case series, interviewer bias can be discounted (Table 11–9).

The association of a factor and a disease may often be restricted to a specific histologic type or other component of the disease spectrum, as determined by objective means. For example, the fact that oat cell pulmonary carcinoma is more positively related to a history of exposure to bis-chloromethyl ether (BCME) than adenocarcinoma of the lung more firmly established the relationship between the two (Pasternak, et al., 1977). When such diagnostic details and their significance are unknown to the interviewer, another check on possible interviewer bias is provided.

The subjects' responses to an interview can also be directly validated by

Table 11–9. The Smoking Habits of Patients in Different Disease Groups, 45–74 Years of Age, Standardized According to the Age Distribution of the Population of England and Wales as of June 30, 1950

DISEASE GROUP	PERCENTAGE OF NONSMOKERS	PERCENT SMOKING DAILY AVERAGE OF CIGARETTES				NUMBER INTERVIEWED
		<5	5–14	15–24	25+	
Males						
Cancer of lung	0.3	4.6	55.9	35.0	24.3	1,224
Patients incorrectly thought to have cancer of lung	5.3	9.9	35.5	37.8	11.4	102
Other respiratory diseases	1.9	9.9	38.3	38.7	11.2	301
Other cancers	4.6	9.4	47.2	26.0	12.8	473
Other diseases	5.6	9.0	44.8	26.9	13.7	875
Females						
Cancer of lung	40.6	13.7	22.0	9.5	14.2	90
Patients incorrectly thought to have cancer of lung	66.9	16.4	12.7	4.2	0.0	45
Other respiratory diseases	66.5	22.4	0.0	11.1	0.0	25
Other cancers	68.4	14.3	11.0	5.0	1.2	294
Other diseases	55.9	22.1	17.5	3.6	0.9	157

Source: Doll and Hill (1952).

comparison with other records. This was shown in a study of the accuracy of recall of the history of contraceptive use. Case-control studies of the relation between oral contraceptive use and a variety of diseases assumed that women recalled their use of oral contraceptives with reasonable accuracy (Collaborative Group for the Study of Stroke in Young Women, 1973; Mann et al., 1975; Thomas, 1972; Vessey and Doll, 1968). This assumption was tested by comparing oral contraceptive histories of seventy-five women attending family planning clinics with information available in the clinic records. It was found that the type of information obtained in the case-control studies was likely to be remembered with reasonable accuracy (Glass et al., 1974). This finding has been confirmed by Stolley et al. (1978).

Most investigators take great pains to prevent bias by rigorously training study interviewers in proper interview methods. Moreover, it is possible to check the interviewers' technique by video-taping the interview or reinterviewing a sample of the subjects to detect information bias at an early stage of a study when corrective measures are possible.

ANALYZING CASE-CONTROL STUDIES

We described the odds ratio in the beginning of this chapter. The comparison of exposure among cases and controls and the calculation of the odds ratio are the unique features in analyzing data from case-control studies. Odds ratios can be calculated for different amounts of exposure, or for subgroups stratified by other risk factors. Analysis of matched pairs is a special case when each pair is a separate strata. Multivariate methods can be used to estimate the effect of several variables on the odds ratio, and one can consider each variable while controlling for the others.

Odds Ratio for Multiple Levels of Exposure

Inferences about the association between a disease and a factor are considerably strengthened if information is available to support a gradient between the degree of exposure (or "dose") to a characteristic and the disease in question. Odds ratios can be computed for each dose of the characteristic. The general approach is to treat the data as a series of 2×2 tables, comparing controls and cases at different levels of exposure, and then calculating the risk at each level. The data from Table 11–7 are presented in Table 11–10, together with the computed odds ratios. The users with different durations of oral contraceptive use are compared with the nonusers, whose risk of breast cancer is set at 1.0. The odds ratios (OR) for users relative to nonusers are:

$$\text{OR } (\leq 1 \text{ year's use}) = \frac{27 \times 273}{26 \times 235} = \frac{7,371}{6,110} = 1.2$$

$$\text{OR } (1\text{–}4 \text{ years' use}) = \frac{43 \times 273}{29 \times 235} = \frac{11,739}{6,815} = 1.7$$

$$\text{OR } (>4 \text{ years' use}) = \frac{46 \times 273}{23 \times 235} = \frac{12,558}{5,405} = 2.3$$

It is possible to employ statistical tests of significance to determine whether or not the obtained relative risks differ from "unity" or 1.0. These tests can be applied to the summary relative risk (Cochran's test) or to all the categories (the Mantel-Haenzel test) (Cochran, 1954; Mantel and Haenszel, 1959) (see Appendix).

Table 11–10.   Relative Risk of Breast Cancer for Smokers and Nonsmokers, by
Duration of Oral Contraceptive Use (Data from Table 11–7)

DURATION OF ORAL CONTRACEPTIVE USE	BREAST CANCER CASES	HOSPITAL CONTROLS	ODDS RATIO (ESTIMATED RELATIVE RISK)
No use	235	273	1.0
≤ 1 Year	27	26	1.2
1–4 Years	43	29	1.7
> 4 Years	46	23	2.3

Source: McPherson et al., 1987.

Matched Cases and Controls

When cases and controls are matched in pairs in order to make the two groups comparable with regard to one or more factors, the fourfold (2 × 2) table takes a form different from that shown in Table 11–1. The status of the cases with regard to the presence or absence of the characteristic is compared with its presence or absence in their respective controls (Table 11–11). The cell in the upper left-hand corner of Table 11–11 contains r number of pairs in which both cases and controls possess the characteristic of interest. The marginal totals (a, b, c, d) represent the entries in the cells of Table 11–11 and the total for the entire table is $\frac{1}{2}N$ pairs where N represents the total number of paired individuals. The calculation of the odds ratio for this table is simple (Kraus, 1958): OR = s/t (provided t is not 0). Both a test of significance and a method of calculating the standard error are presented in the Appendix.

An example of the method of analysis for matched pairs in a case-control study comes from the work of Chow et al. (1990) on the relation between past exposure to *Chlamydia trachomatis* and ectopic pregnancy. Prior *Chlamydia trachomatis* infection had been associated with both tubal infertility and pelvic inflammatory disease, conditions associated with ectopic pregnancy. Chow and

Table 11–11.   Symbolic Representation of Matched Cases and
Controls with and without the Exposure of Interest

| | CONTROLS | | |
	EXPOSED	UNEXPOSED	TOTAL
Exposed	r	s	a*
Unexposed	t	u	c*
Total	b*	d*	½ N

*a, b, c, and d correspond to the cells of Table 11–1.

Table 11–12.   Matched Pair Analysis of a Case-Control Study of the Association
between *Chlamydia trachomatis* and Ectopic Pregnancy

		CONTROLS	
		PAST EXPOSURE TO *C. TRACHOMATIS*	NO EXPOSURE TO *C. TRACHOMATIS*
Cases	Past exposure to *C. trachomatis*	72	109
	No exposure to *C. trachomatis*	36	40

Source: Chow, 1990, personal communication.

her colleagues recruited the cases of ectopic pregnancies from admissions and
the controls from prenatal clinics. The case-control pairs were matched for age
(± 1 year), ethnicity, hospital, and restricted to women whose pregnancy was of
12 to 24 weeks duration. Cases with previous bilateral tubal ligation, ectopic
pregnancy, or an intrauterine device present at the time of conception were
excluded from the study. A total of 257 matched case-control pairs were assembled and each pair was categorized as to past exposure to *Chlamydia trachomatis*
(assessed by antibody titer of $\geq 1:64$). Based on Table 11–11, each pair could be
categorized in one of four ways:

    r. Case exposed and control exposed $(++) = 72$
    s. Case exposed and control not exposed $(+-) = 109$
    t. Case not exposed and control exposed $(-+) = 36$
    u. Case not exposed and control not exposed $(--) = 40$

Group *s* is the group where cases were exposed and controls were not $(+-)$;
group *t* is the group where cases were not exposed, but controls were exposed
$(-+)$. As in the above formula, the odds ratio is estimated as s/t or 109/36 =
3.0 (see Table 11–12). The calculation considers only the discordant pairs, and
this can be explained intuitively: One can see that pairs where both were exposed
or where both were unexposed would give no information about the relationship
of exposure to disease. For example, one could not measure the effect of fluoride
on cavities in a group of pairs that had all received fluoride, or that had all been
unexposed to fluoride (Schlesselman, 1982).

Interrelationships between Risk Factors

Odds ratios can also be used to determine whether interrelationships exist between
various characteristics or risk factors. A case-control study of lung cancer, cigarette smoking, and asbestos exposure among workers in southern Norway exposed

to multiple risk factors provides an example of this (Kjuus et al. 1986). In two neighboring counties in the southern part of Norway, all cases of lung cancer in males during 1979–1983 were ascertained. For each case, a similarly aged control was selected from among the patients in the same geographical area as the case. All men with conditions that would have precluded possible employment in heavy industry were excluded from the study. The 176 cases and 176 controls were interviewed about their history of exposure to asbestos and their smoking habits. The histories were then coded into four categories according to the level of asbestos exposure the person had reported (no exposure, light or sporadic exposure, moderate exposure between 1 and 10 years duration or heavy exposure less than 1 year in duration, and more than 10 years of moderate exposure or more than 1 year of heavy exposure). The relative risks for each category of asbestos exposure and smoking habit are shown in Table 11–13. From these data, it appears that the relative risk increases with an increase in either smoking or asbestos exposure. When the factors are considered together, the odds ratio rises sharply. This suggests that these factors modify and increase each other's effect on the disease.

Effect of Misclassification

Misclassification of both disease and exposure can occur in any type of study. In a case-control study, misclassification of disease would lead to some of the selection biases already discussed; it would alter a person's probability of entering the study. Assuming that selection bias has been dealt with, misclassification of exposure must be addressed in a case-control study. Exposure status usually cannot be measured directly by the researcher in such a study. Instead, the researcher relies on records (e.g., employment records describing work assignments and possible occupational exposures), recall (e.g. employment, residential, smoking, pharmaceutical histories), or even the recall of a close friend or relative, usually a spouse (e.g. diet, smoking, alcohol consumption, exercise). There are two types of misclassification that can occur: (1) differential—where the amount or direction of misclassification is different in the cases and controls, and (2) nondifferential—where the amount and direction of misclassification is the same in cases and controls. Misclassification error can occur in one direction for cases and controls; for example, everyone may underreport their own or their spouse's habitual alcohol consumption. Misclassification can occur in opposite directions; spouses of cirrhosis patients might overreport alcohol consumption, while spouses of other patients might continue to underreport alcohol use. People typically may misreport their abortion histories, smoking histories, number of sexual partners, and income, and this may be all in one direction or not. People may also misreport information because they can't remember their typical breakfast 10 years ago, the number of cigarettes their husbands used to smoke, the length of their menstrual

Table 11–13. Odds Ratio Estimates of the Relative Risks of Lung Cancer for Combined Exposure to Asbestos and Smoking

CIGARETTES SMOKED DAILY	ASBESTOS EXPOSURE			
	NONE	LITTLE	MODERATE	HEAVY
0–4	1.0	1.2	2.7	4.1
5–9	2.9	1.2	7.8	11.9
10–19	9.1	1.9	24.6	37.3
20–29	16.5	19.8	44.6	67.7
≥30	90.3	108.4	243.8	370.2

Source: adapted from Kjuus et al. (1986).

cycle during each decade of life, or how many hours a day they were exposed to silica dust during each year of employment.

Differential misclassification (because the exposure status of cases is more or less likely to be miscategorized than that of the controls) can produce bias in either direction, raising or lowering the estimate of risk (Schlesselman, 1982). Nondifferential misclassification (randomly distributed among cases and controls) generally shifts the odds ratio toward the null hypothesis (OR = 1.0), but exceptions to this can occur (Dosemeci et al., 1990). The effect of misclassification may also depend on how exposure is defined, as a continuous or categorical variable, and if categorical, as a two-level or multilevel variable.

These effects of misclassification emphasize the need to verify the information obtained in a study by every feasible means. Information with respect to previous exposures or characteristics of study individuals may be verified by obtaining records from independent sources (such as hospitals, physicians, schools, military services, and employment records) on either all or a sample of individuals in the study. Disease diagnoses should be verified whenever possible by independent review of medical records, histological slides, electrocardiograms, etc. The degree of verification possible depends upon the factors or characteristics and the diseases being studied. For example, verification of alcohol consumption or of the content of an individual's diet over a period of time poses serious problems of verification. Alternatively, in a health maintenance organization, for instance, records of prior illness or drug prescriptions may be available, eliminating the possibility of misclassification. Another approach is to use antibody titers as an index of past exposure to an infectious agent. This method has been used in case-control studies of hepatitis B infection and primary liver cancer (Szmuness, 1978). Recently, biological markers for some other exposures have been developed. For example, the presence of cotinine, a metabolite of nicotine, in the blood, urine, or saliva can serve as a biomarker of exposure to cigarette smoking; a high level would indicate active smoking, and a low level, exposure to environmental tobacco smoke.

Attributable Fraction

Another measure of association, influenced by the frequency of a characteristic in the population, is the attributable fraction. As noted in Chapter 10, this is the proportion of a disease that can be attributed to an etiological factor; alternatively, it is considered the proportional decrease in the incidence of a disease if the entire population were no longer exposed to the suspected etiological agent. As in cohort studies, the attributable fraction may be estimated in case-control studies as follows:

$$\text{Attributable Fraction (AF)} = \frac{P(OR - 1)}{P(OR - 1) + 1} \times 100\%,$$

where OR = the odds ratio and P = proportion of the total population classified as having the characteristic. The derivation of this formula can be found in the Appendix. Standard errors and confidence limits have been derived for the attributable fraction by Walter (1975, 1978) (see Appendix).

Computations of attributable fraction are also helpful in developing strategies for epidemiologic research, particularly if there are multiple etiological factors (Walter, 1975). In the study of past *Chlamydia trachomatis* infection and ectopic pregnancy, for example, the attributable fraction for past chlamydial infection was 47 percent, while that for douching (an independent risk factor) was 45 percent (Chow et al., 1990). These data suggest the need for further investigation of douching practices in relation to ectopic pregnancy occurrence, while underscoring the need for control of chlamydial infections to prevent ectopic pregnancies.

Regression Models and Adjustment for Confounding Variables

In a case-control study, several variables may be studied as potential risk factors, variables thought to influence the outcome (occurrence of disease). As will be discussed in Chapter 12, it is always possible that these variables may be **confounded** with one another. For example, in a case-control study of lung cancer, exposures of interest may include cigarette smoking, exposure to asbestos, and use of alcohol. Which of these exposures are associated with lung cancer and which are not (but are associated with one another)? The epidemiologist can deal with this problem by using **multivariate analysis,** a set of techniques for studying the effects of several factors simultaneously (Kleinbaum et al., 1982). These techniques range from simple cross-classification and adjustment to more complex methods of statistical regression analysis.

Various models have been used by epidemiologists, such as "multiple logistic," "log-linear," "multiple linear," and "simple linear" regression. These techniques permit the investigator to determine which of the variables has an independent association with the outcome, to determine which variables interact among themselves, and to quantify the relative contribution of each variable or combination of variables to the risk of the disease. Multivariate analysis does not necessarily distinguish causal from noncausal associations, but it may give indications about the relative strengths of the independent and joint effects of multiple exposures.

ADVANTAGES AND DISADVANTAGES OF CASE-CONTROL STUDIES

Advantages

The case-control study can be used to test hypotheses concerned with the long-term effects of an exposure on a disease, and the study can often be completed quickly. For example, in one to two years data can be collected about 20 or 30 years of exposure to an environmental or occupational hazard.

The case-control study can also be used to test hypotheses about rare diseases or diseases that have long latency periods. The first case-control study estimating the association between diethylstilbestrol (DES) and adenocarcinoma of the vagina in young women used only 8 cases and 32 controls (Herbst et al., 1971). The disease was very rare (about 10 cases in 10 million young women) and 15 to 20 years elapsed between exposure and disease, but the case-control study identified the risk factor and estimated the relative risk. In Table 11–14 one may see how the rareness of disease influences the number of subjects needed in cohort or case-control studies and the advantage of a case-control study for studying rare conditions.

The case-control study is well suited to the study of adverse effects of a drug or treatment, or of a new disease where efficient identification of a risk factor can lead to prompt public health intervention.

The case-control study can be relatively inexpensive because it may use fewer study subjects and take a shorter period of time than some other designs. It also allows examination of several risk factors for a single disease.

Disadvantages

It is sometimes difficult to find an appropriate control group, for theoretical or practical reasons. For example, what is the appropriate control group for auto accident victims? What is the appropriate control group for tennis players with a particular injury? Will there be enough subjects available for a control group?

It is sometimes difficult to decide if the exposure preceded the disease. In

Table 11–14. Sample Size Requirements for Cohort and Case-Control Studies*

DISEASE INCIDENCE IN UNEXPOSED GROUP	FREQUENCY OF ATTRIBUTE DETECTABLE IN POPULATION (%)	RELATIVE RISK	SAMPLE SIZE NEEDED IN EACH GROUP	
			COHORT STUDY	CASE-CONTROL STUDY
1/1,000	50	1.2	576,732	2,535
		2.0	31,443	177
		4.0	5,815	48
1/100	50	1.2	57,100	2,535
		2.0	3,100	177
		4.0	567	48
1/10	50	1.2	5,137	2,535
		2.0	266	177
		4.0	42	48

*Power = 90%; alpha = 5%.
Source: Kahn and Sempos (1989).

studying diarrhea among breast-fed or formula-fed babies, one would want to know if diarrhea led to cessation of breast feeding, or if cessation of breast feeding led to an episode of diarrhea. Similarly, in a study of heart disease among letter carriers, one would like to know whether healthy people choose to become letter carriers or whether letter carrying (and walking each day) leads to healthier cardiovascular systems.

Case-control studies are subject to a number of biases, especially survival biases, selection biases, recall biases, and misclassification. Well-designed studies can sometimes minimize the introduction of biases, but the potential for biases must be considered for each study question. Case-control studies frequently rely on information collected from living cases of the disease of interest. If the deceased cases are different from the surviving cases, a bias may be introduced into the study.

Case-control studies do not actually measure incidence of disease in the population at risk, although estimates can sometimes be made (when all cases of the disease are known, and the population at risk is known).

SUMMARY

In a case-control study, the investigator compares the history of past exposure to a factor or presence of a characteristic among those persons with a given disease or condition (cases) and among those who do not have the disease or condition (controls). The proportion of those exposed among the cases is compared with that among the controls. If these proportions are different, then an association exists between the factor and the disease. Cases can be ascertained from hospitals, clinics, disease registries, or during a prevalence or incidence survey in a population. Controls can likewise be sampled from hospitals, clinics, or a random sample of the population. Care must be exercised in the case and control selection methods, because selection biases can lead to spurious associations. An alternative approach to control selection is to match each control to each case, based on factors thought to be related to the exposure of interest and the disease. In the process of matching, the investigator loses representativeness, i.e., the ability to generalize the findings to the general population, but gains greater comparability among the cases and controls. Unbiased collection of data from both cases and controls is necessary. Biases can occur in recalling past exposures.

The measure of the strength of an association in a case-control study is the odds ratio estimate of the relative risk of developing the disease for those who have been exposed compared with that for those not exposed. Odds ratios can be calculated for both matched and unmatched designs. Misclassification of either the presence or absence of disease, or of exposure status, can affect the estimate of the relative risk. Confounding factors can also affect the estimate of the relative risk. Techniques such as the Mantel-Haenszel test and logistic regression can be used to adjust for confounding factors in the data analysis. However, such statistical techniques cannot make up for errors in study design or data collection. Another measure of association is the attributable fraction, which measures the proportion of disease occurrence that is associated with the factor of interest.

Case-control studies have many advantages and disadvantages compared with cohort studies (Table 11–15). Among the advantages are their lower costs, shorter time to completion, and the ability to examine the association of many

Table 11–15. Advantages and Disadvantages of Case-Control Studies

---

Advantages
1. Generally a short study period.
2. One may study rare diseases.
3. Inexpensive.
4. One may study several risk factors for a single disease.
5. Useful for studying adverse drug reactions or new diseases.

Disadvantages

1. Sometimes difficult to choose appropriate control.
2. Sometimes difficult to determine if exposure preceded the disease.
3. Prone to biases in selection and information.
4. One is usually unable to calculate incidence rates.

---

factors with a given disease. Among their disadvantages are the potential for bias in case and control selection, the potential for recall bias during data collection, and the possible bias associated with investigating survivors of a disease.

STUDY PROBLEMS

1. What would be an appropriate control group (or groups) for the following conditions (mention possible exclusions):
   (a) Babies born at very low birth weight ($\leq$1500 grams).
   (b) Infants with chronic ear infections.
   (c) Transplant patients who reject a transplant.
   (d) Russian roulette suicide victims.

2. Marzuk et al. (1992) conducted a case-control study of cocaine and alcohol use as risk factors for suicide by Russian roulette. The controls were handgun suicides. Toxicological analyses were performed and the data below were obtained. The authors did not calculate an odds ratio, but you can. Calculate the odds ratios and write one sentence for each odds ratio explaining its meaning.

(a)	DRUGS OR ALCOHOL PRESENT IN BLOOD	NO DRUGS OR ALCOHOL IN BLOOD	TOTAL
Russian roulette suicide victims	11	3	14
Handgun suicide victims	33	21	54
Total	44	24	68

(b)	COCAINE DETECTED IN BLOOD	NO COCAINE DETECTED IN BLOOD	TOTAL
Russian roulette suicide victims	9	5	14
Handgun suicide victims	19	35	54
Total	28	40	68

3. Name an advantage and a disadvantage of using a case-control study design to test the hypothesis that cocaine use increases the probability of death from Russian roulette.

4. The recent controversy over silicone breast implants began with the observation of breast cancer among women with the implants.

    (a) What is the advantage in using a case-control study to test the hypothesis that silicone breast implants are associated with breast cancer?

    (b) Who should be the cases in such a study?

    (c) What groups would make appropriate controls?

    (d) What variables might one use to select the control group?

    (e) What variables might be useful in group or pair matching?

    (f) What would be the problem in choosing many variables for matching?

    (g) How could one collect information about women's silicone breast implants?

    (h) What problems arise in collecting the women's medical histories?

REFERENCES

Antunes, C.M.F., Stolley, P. D., Rosensheim, N. B., Davies, J. L., Tonascia, J. A., Brown, C., Burnett, L., Rutledge, A., Pokempner, M. and Garcia, R. 1979. "Endometrial cancer and estrogen use." *New Engl. J. Med.* 300:9–13.

Berkson, J. 1946. "Limitations of the application of fourfold table analysis to hospital data." *Biometrics* 2:47–53.

Bross, I.D.J., and Tidings, J. 1973. "Another look at coffee drinking and cancer of the urinary bladder." *Prev. Med.* 2:445–451.

Bross, I.D.J. 1968. "Effect of filter cigarettes on the risk of lung cancer." *Nat. Cancer Inst. Monogr.* 28:35–40.

Cancer and Steroid Hormone Study of the Centers for Disease Control and the National Institute of Child Health and Human Development. 1987. "The reduction in risk of ovarian cancer associated with oral contraceptive use." *NEJM* 316:650–655.

Chow, J. M., Yonekura, M. L., Richwald, G. A., Greenland, S., Sweet, R. L., Schachter, J. 1990. "The association between *Chlamydia trachomatis* and ectopic pregnancy." *JAMA* 263(23):3164–3167.

Cochran, W. G. 1954. "Some methods of strengthening the common χ^2 tests." *Biometrics* 10:417–451.

Collaborative Group for the Study of Stroke in Young Women. 1973. "Oral contraception and increased risk of cerebral ischemia or thrombosis." *New Engl. J. Med.* 288:871–878.

Cornfield, J. 1951. "A method of estimating comparative rates from clinical data. Applications to cancer of the lung, breast and cervix." *J. Natl. Cancer Inst.* 11:1269–1275.

Doll, R. and Hill, A. B. 1952. "A study of the aetiology of carcinoma of the lung." *Brit. Med. J.* 2:1271–1286.

Dosemeci, M., Wacholder, S. and Lubin, J. H. 1990. "Does nondifferential misclassification of exposure always bias a true effect toward the null value?" *Am. J. Epidemiol.* 132(4):746–748.

Gail, M., Williams, R., Byar, D. P., and Brown, C. 1976. "How many controls?" *J. of Chronic Disease* 29:723–731.

Glass, R., Johnson, B., and Vessey, M. 1974. "Accuracy of recall of histories of oral contraceptive use." *Brit. J. Prev. Med.* 28:273–275.

Guy, W. A. 1856. "On the nature and extent of the benefits conferred by hospitals on the working classes and the poor." *J. Roy. Stat. Soc.* 19:12–27.

Herbst, A. L., Ulfelder, H. and Poskanzer, D. C. 1971. "Association of maternal stilbestrol therapy with tumor appearance in young women." *NEJM* 284(16):878–881.

Hurwitz, E. S., Barrett, M. J., Bregman, D., et al. 1987. "Public health service study of Reye's Syndrome and medications: Report of the main study." *JAMA* 257(14):1905–1911.

Kahn, H. A. and Sempos, C. T. 1989. *Statistical Methods in Epidemiology.* New York: Oxford University Press.

Kjuus, H., Skjaerven, R., Langard, S., Lien, J. T., Aamodt, T. 1986. "A case-referent study of lung cancer, occupational exposures and smoking. II: Role of asbestos exposure." *Scand. J. Work Environ. Health* 12:203–209.

Kleinbaum, D. G., Kupper, L. L., Morgenstern, H. 1982. *Epidemiologic Research.* Belmont, Calif.: Lifetime Learning Publications.

Kraus, A. S. 1954. "The use of hospital data in studying the association between a characteristic and a disease." *Pub. Health Rep.* 69:1211–1214.

———. 1958. "The Use of Family Members as Controls in the Study of the Possible Etiologic Factors of a Disease." Sc.D. Thesis, Graduate School of Public Health, University of Pittsburgh.

Levin, M. I., Goldstein, H., and Gerhardt, P. R. 1950. "Cancer and tobacco smoking: A preliminary report." *JAMA* 143:336–338.

Levin, M. I., Kraus, A. S., Goldberg, I. D., and Gerhardt, P. R. 1955. "Problems in the study of occupation and smoking in relation to lung cancer." *Cancer* 8:932–936.

Lilienfeld, A. M. 1956. "The relationship of cancer of the female breast to artificial menopause and marital status." *Cancer* 9:927–934.

Mainland, D. 1953. "Risk of fallacious conclusions from autopsy data on incidence of disease with applications to heart disease." *Amer. Heart J.* 45:644–654.

Mann, J. I., Vessey, M. P., Thorogood, M., and Doll, R. 1975. "Myocardial infarction in young women with special reference to oral contraceptive practice." *Brit. Med. J.* 2:241–245.

Mantel, N., and Haenszel, W. E. 1959. "Statistical aspects of the analysis of data from retrospective studies of disease." *J. Natl. Cancer Inst.* 22:719–748.

Marzuk, P. M., Tardiff, K., Smyth, D., Stajic, M., Leon, A. C. 1992. "Cocaine use, risk taking and fatal Russian Roulette." *JAMA* 267(19):2635–2637.

McMahan, C. A. 1962. "Age-sex distribution of selected groups of human autopsied cases." *Arch. Path.* 73:40–47.

McPherson, K., Vessey, M. P., Neil, A., Doll, R., Jones, L., Roberts, M. 1987. "Early oral contraceptive use and breast cancer: results of another case-control study." *Br. J. Cancer* 56:653–660.

Pasternak, B., Shore, R. E., Albert, R. E. 1977. "Occupational exposure to chloromethyl ethers." *J. Occupational Medicine* 19:741–746.

Schlesselman, J. J. 1982. *Case-Control Studies: Design, Conduct, Analysis.* New York: Oxford University Press.

Snedecor, G. W., and Cochran, W. G. 1967. *Statistical Methods* 6th ed. Ames, Iowa: The Iowa State University Press.

Solomon, H. A., Priore, R. I., and Bross, I.D.J. 1968. "Cigarette smoking and periodontal disease." *J. Amer. Dent. Assoc.* 77:1081–1084.

Stolley, P. D., Tonascia, J. A., Sartwell, P. E., Tockman, M. S., Tonascia, S., Rutledge, A., and Schinnar, R. 1978. "Agreement rates between oral contraceptive users and prescribers in relation to drug use histories." *Am. J. Epid.* 107:226–235.

Szmuness, W. 1978. "Hepatocellular carcinoma and the hepatitis B virus: Evidence for a causal association." *Prog. Med. Virol.* 24:40–69.

Thomas, D. B. 1972. "Relationship of oral contraceptives to cervical carcinogenesis." *Obstet. Gynec.* 40:508–518.

Vessey, M. P., and Doll, R. 1968. "Investigation of relation between use of oral contraceptives and thromboembolic disease." *Brit. Med. J.* 2:199–205.

Waife, S. O., Lucchesi, P. F., and Sigmond, B. 1952. "Significance of mortality statistics in medical research: Analysis of 1,000 deaths at Philadelphia General Hospital." *Ann. Intern. Med.* 37:332–337.

Walter, S. D. 1975. "The distribution of Levin's measure of attributable risk." *Biometrics* 62:371–374.

———. 1978. "Calculation of attributable risk from epidemiological data." *Int. J. Epid.* 7:175–182.

Winkelstein Jr., W., Stenchever, M. A., and Lilienfeld, A. M. 1958. "Occurrence of pregnancy, abortion, and artificial menopause among women with coronary artery disease: A preliminary study." *J. Chron. Dis.* 7:273–286.

IV

USING EPIDEMIOLOGIC DATA

This final section deals with the use of epidemiologic data. The means by which the results of epidemiologic studies, demographic studies, and toxicological and clinical findings are assembled into a consistent biological inference are discussed in Chapter 12. It is important to recognize that the aggregate of available data on the relationship between a factor and a disease must be integrated before a biological inference is derived. This means that the epidemiologist often must venture into other scientific disciplines. It also means that the process of deriving a biological inference may be a subjective one in which the evidence is weighed in order to determine whether a causal relationship exists. The process of epidemiologic reasoning to achieve this purpose is considered in Chapter 12.

The clinical uses of epidemiologic data are discussed in Chapter 13. The application of decision analysis to clinical medicine and policy-making is illustrated. We try to show how epidemiology can help physicians and other health care providers review reports in the clinical literature critically and we provide a checklist for this purpose. Finally, the use of epidemiologic methods in describing the full spectrum and natural history of disease and in studying disease etiology is briefly outlined.

12

DERIVING BIOLOGICAL INFERENCES FROM EPIDEMIOLOGIC STUDIES

> I cannot give any scientist of any age any better advice
> than this: The intensity of the conviction that a hypothesis
> is true has no bearing on whether it is true or not.
> Sir Peter Medawar, 1979

The demonstration of a statistical relationship between a disease and a biological or psychosocial characteristic is but the first step in the epidemiologic analysis of its etiology and/or natural history. The second step is to ascertain the meaning of the relationship. This chapter will deal with the inferences about a disease's etiology that can be derived from epidemiologic observations and the reasoning by which epidemiologists select the most plausible one. Several elements in this process have been discussed previously, but here they are brought together into a whole. Broadly speaking, a series of reported statistical associations can be explained as:

1. Artifactual (spurious).
2. Due to association of interrelated but non-causal variables.
3. Due to uncontrolled confounding.
4. Causal or etiological.

ARTIFACTUAL ASSOCIATIONS

The possibility that an observed association represents a statistical artifact has been pointed out repeatedly in this book. As indicated in Chapter 11, an artifactual association can result from biased methods of selecting cases and controls. This point can be illustrated by the objections raised to certain case-control studies of exogenous estrogens and endometrial cancer. It was argued that the users of exogenous estrogen, having had to see a physician for their prescriptions, would be more closely observed than the controls and therefore would be more likely to have endometrial cancer diagnosed than those who did not use estrogen. (This turned out not to be the case.) A spurious association may also arise from biased methods of recording observations or obtaining information by interview. This is illustrated in its simplest form by a fictional example. Suppose that in a case-control study of the possible relationship between automobile driving and "slipped discs" (herniated lumbar vertebral discs), an investigator with a pre-conceived notion that automobile driving is of etiological importance asks the patients, "You frequently drive an automobile, don't you?" and the controls, "You don't drive an automobile frequently, do you?" This difference in phrasing the question could lead to a difference in the responses of cases and controls, resulting in an artifactual statistical association between automobile driving and slipped discs.

Errors in the conduct or design of a study can also introduce artifactual errors through nonrepresentative study groups, misclassification of exposure or disease, measurement errors, nonresponse or loss to follow-up, and observer biases. Well-designed studies can avoid most of these problems or even measure the effect of misclassification and of loss to follow-up.

ASSOCIATIONS DUE TO INTERRELATED BUT NON-CAUSAL VARIABLES

An association between two or more variables can be observed and still be non-causal because many variables can occur together without being a part of the causal chain. For example, currently in the United States, cigarette smoking is associated with lower educational status, "blue-collar" occupational status, and relative poverty. But only cigarette smoking is truly causal of lung cancer; the associations with cigarette smoking just mentioned will be detected with an epidemiologic study of the etiology of lung cancer but are interrelated with smoking rather than a cause of the tumor. Examination of these interrelated associations is useful as they may suggest ways to reduce exposure to the causal variable, in this case, smoking.

CONFOUNDING

If any factor either increasing or decreasing the risk of a disease besides the characteristic or exposure under study is unequally distributed in the groups that are being compared with regard to the disease, this itself will give rise to differences in disease frequency in the compared groups. Such distortion, termed *con-*

founding, leads to an invalid comparison. The extraneous variable resulting in a confounded comparison is a **confounding variable** (confounding factor) or a ''confounder.''

The relationship between the confounding factor (CF), the etiological factor (E), and the disease or outcome of interest (D) is shown in Figure 12–1. The confounding variable is associated with both the etiological factor and the disease. For simplicity, this illustration uses only one confounding factor and one etiological factor, but there may be many confounding variables and etiological factors. The above discussion can be extended to such multivariate situations. However, a complete discussion of such situations is beyond the scope of this book; several references for dealing with more than one confounding variable and/or etiological factor are given in the Appendix.

An example of a confounded comparison is provided by consumption of alcoholic beverages, cigarette smoking, and lung cancer. Cigarette smoking is an etiological factor for lung cancer. Persons who smoke cigarettes also tend to drink more alcoholic beverages than those who do not smoke; and those who smoke more cigarettes tend to drink more than those who smoke fewer cigarettes. Hence, cigarette smoking might be a confounding variable in a study of the relationship between alcohol consumption and lung cancer.

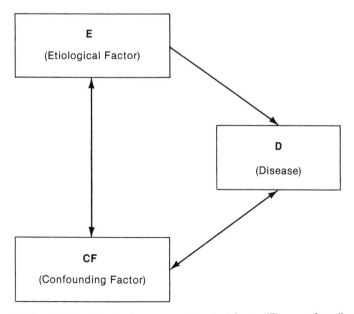

Figure 12–1.   Relationships between an etiological factor (E), a confounding factor (CF), and a disease (D).

Another example was given in Chapter 4, in the comparison of mortality among residents of Florida and Alaska. In that instance, age (C) was a confounding variable in evaluating the effect of place of residence (E) on mortality (D). The possible presence of confounding must be considered when conducting an epidemiologic study, particularly during its design and the analysis of its data, and when assessing the results of an epidemiologic study reported in the literature.

Three methods can be used to address the issue of confounding in an epidemiologic study: (1) the study can be restricted to a specific population group, minimizing the presence of potential confounding variables; (2) the study participants can be *matched* for the potential confounding variable or (3) information can be collected on that variable during the study and the analysis adjusted for its possible effect. Reports in the literature can often be useful in determining what the potential confounding variables might be in a given study so that data on them can be collected. If no data about a possible confounding variable are collected, then the epidemiologist may not be able to disentangle the possibly distorting effects of the confounding.

In analyzing the data collected during a study, one must determine whether

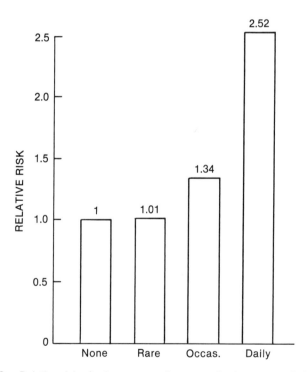

Figure 12-2.   Relative risks for lung cancer in women by frequency of alcohol consumption. *Source:* Hirayama (1990).

or not a variable is a confounder in the study data set. If the variable is a confounder, then the distortion of effect created by its presence must be controlled statistically in the analysis. The statistical approach to the assessment of confounding is to measure the overall association (using either odds radios or relative risks) between exposure and disease and the change in this value after control for a variable (Miettinen, 1974; Kleinbaum et al., 1982; Schlesselman, 1982).

In stratified analyses, data are broken down into levels of one or more variables and analyzed by level; summary statistics then can be used. One common technique for estimating a summary relative risk across strata is the Mantel-Haenszel approach (Mantel and Haenszel, 1959, 1960; Kahn and Sempos, 1989). In this method, each stratum is assigned an appropriate weight. These weights are then used to calculate the summary relative risk. Multivariate analysis techniques incude both multiple and logistic regression and log-linear models. In these approaches, the epidemiologist mathematically models the occurrence of disease based upon the presence or absence of possible risk factors and confounders. These techniques allow several independent variables (potential confounders) to be in the model simultaneously. In general, control for confounding is technical

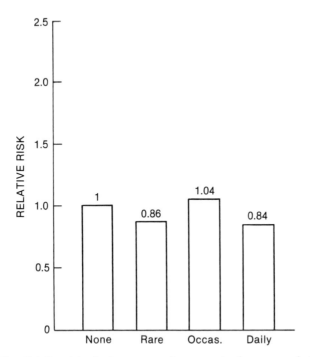

Figure 12-3. Relative risks for lung cancer in women by frequency of alcohol consumption, adjusted for cigarette smoking. *Source:* Hirayama (1990).

but straightforward; more difficult is deciding which variables are to be considered potential confounders.

An example of the analysis of data to reveal confounding comes from a cohort study by Hirayama (1990). He found that the relative risk for lung cancer in women who consume alcoholic beverages increased with ascending consumption (Figure 12–2). This indicates that consumption of alcoholic beverages is associated with the risk of developing lung cancer. However, when the data were adjusted for differences in cigarette smoking patterns among those persons in the different alcohol consumption categories, the association between alcohol consumption and lung cancer disappeared (Figure 12–3). In this instance, cigarette smoking was a confounding variable. Its presence misled the investigators about the role of alcohol in the development of lung cancer until they unravelled the confounding.

Concerns about confounding also arise when interpreting the results of epidemiologic studies reported in the literature. One must ask whether studies showing a relationship between a risk factor and a disease have controlled for potential confounders in their design or analysis. If the study did not adequately control for the presence of confounding variables, the inferences drawn from the results may not be well founded. A study examining a new risk factor for lung cancer, for instance, would have to show that differences in smoking do not explain the relationship between the new risk factor and lung cancer. Studies in which there was inadequate control of all known confounders may be criticized on those grounds; their results may be explained by an unequal distribution of extraneous variables in the study groups and not by the effect of exposure on disease.

It is possible that risk factors may interact in their biological effect. For example, exposures to asbestos fibers and cigarette smoking interact to cause lung cancer at a greater rate than either would individually. Some epidemiologists refer to this phenomenon as "effect modification." Such interactions must be distinguished from confounding, as was illustrated with the associations between cigarette smoking, alcohol consumption, and lung cancer (Figures 12–2 and 12–3). Since there was no relationship between alcohol consumption and lung cancer *after* controlling for the effect of cigarette smoking, there was *no* interaction between cigarette smoking and alcohol consumption to produce lung cancer. Hence, cigarette smoking *confounded* the relationship between alcohol consumption and lung cancer, that is, created the appearance of a causal relationship where none existed. Since there is no causal relationship, there can be no interaction between these two variables (alcohol consumption and cigarette smoking).

As with confounding, there is much debate about the appropriate way to assess and analyze interaction. When interaction is found in a data set, it should be described. One may point out that men and women showed different responses to a treatment or that children in a particular age group were especially prone to accidents.

CAUSAL ASSOCIATIONS

The Evolution of Causal Thinking in Epidemiology

Some investigators have held the view that a factor must be both necessary and sufficient for the occurrence of a disease before it be considered the cause of that disease. This is the logician's definition of "cause." As one might intuitively guess, *necessary* refers to the fact that the factor must be present for the disease to occur, while *sufficient* means that the factor alone can lead to the disease (but the factor's presence does not *always* result in the disease's occurrence). The concept of "necessary *and* sufficient" implies that there must be a one-to-one relationship between the factor and the disease; that is, whenever the factor is present, the disease must occur, and whenever the disease occurs, the factor must be present. Even in infectious diseases, however, a microorganism is not necessary and sufficient for the development of disease; many environmental and host factors are also involved. For example, the tubercle bacillus is a necessary but not a sufficient factor in the development of tuberculosis; additional factors usually included under the term "susceptibility" are also important.

The classical rules for determining whether a microorganism can be regarded as a causal agent of an infectious disease are collectively known as the "Henle-Koch postulates." Although the wording of these postulates varies, they can be simply stated as follows:

1. The organism must be found in all cases of the disease in question.
2. It must be possible to isolate the organism from patients with the disease and to grow it in pure culture.
3. When the pure culture is inoculated into susceptible animals or humans, it must reproduce the disease.

To be considered a causal agent under these requirements, a microorganism must be a necessary condition for the occurrence of disease in humans but need not be sufficient.

An example of sufficient cause for the development of disease is given in Figure 12–4. Each of the factors A_1, A_2, A_3, and so on is sufficient to induce the cellular events (B) resulting in the development of disease (C). None of these factors, however, is necessary for the development of the disease since any of

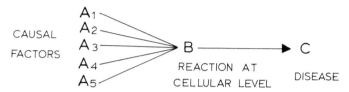

Figure 12–4. Diagrammatic representation of a causal relationship with multiple independent (sufficient) etiological factors.

them is sufficient to produce the cellular changes. In Figure 12–5, all three causal factors (A_1, A_2, and A_3) are necessary for the induction of the cellular reactions (B) that result in disease (C). None of these three factors is sufficient for the development of the disease as all three must be present to initiate the cellular reactions.

Evans (1976) has developed a unified concept of causation that parallels the Henle-Koch postulates and is generally applicable to both infectious and noninfectious diseases.

1. The prevalence of the disease should be significantly higher in those exposed to the hyothesized cause than in controls not so exposed (the cause may be present in the external environment or as a defect in host responses).
2. Exposure to the hypothesized cause should be more frequent among those with the disease than in controls without the disease when all other risk factors are held constant.
3. Incidence of the disease should be significantly higher in those exposed to the cause than in those not so exposed, as shown by prospective studies.
4. Temporally, the disease should follow exposure to the hypothesized cause.
5. A spectrum of host responses should follow exposure to the hypothesized agent along a logical biologic gradient from mild to severe.
6. A measurable host response following exposure to the hypothesized cause should have a high probability of appearing in those lacking the response before exposure (e.g., antibody, cancer cells), or should

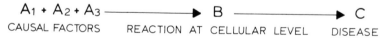

Figure 12–5. Diagrammatic representation of a causal relationship with three cumulative (necessary) causal factors.

increase in magnitude if present before exposure; this response pattern should occur infrequently in persons not so exposed.

7. Experimental reproduction of the disease should occur more frequently in animals or humans appropriately exposed to the hypothesized cause than in those not so exposed; this exposure may be deliberate in volunteers, experimentally induced in the laboratory, or demonstrated in a controlled regulation of natural exposure.

8. Elimination or modification of the hypothesized cause or of the vector carrying it should decrease the incidence of the disease (e.g., control of polluted water, removal of tar from cigarettes).

9. Prevention or modification of the host's response on exposure to the hypothesized cause should decrease or eliminate the disease (e.g., immunization).

10. All of the relationships and findings should make biologic and epidemiologic sense.

Assessing Causality

The epidemiologist applies criteria of causality to the research before recommending clinical or public health actions. These criteria need not be satisfied in every way before causality can be inferred. Rather, they provide a framework for deriving a biological inference from epidemiologic and other scientific data. In practice, *a relationship is considered causal whenever evidence indicates that the factors form part of the complex of circumstances which increases the probability of the occurrence of disease and that a diminution of one or more of these factors decreases the frequency of the disease.* The etiologic factor need not be the only cause of the disease, and it may have effects on other diseases.

The following concepts are used by epidemiologists in making a causal inference:

- Strength of association
- Consistency of the observed association
- Specificity of the association
- Temporal sequence of events
- Dose-response relationship
- Biological plausibility of the observed association
- Experimental evidence

Strength of association

The strength of association is measured by the relative risk (or odds ratio estimate of the relative risk). A strong association between exposure and outcome gives support to a causal hypothesis. When a weak association is found (for example, a relative risk of 1.2 to 1.5), other information is needed to support causality. Repeated findings of a weak association in well-conducted studies can still lead to effective public health action. When an exposure affects many people and the outcome is extremely adverse, a small increase in risk can be of major concern to public health officials. Action may be taken to lower the exposure and reduce the risk for large segments of the population. Strength of association supports a hypothesis of causality, but weak associations supported by other evidence of causality are sometimes equally important.

Consistency of the observed association

Confirmation by repeated findings of an association in case-control and cohort studies in different population groups and different settings strengthens the inference of a causal connection. Finding such consistency is logically equivalent to the replication of results in laboratory experiments under a variety of environmental or biological conditions.

Consistency of association can be illustrated by data from many studies of the relationship of oral contraceptives to cardiovascular disease. Many cohort and case-control studies have shown an increased risk of cardiovascular disease associated with oral contraceptive use in a variety of settings and population groups (Vessey, 1978).

Specificity of the association

It was formerly thought that to be causal, a one-to-one relationship should exist between the exposure and the disease; one exposure should cause one disease, and no other exposures should cause the disease. This has its roots in the bacteriological model where one microorganism is associated with one disease. In the study of chronic diseases, less emphasis has been given to specificity as a criterion of causality. The development of cancer is associated with a number of exposures, many of which are accepted as causal. Conversely, exposures such as smoking are associated with a number of adverse outcomes from cancer and cardiovascular disease to birth problems, and these associations are accepted as causal by the medical and public health communities. Specificity of a relationship between exposure and outcome strengthens confidence in a causal inference, but lack of specificity does not rule out causality.

Temporal sequence of events

It seems obvious that in order for an exposure to cause an event (disease), it must precede and not follow the disease. In many cases, the temporal sequence of events is clear-cut. One example is the study of prenatal exposures and malformations; it is usually easy to document that an exposure precedes the birth of the malformed baby. However, for many other associations the temporal relationship is subject to debate.

In studying the relationship between age when breast-feeding ceases and infections of the baby, for instance, some researchers claim that longer duration of breast-feeding leads to fewer infections, but others claim that illness of the child leads to a cessation of breast-feeding. Which came first, the illness or the weaning? A cohort study design can resolve the issue of temporality, but for many study questions prospective studies are difficult or impossible to carry out.

Dose-response relationships

If a factor is of causal importance in the occurrence of a disease, then the risk of developing the disease shoud be related to the degree of exposure to the factor, i.e., a dose-response relationship should exist. The dose-response relationship between serum cholesterol level and the risk of coronary heart disease is an example. Another example is the relationship between duration of estrogen use and risk of endometrial cancer. Several studies also suggest that low-dose estrogen contraceptives carry a lower risk of venous thromboembolism than do higher-dose estrogens.

An observed dose-response relationship strengthens a causal hypothesis. Unfortunately, it is sometimes difficult to quantify an exposure in terms of a dosage or gradient. Dosage and duration of exposure are often interchanged in study designs, and both may cause a gradient in disease frequencies. Dosage can refer to the amount of a given exposure in a given time period, as in the number of cigarettes smoked per day, the amount of a hazardous chemical or particle in the work environment, or the amount of a drug taken each day. Information on actual dosage is often not available, so duration of exposure is substituted, as in years of cigarette smoking, years working in a given occupational environment, or length of time using a drug. Use of duration as a proxy for dosage necessitates an analysis that accounts for time; people with longer exposure times may have a greater time period in which to develop or discover the disease.

Biological plausibility of the observed association

A causal hypothesis must be viewed in the light of its biological plausibility. A causal association between ingrown toenails and leukemia, to take an absurd example, would be highly improbable. On the other hand, an association that does not appear biologically credible at one time may eventually prove to be so; indeed, the observation of a seemingly implausible association may actually represent the beginning of an extension of our knowledge. The established statistical association between circulatory diseases and oral contraceptive use is an excellent example of this. At first, there was no known physiological mechanism by which hormones could so profoundly affect the circulatory system. Yet, the statistical association was present, and possible physiological mechanisms were later discovered, such as alteration of the clotting cascade, increased platelet adhesiveness, and direct effects on the arterial wall. It becomes important, therefore, to further investigate associations even if they are initially thought to be biologically implausible. The cigarette smoking–lung cancer relationship was initially considered biologically implausible by some, but carcinogens in cigarettes were identified, which lent biological plausibility to the observed association.

The ability to produce a particular disease in animals by exposing them to possible etiologic agents considerably enhances the causal hypothesis. Though one must be cautious in generalizing from the results of animal experiments to the human condition, this may be a relatively minor problem if the results of both animal experiments and epidemiologic studies in human populations are consistent. Animal experiments can also be valuable in determining the intermediate biological mechanisms that are involved in a disease, thereby providing the basis for seeking similar mechanisms in humans. Darwin's signal contribution to biological thinking was that the human species is not so unique a biological phenomenon as we may like to think; modern molecular biology confirms the unity of human and other animal species.

Experimental evidence

The randomized clinical trial (RCT) is the closest approximation in epidemiology to an experiment, and a well-run trial may confirm a causal relationship between an exposure and an outcome. The "exposure" is generally a drug, treatment, or procedure, and the outcome is reduction of disease or mortality. The Lipid Research Clinics Trial demonstrated that a pharmacological reduction in serum cholesterol led to lower heart disease, and other clinical trials have shown that pharmacologic lowering of blood pressure also reduces heart disease. Similar comments apply to the results of community trials. Ethics prevent the conduct of a trial of an exposure that is thought to have deleterious effects, and thus the randomized clinical trial and the community trial are limited to a subset of study questions related to potentially beneficial effects of an exposure.

Some situations approximate an experiment without the benefit of randomized, concurrent controls. The efficacy of inner-city comprehensive-care programs in reducing the incidence of rheumatic fever was demonstrated by comparing neighborhoods in a city that were simlar to one another except for their eligibility for the programs, but the populations may have differed in ways not known or documented in the study (Gordis, 1973). Conversely, removal or reduction of an exposure may result in a decrease in disease. The decrease in smoking among physicians led to a decrease in lung cancer among physicians while rates in the general population continued to rise. The decline in the use of isoprenaline in England in the 1960s led to a decline in asthma-related deaths.

SUMMARY

One of the foremost biometricians of the twentieth century, A. Bradford Hill (1937), noted the importance of common sense in developing inferences. He summarized the questions that should guide a consideration of causality as follows: "Is there any other way of explaining the set of facts before us, is there any other answer more likely than cause and effect?" An association between exposure and outcome can be evaluated within the context of epidemiologic criteria of causality; with common sense, reasonable inferences may be made and actions taken.

Epidemiologic inferences lead to action, to changes in clinical practice, public policy, legislation, health education, or new research directions. Health care providers no longer prescribe diethylstilbestrol (DES) to prevent miscarriages, they now use blood pressure–lowering agents to treat patients with moderate hypertension, and they now have evidence that regular sigmoidoscopic examinations can lower colon cancer mortality.

An example of the role of epidemiologic data in the development of public policy is the recent legislation in the United States regulating where people may smoke to protect citizens from exposure to environmental tobacco smoke. Health education efforts emphasize the use of condoms in preventing the spread of AIDS, the need to reduce alcohol intake during pregnancy to prevent fetal-alcohol syndrome, the use of seat belts to reduce auto accident injuries, and the role of low-fat diets in reducing heart disease.

Experimentation and the determination of biological mechanisms provide the most direct evidence of a causal relationship between a factor and a disease. Epidemiologic studies can provide very strong support for hypotheses of either a causal or an indirect association. However, inferences from such studies are not made in isolation; they must take into account all relevant biological information. Epidemiologic and other evidence can accumulate to the point where a causal hypothesis becomes highly probable. Unfortunately, it is not yet possible to quantitate the degree of probability achieved by all the evidence for a specific hypothesis about the cause of a disease, so an element of subjectivity remains. Nevertheless, a causal hypothesis can be sufficiently probable to provide a reasonable basis for successful preventive and public health action, as the history of public health amply demonstrates.

STUDY PROBLEMS

1. Name two important ways to control for confounding when designing a study.
2. What options are there for controlling confounding in the analysis stage?

3. What is the difference between biological significance and statistical significance?

4. Name three concepts that are useful in assessing causality.

REFERENCES

Evans, A. S. 1976. "Causation and disease: The Henle-Koch postulates revisited." *Yale J. Biol. Med.* 49:175–195.

Gordis, L. 1973. "Effectiveness of comprehensive-care programs in preventing rheumatic fever." *New Engl. J. Med.* 289:331–335.

Hill, A. B. 1971. Statistical Evidence and Inference. In *Principles of Medical Statistics.* New York: Oxford University Press, 309–323.

Hirayama, T. 1990. *Life-style and mortality: a large-scale census-based cohort study in Japan.* Basel: S. Karger.

Kahn, H. A., and Sempos, C. T. 1989. *Statistical Methods in Epidemiology.* New York: Oxford University Press.

Kleinbaum, D. G., Kupper, L. L., and Morgenstern, H. 1982. *Epidemiologic Research.* Belmont, Calif.: Lifetime Learning Publications.

Mantel, N., Haenszel, W. 1959. Statistical aspects of the analysis of data from retrospective studies of disease. *Journal of the National Cancer Institute* 22:719–748.

Miettinen, O. 1974. "Confounding and effect modification." *Am. J. Epidemiol.* 100:350–353.

Schlesselman, J. J. 1982. *Case-Control Studies.* New York: Oxford University Press.

Vessey, M. P., and Mann, J. I. 1978. "Female sex hormones and thrombosis: Epidemiological aspects." *Brit. Med. Bull.* 34:157–162.

13

EPIDEMIOLOGY IN CLINICAL PRACTICE

with the Assistance of Tamar Lasky, Ph.D., M.S.P.H.

Clinicians apply the principles of epidemiology to everyday practice in three main ways: (1) clinical decision making, (2) reading and interpreting medical literature, (3) describing and understanding the etiology of disease.

In the first category are the decisions to order diagnostic tests or procedures, assign a diagnosis, and recommend a treatment. Second, physicians who can intelligently and efficiently read the literature will make the best use of new information in providing optimal care to their patients. Finally, clinicians with an understanding of epidemiology are better able to identify disease entities, suggest etiologic hypotheses, monitor and evaluate the safety of drugs and other therapies, find the causes of local epidemics and institute preventive measures, and participate in collaborative research. These related concerns are the domain of what is sometimes called clinical epidemiology, though not its exclusive domain (Fletcher et al., 1988; Sackett et al., 1991; Schuman, 1986; Weiss, 1986).

CLINICAL DECISION MAKING

In all aspects of medical practice, the physician faces a series of choices—choices that are made in a specific context for a particular patient. Despite the intention to provide well-reasoned care, however, patterns of diagnosis and treatment are sometimes less than optimal.

One classical example is that of the diagnosis of tonsillitis and referral for tonsillectomy and adenoidectomy (Bakwin, 1945). Three groups of pediatricians had an opportunity to screen a group of children for tonsillectomy. The first group referred 174 out of 389 children (45 percent) for tonsillectomy. The "healthy" remaining 215 children were examined by the second group of physicians. They recommended tonsillectomy for 99 of these children (46 percent). The third group of physicians examined the remaining 116 children and referred 51 (44 percent) of them for tonsillectomy. The pediatricians referred approximately the same proportion of children for tonsillectomy, which perhaps reflected habit, expectations, carelessness, and a lack of objective and validated criteria for surgery (Figure 13–1).

Sackett et al. (1991) compared university hospital physicians with family physicians treating the same group of 230 hypertensive patients. All the patients were recommended for treatment by the university group, but only two-thirds of the family physicians started the patients on antihypertensive drug regimens. Three factors predicted the decision of family physicians to prescribe antihypertensives. First and third were the patient's diastolic blood pressure (as it should

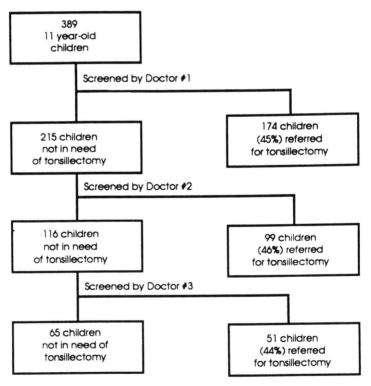

Figure 13–1. Patterns of tonsillectomy referrals in three groups of pediatricians. *Source:* Bakwin (1945).

have been) and evidence of target organ damage, but second was the physician's year of graduation from medical school. More recent graduates were more likely to treat for hypertension, reflecting advances in research findings and teaching. This study illustrates the well-known problem of keeping up to date in medicine and perhaps other factors.

Epidemiologic research can be used to analyze decision-making behavior (factors influencing a clinician's decision to use a test, procedure, or treatment), and it helps clinicians improve their decision-making skills. After reviewing the literature, a clinician may wish to apply research findings to an individual patient; however, information about a study population is sometimes difficult to use in this way. The decision to order a diagnostic test may vary with the patient's characteristics (e.g., age, other medical conditions), the availability of treatment options, and the risks of injury or side effects associated with a procedure. Similarly, the decision to order a treatment must be weighed against the probability that the treatment works, that side effects are likely or unlikely, and that the patient will comply with the course of treatment. This decision-making process has both objective and subjective aspects. The probability that the procedure will work or that the patient will die in surgery, for instance, can be derived from the literature. But what value does the patient assign to the risks and benefits of a diagnostic test, procedure, or treatment? Thus, there is also a "subjective" aspect to clinical decision-making.

Decision Analysis

Decision analysis is an approach that can help the clinician deal with such situations, weighing the probabilities of various outcomes with the subjective value accorded to them by the patient. The selection and interpretation of diagnostic tests involves the application of probability theory, whether applied consciously or unconsciously. When a test is ordered for a patient, the physician has some sense of the probability that the results will be positive and thus help establish the correct diagnosis. If that probability (on a scale of 0.0 to 1.0) were close to 0.0, there would usually be little point in performing the test. Similarly, if the clinician is so sure of the diagnosis that the test has a 1.0 probability of being positive, again there would be little point to ordering the test as the diagnosis is established without benefit of the test. It is between these extremes of expecting a surely negative or surely positive test result that most clinical decision-making lies, and in these situations decision analysis may be helpful.

Descriptions of decision analysis include variations on the following steps as adapted from Sackett et al., (1991) and Pauker (1991).

1. *Frame the question in terms of specific choices that are mutually exclusive and exhaustive.* This means that a physician should consider all treatments, the possibility of no treatment, and, if appropriate, the possibility of combined treatments. Decision analysis forces one to think through, and define, the full range of choices.

2. *Create a decision tree.* One must structure the problem by diagramming the decision tree for the specific clinical question, showing the clinical options and the possible outcomes of each option. The decision tree for a question about ordering a diagnostic test will have different branches than the decision tree for a question about treatment.

3. *Assign probabilities to the outcomes.* Here one relies on the literature and one's experience to estimate probabilities for branches and points of the decision tree. In deciding on the probability of various outcomes, a clinician may use information about the prevalence of a disease, the sensitivity and specificity of a diagnostic test, the probability of side effects of a procedure or treatment, the probability that a treatment will cure or prevent a disease, etc.

4. *Assign utilities to the outcomes.* The outcomes can include loss of life, complete recovery, and the risks of side effects. The utilities (relative values) are subjective and any scale can be used (e.g., years of survival, dollars spent, or an arbitrary scale of 0 to 100). It is usually easy to assign the lowest value to death and the highest value to complete healthy recovery, but it is not always easy to place intermediate outcomes on the scale. The risks and side effects of procedures and treatments have different meanings for different people. Sometimes the patient can help assign values to intermediate outcomes in discussions with his or her physician or in response to direct questions such as, "On a scale of 0 to 100, how would you rate the following side effect to a treatment for your condition?" The patient has to live with one of the outcomes and knows how he or she feels about them. Of course, the physician can consult with other physicians, social workers, or groups of patients in developing values for outcomes. As shown below, the subjectivity and variability in assigning values makes decision analysis adaptable for different contexts.

5. *Calculate the expected utility.* One calculates back from the outcomes to the first choices on the decision tree. The probability of an outcome is multiplied by the value (subjectively assigned) and then averaged with the product calculated for other outcomes in the same decision branch (see example below).

6. *Perform sensitivity analysis.* Depending on the specifics of a decision tree, one might do the analysis again under different assumptions. For example, one might vary the values assigned to outcomes to see how one's subjective judgment changes the overall analysis. This helps clarify the contribution of different factors to the ultimate decision.

An Example of Decision Analysis

We present an example of decision analysis below, following the steps just described.

1. *Frame the question.* In this example, we ask the question, "Should anti-hypertensive treatment be given to prevent stroke in patients over 60 with no symptoms other than isolated systolic hypertension (ISH—systolic blood pressure 160–219 mm Hg and diastolic blood pressure less than 90 mm Hg)?" This question arose from reading the results of a multicenter, randomized, controlled clinical trial which showed that treated patients aged 60 and over had a reduced risk of stroke compared to untreated patients (SHEP Cooperative Research Group, 1991). The authors stated that the trial demonstrated the efficacy of active anti-hypertensive drug treatment in preventing stroke in persons aged 60 and older with ISH, but they did not say whether a clinician should prescribe the treatment regimen (a combination plan of chlorthalidone and atenolol or reserpine) to all patients similar to those in the trial. One physician may be enthusiastic about treating this group, but another physician may be reluctant to prescribe long-term medication to a fairly healthy group of patients. Is there an objective way to decide this clinical question?

2. *Create a decision tree.* The decision tree in Figure 13–2 shows the two choices facing the clinician who diagnoses ISH in a patient. The physician can treat the hypertension with drugs or decide not to treat. This decision is controlled by the clinician (and the patient) and is represented by a square. In this example we have identified three possible outcomes for patients. They can suffer a stroke, they can experience intolerable symptoms (some of which may be associated with the treatment), or they can live free of stroke and intolerable symptoms.

3. *Assign probabilities to the possible outcomes.* In this case probabilities are derived from the paper that presented the results of the trial. The authors reported that 5.2 percent of the treated group experienced a stroke, compared to 8.2 percent of the placebo group. This is expressed as a probability of .052 of stroke if treated and .082 if not treated. The authors also reported the prevalence of symptoms characterized as intolerable by the patients. These symptoms included faintness, loss of consciousness, chest pain, trouble with memory, problems with sexual function, and nausea or vomiting. In the treatment group, 28.1 percent experienced intolerable symptoms compared to 20.8 percent in the placebo group. These prevalence data can be used to represent the probability of experiencing intolerable symptoms. We assigned a probability of .281 to the treated group and .208 to the untreated group. The people who did not experience stroke or intolerable symptoms were considered to be healthy and symptom-free

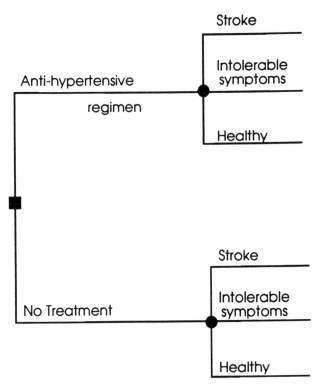

Figure 13–2. A decision tree.

in this analysis. The probability of being healthy and symptom free was 1.00 minus the probability of stroke and the probability of intolerable symptoms, or .667 in the treatment group and .710 in the untreated group.

    4. *Assign a utility to each possible outcome.* In this example, we assigned the value of 0 to stroke and 100 to a healthy, symptom-free condition. How does one assign a value to having intolerable symptoms? Some of the symptoms described could greatly reduce the quality of life, necessitating job and activity changes (less driving, less eating out, etc.), so we assigned a value of 50 to these symptoms.

    5. *Calculate the expected utilities.* In the group of patients receiving anti-hypertensive treatment, the probabilities of each outcome were as follows: .052 for stroke, .281 for intolerable symptoms, and .667 for a healthy symptom-free status. Each probability is multiplied by its utility as follow:

Stroke	.052 (0) = 0
Intolerable symptoms	.281 (50) = 14.05
Healthy, symptom-free	.667 (100) = 66.70

One then sums the three products (80.75) and averages them. In this case one divides by three, even though one product is zero, and the expected utility is 26.92 for treating with antihypertensives (Figure 13–3). Similar calculations for not treating yield an expected utility of 27.13, slightly higher than treating. This suggests that it is a toss-up whether to treat or not.

6. *Perform sensitivity analysis.* We can do the analysis again assigning a value of 75 to the outcome of intolerable symptoms (Figure 13–4). The expected utilities are then 29.26 for treatment and 28.87 for no treatment. It is again very close, confirming the previous analysis that the decision to treat is a toss-up.

In our example we did not separate stroke resulting in death from nonfatal stroke, consider nonstroke fatal events or heart disease, or include the economic cost of treatment. We simplified the options in order to illustrate the principle, but more complex anlayses are possible. Even this simplified decision analysis of the SHEP study helped put the authors' findings in clinical perspective. That

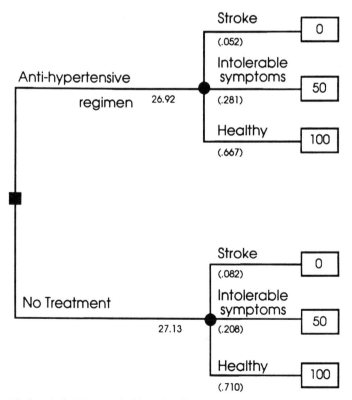

Figure 13–3. A decision tree with probabilities, values, and calculated utilities.

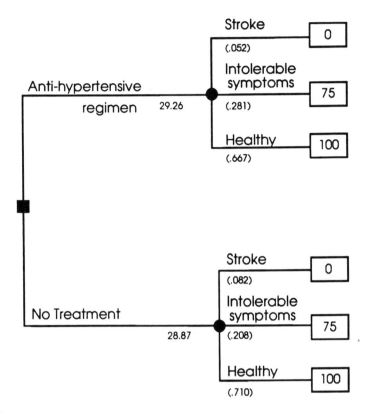

Figure 13–4.   A decision tree with different values than Figure 13–3, and recalculated utilities.

is, after a clinical trial has been conducted among many patients, the results of the clinical trial can be used in decision analysis to decide an individual's course of treatment. The medical risks and benefits of treatment can be balanced against cost and the patient's personal preferences. The significant finding of a reduced risk of stroke does not necessarily mean that physicians should place all their healthy elderly patients with isolated systolic hypertension on treatment. Our analysis suggests that the choice of treatment can be viewed as an option for physicians and patients and depends on the circumstances and the patient's preferences.

Decision analysis can be a cumbersome tool. It is limited by our ability to describe outcomes and probabilities and to assign subjective values to outcomes. It can help a physician, researcher, or policymaker think through a decision, gain understanding of the factors affecting a decision, and place the clinical decision in a broader context. Researchers can use this tool to develop guidelines for clinicians to follow, and policymakers can use it in making recommendations.

READING AND INTERPRETING SCIENTIFIC LITERATURE

The epidemiologic principles presented in this book can contribute to a critical reading of clinical research literature (Stolley and Davies, 1980; Sackett et al., 1991). Whether one wishes to learn more about the value of a diagnostic test, evaluate a new therapy, or determine the etiology of a disease, epidemiologic principles can be of clinical use. The suggestions that follow may be helpful in reading or writing clinical and epidemiological research papers.

Identifying the Study Problem

The title, abstract, and introductory paragraph should state the study's objectives. The reader may ask, ''What is the study hypothesis? What is the main exposure of interest? What is the disease or condition being studied?'' ''Exposure'' can refer to beneficial or detrimental factors, behavioral patterns, treatments, procedures, or drugs suspected of causing adverse effects. Many studies focus on more than one risk factor or disease, and the paper should identify them.

In Chapters 4, 5, 6, and 7 we discussed the variety of disease outcomes studied by epidemiologists and the difference between morbidity and mortality as endpoints in a study. A reader should be able to identify the illness or cause of death that is the focus of the study and the criteria for categorizing patients into disease categories. For example, a report of a study of hypertension should describe the blood pressure levels used to determine which patients were considered hypertensive. Similarly, a report of a study whose major focus is a reduction in blood pressure should specify the exact amount or percent decline that was considered a meaningful decrease in blood pressure.

Describing the Study Design

In Chapter 8, 9, 10, and 11 we described the study designs used in epidemiologic studies. Each study design—randomized clinical trial, community trial, cohort study, and case-control study—has its value and is appropriate for particular types of study questions. The randomized clinical trial is usually the best design to supply the information needed to determine the efficacy of a treatment. More and more, screening measures and diagnostic tests are also being evaluated by clinical trials to determine whether early detection of a condition (e.g., breast cancer by mammography) leads to an improvement in morbidity or mortality. Case-control studies are a cost-efficient way to investigate a new disease, an increase in a known disease, or a suspected adverse reaction to a drug or procedure because the researcher may examine several suspected risk factors and test hypotheses about their causal association with the disease of interest. Community trials are well suited to the testing of interventions that affect a community at large, such as changes in driving, drinking, or gun control laws, public education campaigns, or changes in pollutant emissions.

Cohort studies, reconstructed from records or conducted prospectively, are often useful in understanding the etiology of disease or the consequences of certain suspect exposures. The reader of a report describing a cohort study knows that certain selection biases have been avoided; incidence rates may be calculated, and a description of more than one health outcome is possible. Cohort studies are particularly suited to the investigation of etiology because exposure to suspected agents can be documented and then tracked over time to determine the "disease destiny" of the exposed and unexposed populations. The control of potential confounders and the investigation of possible biases can often be more thoroughly handled in a cohort study than is possible with other observational designs. It is particularly easy to study cohorts of pregnant women or infants to observe birth or childhood outcomes because patients are available and the follow-up time period is relatively short. The cohort design can also be used in occupational studies, nutritional studies, studies of the elderly, and many other areas.

Describing the Study Sample

Many questions may be raised about the sample described in an article. In general, the reader wishes to know if the sample has been chosen in a way that minimizes bias, if results can be generalized to other patients, and if the sample is large enough to allow the appropriate statistical analyses and to provide adequate statistical power to answer the question posed. A critical reader should look for descriptions of the sample selection process, the characteristics of the study sample (age, gender, ethnicity, etc.) and the sample size calculations.

Throughout this book we have stressed the importance of sample selection, whether in studies relying on routinely collected data such as death certificates or in studies that actively recruit subjects. If the researchers used death certificates to identify cases, did they address the possibility of any coding changes that took place during the study period or in the geographic areas where the study was conducted? If the researchers identified patients in prenatal clinics for a cohort study, did they consider the characteristics of pregnant women not attending those clinics? Did the researchers describe the eligibility criteria, the people who were excluded from the study, and the nonrespondents?

A good description of the study sample will allow a reader to consider the possible introduction of bias, and it will also allow the critical reader to decide what generalizations can be made from the data. Reports of most studies provide information about the age and gender of the study subjects, but more information is often useful. In a study of mammography screening among older women, it might be useful to know if the patients were using replacement estrogens, had a family history of breast cancer, or were smokers. Such specific information allows the reader to apply the study findings to the appropriate population of patients.

Many researchers do not report their sample size calculations; that is, they do not describe the sample sizes needed to detect a given difference with a specified probability that the observed difference is not due to chance, and they do not describe the probability that an observation of no difference is not due to too small a sample (alpha and beta). This is particularly relevant when reading articles about drug safety. Studies with small sample sizes will often conclude that a new drug is as safe as a previously used drug although the study may be too small to detect clinically meaningful differences in safety between the new and old drugs.

Data Analysis

A general reader may be reluctant to critique the data analysis, but some simple questions can help the reader sift out the studies that employ appropriate statistical techniques. Epidemiologists prefer to use relative measures of effect or association such as relative risk or the odds ratio. Many researchers do not calculate such a measure. Authors often include the necessary data for the reader who wishes to calculate a relative risk or an odds ratio, but the authors should carry out the analysis. Confidence intervals allow a reader to know if the measure of effect may be attributed to chance variation or if an association is likely or unlikely to be due to chance. The authors should address the subject of confounding by describing the variables that are generally thought to be confounders, their efforts to collect data on possible confounders, and the results of analyses of confounding variables.

Inferences

The researchers' conclusions may not be justified by the study results. A common example is the finding of a trend which is not statistically significant and which the authors interpret as supporting a particular point of view. In the discussion, authors often address issues of bias or confounding and their possible effects on the study findings. The reader may or may not be convinced by the authors' arguments and conclusions. When the reseachers' conclusions go beyond the study findings, the reader may apply the criteria of causality to their argument. Does the study show an association that is strong? Is it consistent with other studies? Is the temporal sequence logical? Are the results biologically plausible? Can the association be explained by bias in study design or by confounding?

Most often a study will be conducted in a specific population characterized by age, gender, social class, or medical condition, and the reader may wonder whether the findings can be applied to patients who differ from the study sample. The authors should address this issue and describe how widely the inferences from their study can be justifiably applied. An author may suggest, for example, that a screening test will be useful for patients five years younger than the patients in the study group and may then explain the reasoning behind this recommendation. A reader should sort out the firm conclusions from the suggested possibilities and keep in mind the applications to his or her clinical practice. Table 13–1 provides a useful checklist for the reader of medical papers.

Table 13–1.   Guide to Reading the Literature

Identify the study problem

   What is the study hypothesis?
   What is the exposure (risk factor, treatment, cause)?
   What is the outcome (physiologic measurement, disease, death)?

Describe the study design

   What design was used (clinical trial, case-control study, etc.)?
   Is the design appropriate to the study question?

Describe the study sample

   How was the sample selected?
   Are inclusion and exclusion criteria described?
   Do the authors describe those that refused to participate or were lost to follow-up?
   What size samples were used?
   Do the authors discuss the sample size calculations?

Data analysis

   Do the authors calculate a measure of effect (OR, RR or other)? What was it?
   Do they calculate confidence intervals for the measure of effect? What was it?
   Does the analysis assess and control for confounding? What were the results?

Inferences

   What are the study results (what do the numbers say)?
   What are the authors' conclusions (do they differ from what the numbers say)?
   Does their discussion convince the reader to accept their conclusions?
   Are the authors' conclusions supported by the criteria of causality?
   Can the results be generalized beyond the study group? To which groups?
   To what group of your patients can you apply the study results?
   What changes would you make in your practice as a result of the study?

DESCRIBING AND UNDERSTANDING THE ETIOLOGY OF DISEASE

It is a humbling experience to read older textbooks of medicine. Statements that are now known to be incorrect were often written with great certainty and authority. One wonders which of today's certainties will be overturned tomorrow. Consider the following example from the early 1960s.

The 11th edition of *Cecil-Loeb Textbook of Medicine* contains this description of the migraine sufferer:

> Patients with migraine headaches are anxious, striving, perfectionistic, order-loving, rigid persons, who, during periods of threat or conflict, become progressively more tense, resentful and fatigued. . . . The person with migraine attempts to gain approval by doing more and better work than his fellows by "application" and "hard work," and to gain security by holding to a stable environment (Beeson and McDermott, 1963).

This description of the "typical" migraine patient was derived from the experience of the author, Harold Wolff, a well-known neurologist, in examining and treating patients who attended his headache clinic in New York City. The headache sufferers who elected to go to a specialty clinic at a large medical center may have been a highly selected sample of all migrainous individuals. They may have represented those hard-driving and compulsive people who hate to lose a day of work from headaches.

Several community surveys of migraine have been conducted since Harold Wolff wrote the above passage, and they do not support the generalizations he drew from the skewed sample attending his clinic (Linet and Stewart, 1984). Instead, they reveal migraine to be a common disorder affecting about 10 to 15 percent of the population and all sorts of personality types; indeed, no particular personality type can be identified as being at special risk of migraine.

If we learn the cause of a disease, or the risk factors, we are usually in a better position to treat or prevent it. An apparently new disease was identified in 1989 and was labeled the eosinophilia-myalgia syndrome (EMS). In the first cluster of cases in New Mexico, a striking eosinophilia and severe muscle aching (myalgia) were noted. Many of the patients were women 30 to 60 years old, and the diagnosis of trichinosis was excluded during the course of the clinical investigation. Some patients experienced skin rashes, peripheral edema, various neuropathies, and respiratory symptoms. Quickly organized case-control studies revealed that all the patients had taken the food supplement L-tryptophan, an amino acid sold in health food stores for the relief of insomnia and depression; few of the controls consumed L-tryptophan (Eidson et al., 1990). Further investigations showed that the L-tryptophan implicated in the disease all came from a single Japanese manufacturer (Slutsker et al, 1990; Belongia et al., 1990). The eosinophilia-myalgia syndrome was due to an as yet unidentified contaminant.

The story of subacute myelo-optic neuropathy (SMON) is another example of an epidemiologic investigation that had immediate relevance to clinical practice. During the years 1956 to 1970, over 10,000 cases of this new syndrome were described in Japan. The patients showed peripheral neuropathy and myelopathy, ranging from minimal dysesthesia to death and including optic atrophy (Oakley, 1973).

The disease occurred most frequently in the summer. Because of its seasonal pattern, some scientists concluded that the epidemic was caused by a virus. It took a decade of multidisciplinary investigation to identify halogenated hydroxyquinolines as the causal agent. These drugs had been sold over the counter for the treatment of intestinal amebiasis and diarrhea. The sales of hydroxyquinolines increased with the seasonal increase in diarrhea, producing a seasonal increase in the incidence of SMON. After the halogenated hydroxyquinolines were removed from the market, the incidence of SMON declined sharply (Figure 13–5).

Clinical practitioners can contribute to epidemiologic research. Schuman (1986) has written a useful guide for clinicians who want to relate their observations in the course of practice to the larger world of medical research. Clinicians practicing in university medical centers can easily become involved in collabo-

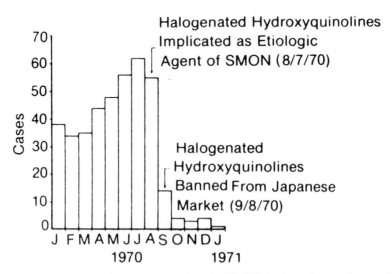

Figure 13–5. Cases of subacute myelo-optic (SMON) in Japan by month reported. *Source:* Oakley, 1973.

rative studies, but physicians in individual practices can also join or start studies. They can initiate research by observing and describing trends in their own practices, consulting with other specialists, and identifying issues to study.

Schuman points out the number of syndromes, diseases, and adverse drug reactions that were first noticed by an alert clinician. For instance, Pittman was first in the United States to recognize optic atrophy in a child treated with diiodohydroxyquin for diarrhea, and his subsequent persistence in identifying cases led to warning labels and the eventual withdrawal of the drug from the market (Pittman and Westphal, 1974). Schuman himself identified a previously unnoticed osteosarcomal malformation syndrome (now called Schuman-Burton syndrome) based on observations he made in a home visit with a physician in training. The history of epidemiology is filled with examples of observant physicians whose curiosity and persistence led to the discovery of important associations, such as Gregg's discovery in 1941 of the association between rubella exposure during pregnancy and congenital malformations, and the association between smoking and lung cancer about which Wynder published his landmark paper while still a medical student (Wynder and Graham, 1950).

In clinical practice a physician may notice trends in patient compliance, new patient characteristics, adverse drug reactions, and associations between exposures and diseases. Reporting such observations may lead to further studies and produce information that is useful to the medical community at large.

SUMMARY

Epidemiologic principles can be applied by the clinician in clinical decision making, in clinical research, and in reading and interpreting the literature. Ideally, a critical reading of the literature should inform practice, and clinical experience can in turn lead to research questions. The interrelationship between practice and research can improve the quality of care and increase the probability that clinical decisions will benefit and not harm the patient. An alert physician can add to medical knowledge by identifying unknown diseases, syndromes, or previously unsuspected associations and by identifying possible causal factors.

STUDY PROBLEMS

1. Describe a way in which decision analysis can be applied to clinical practice.
2. Decision analysis can be useful in many situations, but it also has a number of limitations. Name one of the limitations.

3. When reading the literature, a critical reader should look for information about the study reported. Name three things that should be described in the report of a study.

4. Why is a discussion of bias essential to any article describing a study and its results?

5. Name two ways that a clinician can participate in epidemiologic research.

REFERENCES

Bakwin, H. 1945. "Pseudodoxia pediatrica." *NEJM* 232:691–697.

Beeson, P. B. and McDermott, W., eds. 1963. *Cecil-Loeb Textbook of Medicine,* 11th edition. Philadelphia: W.B. Saunders.

Belongia, E. A., Hedberg, C. W., Gleich, G. J., et al. 1990. "An investigation of the cause of eosinophilia-myalgia syndrome associated with tryptophan use." *NEJM* 323:357–365.

Eidson, M., Philen, R. M., Sewell, C. M., Voorhees, R. and Kilbourne, E. M. 1990. "L-tryptophan and eosinophilia-myalgia syndrome in New Mexico." *Lancet* 355:645–648.

Fletcher, R. H., Fletcher, S. W. and Wagner, E. 1988. *Clinical Epidemiology: The Essentials.* Baltimore: Williams & Wilkins.

Gregg, N. W. 1941. "Congenital cataract following German Measles in the mother." *Trans. Ophthalmol. Soc. Aust.* 3:35.

Linet, M. S. and Stewart, W. F. 1984. "Migraine headache: epidemiologic perspectives." *Epidemiologic Reviews* Vol. 6:107–139.

Oakley, Jr., G. P. 1973. "The neurotoxicity of the halogenated hydroxyquinolines." *JAMA* 225(4):395–397.

Pauker, S. G. Clinical Decision Making. In: Wyngaarden, J. B., Lloyd, H., Smith, J., Bennett, J. C., ed. Cecil Textbook of Medicine. 19th ed. Philadelphia: W.B. Saunders Company, 1992: vol 1: pp. 68–73.

Pittman, F. E. and Westphal, M. C. 1974. "Optic atrophy following treatment with di-iodohydroxyquin." *Pediatrics* 54:81–83.

Sackett, D. L., Haynes, R. B., and Tugwell, P. 1991. *Clinical Epidemiology: A Basic Science for Clinical Medicine,* 2nd edition. Boston: Little, Brown & Co.

Schuman, S. H. 1986. *Practice-Based Epidemiology.* New York: Gordon and Breach Science Publications.

SHEP Cooperative Research Group. 1991. "Prevention of stroke by antihypertensive drug treatment in older persons with isolated systolic hypertension." *JAMA* 265(24):3255–3264.

Slutsker, L., Hoesly, F. C., Miller, L., Williams, L. P., Watson, J. C., Fleming, D. W. 1990. "Eosinophilia-myalgia syndrome associated with exposure to tryptophan from a single manufacturer." *JAMA* 264:213–217.

Stolley, P. D., Davies, J. L. 1980. "Reading the Medical Literature." In *The Physician's*

Practice, Eisenberg, J. M., and Williams, S. V., with Smith, E. S., eds. New York: John Wiley & Sons.

Weiss, Noel S. 1986. *Clinical Epidemiology: The Study of the Outcome of Illness.* New York: Oxford University Press.

Wynder, E. L. and Graham, E. A. 1950. "Tobacco smoking as a possible etiologic factor in bronchiogenic carcinoma." *JAMA* 143:329–336.

Appendix

SELECTED STATISTICAL PROCEDURES

This appendix describes some of the statistical tools and concepts that epidemiologists use. The methods selected are limited to those that can be applied to most studies and that do not require elaborate computing devices. The discussion is condensed and certain technical aspects have been omitted or only briefly described. More detailed expositions of these methods can be found in many textbooks of biostatistics.

SAMPLING OF A POPULATION

Some General Considerations

In most epidemiologic studies, it is necessary to deal with a sample of the population or a subgroup of a population about whose members certain information is desired. The population may be an entire community, the male members of the community, or another subgroup of the community that has a certain characteristic such as gender, race, or religion. Hospital inpatients can also be regarded as a population from which a sample may be taken. The sample does not have to be individuals, but may consist of households, families, or blocks in a city.

When a list of all members of the population is available, the selection of a representative sample is relatively simple. However, it is important to make certain that any available list of names, households, or addresses is indeed complete. The investigator should determine how the list was obtained and maintained, to make sure that duplicates and mistaken entries were removed and that necessary additions were made. Most routinely obtained lists that have not been developed for specific research purposes will reveal one or more deficiencies.

The members of the population list from which a sample is selected will be referred to as the sampling unit. If it is a list of names of individuals, each name is the sampling unit; if of addresses, each address is the sampling unit.

Samples are selected from a population and their characteristics are studied so that one can make inferences from the sample about the population from which it is derived. In other words, the investigator wants the sample to be representative of the population.

Samples may be selected in a variety of ways: the recommended method is known as *probability sampling,* in which each sampling unit has a known probability of being selected. This allows one to derive inferences from the sample about the population with a measurable degree of precision. There are various methods of probability sampling, and they will be discussed below.

Other sampling procedures are of limited or no value in epidemiology since the probability by which a sampling unit enters the sample is not known. Therefore, no statistical assessment can be made of the accuracy of the characteristics of the selected sample in representing the population. Also, unlike probability sampling, there is no objective assurance that potential biases have not entered into the method of selecting the sample. The following are some examples of these sampling procedures:

1. The sample is chosen haphazardly, as in many laboratory experiments where experimental animals are chosen as the investigator can catch and remove them from a cage.
2. An investigator may select individuals who, in his opinion, are typical of the population being studied. The disadvantage of this method is that one really does not know if there are differences between these ''typical'' or ''representative'' individuals and the population, so that generalizations made from the sample may be incorrect.
3. The sample consists of self-selected individuals such as those who have volunteered for an experiment, series of measurements, or interview.

Such methods may be used in exploratory epidemiologic studies to obtain a ''quick and dirty'' look at the problem being investigated. They could provide some information about the population, serving as a basis for planning more adequate studies.

Selecting a Probability Sample

For probability sampling it is necessary to have a complete list of the sampling units of the total population, whether the units are individual persons, households, addresses, blocks, etc. as the specific study requires. If some type of list is available, it may have to be revised; if not available, it is necessary to prepare a list and this usually requires ingenuity and work.

The simplest form of probability sampling is simple random sampling in which each unit in the population list has an equal probability of being selected for the sample. To select a simple random sample the investigator (1) makes a numbered list of the units in the population that he wants to sample; (2) decides on the size of the sample, a matter which is beyond the scope of this book but is discussed in most texts on statistics and sampling, e.g., Cochran (1977); and (3) selects the required number of sampling units using a table of random numbers. Such tables of random numbers are found in most books of statistical tables or texts on statistics. Table A–1 is a table of 1,000 random digits from Snedecor and Cochran (1967) for illustrative purposes.

If such a table is not available and the size of the population to be sampled is not too large, one can write the numbers 1 to N on small cards, place them in a bowl, and mix them thoroughly. If the size of the sample to be selected is n, the cards are selected from the bowl in succession until n cards are drawn. These cards are not returned to the bowl after being drawn. The different numbers are

Table A–1.   One Thousand Random Digits

	00–04	05–09	10–14	15–19	20–24	25–29	30–34	35–39	40–44	45–49
00	54463	22662	65905	70639	79365	67382	29085	69831	47058	08186
01	15389	85205	18850	39226	42249	90669	96325	23248	60933	26927
02	85941	40756	82414	02015	13858	78030	16269	65978	01385	15345
03	61149	69440	11286	88218	58925	03638	52862	62733	33451	77455
04	05219	81619	10651	67079	92511	59888	84502	72095	83463	75577
05	41417	98326	87719	92294	46614	50948	64886	20002	97365	30976
06	28357	94070	20652	35774	16249	75019	21145	05217	47286	76305
07	17783	00015	10806	83091	91530	36466	39981	62481	49177	75779
08	40950	84820	29881	85966	62800	70326	84740	62660	77379	90279
09	82995	64157	66164	41180	10089	41757	78258	96488	88629	37231
10	96754	17676	55659	44105	47361	34833	86679	23930	53249	27083
11	34357	88040	53364	71726	45690	66334	60332	22554	90600	71113
12	06318	37403	49927	57715	50423	67372	63116	48888	21505	80182
13	62111	52820	07243	79931	89292	84767	85693	73947	22278	11551
14	47534	09243	67879	00544	23410	12740	02540	54440	32949	13491
15	98614	75993	84460	62846	59844	14922	48730	73443	48167	34770
16	24856	03648	44898	09351	98795	18644	39765	71058	90368	44104
17	96887	12479	80621	66223	86085	78285	02432	53342	42846	94771
18	90801	21472	42815	77408	37390	76766	52615	32141	30268	18106
19	55165	77312	83666	36028	28420	70219	81369	41943	47366	41067

Source: Snedecor and Cochran (1967). Reprinted by permission from *Statistical Methods* by George W. Snedecor and William G. Cochran, 6th ed. © 1967 by The Iowa State University Press, South State Avenue, Ames, Iowa 50010.

recorded and the correspondingly numbered sampling units in the population are then selected. Mixing the cards provides equal probability of selection and assures randomness. However, since mixing and selection may not be done properly, it is better to use a table of random numbers.

To illustrate the use of these tables, assume that the investigator has a population of 900 case records and a simple random sample of 250 records is desired for a study. The records are numbered from 1 to 900, and a table such as A–1 is entered in a variety of ways, either from the beginning, or by arbitrarily placing a pencil at any number in the table, or by selecting certain columns. Since $N = 900$, it is only necessary to select random numbers composed of three digits. The investigator can go down columns 15–17, for instance, selecting the numbers between 001 and 900 until 250 have been selected. Any number greater than 900 is discarded, as well as any number that is repeated. Since these three columns will not provide all the 250 numbers, another set of three columns, e.g., 30–32, can be used to repeat the procedure. If large sample sizes are required, the most practical method is to use a larger table and select all eligible numbers. The Rand Corporation (1955) has published a table of one million digits, and Kendall and Smith (1938) one of 100,000 digits. Books with smaller tables usually provide instructions as to the most convenient method of using the table.

Simple random sampling may become tedious if the sample and population are large. Suppose an investigator has a list of 250,000 inhabitants or file cards and wants to choose a sample of 1,000. A method of sampling that is used more frequently than simple random sampling in such cases is systematic sampling. To select a systematic sample, two things are needed: a sampling interval and a random start. For example, if $N = 250,000$ and $n = 1,000$, one divides 250,000 by 1,000, which equals 250. Beginning with a random number between 1 and 250 (random start), one selects every 250th number thereafter. Thus if the random number is 125, the next number would be 375, then 625, etc. If n does not divide evenly into N, one selects the nearest whole number. One advantage of systematic sampling is that it spreads the sample more evenly over the population. It is conceivable, however, that the systematic sample may be biased if there is a periodicity or systematic ordering in the population list, e.g., it may always be a corner household.

Certain assumptions must be made about the characteristics of the population to be sampled in order to estimate the sampling error. A full discussion of these problems and their solutions can be found in Cochran (1977).

It should be emphasized that the listings of the population must have the same units as the desired sample, e.g., samples of individuals from lists of persons and samples of households from household lists. If a household list is available to the investigator but a simple random sample of persons is desired, there are additional considerations. If the investigator selects a simple random sample of *n* households and interviews or examines one person per household, the resulting sample of *n* persons will not be a simple random sample since individuals in smaller households will have a greater chance of being selected than those in larger households. Thus, each individual would not have had an equal probability of being selected for the sample. If the factor being studied is related to the size of the household, a biased sample will result. More complex methods can be used to obtain an unbiased sample in such situations and some of these will be mentioned below, but again the interested reader should consult Cochran (1977).

The population to be sampled can be divided into subgroups or *strata* by one or more characteristics, such as age, gender, or severity of disease, and within each stratum a random sample can be selected. This procedure is known as *stratified sampling* and it has several advantages. It reduces sampling variability by eliminating variation with respect to the characteristic by which the strata are constructed and if the strata are more uniform than the total population with respect to other factors. It also has the advantage of allowing one to use different sampling fractions (percent of individuals in the strata that is being selected for the sample) in the different strata since it is possible to obtain larger fractions in strata with a smaller number of units.

Sampling where no population lists exist

In many areas where epidemiologic studies are needed, there is no satisfactory population list of individuals. Frequently, lists of various groupings of individuals are available or can be compiled. These groups are socially or politically defined clusterings of individuals, such as households, addresses of buildings, city blocks, or census enumeration districts. When such lists are available or when they can be readily compiled, two methods may be used to select the desired sample of individuals:

1. A random sample of clusters is selected and all individuals in the cluster are included in the study. This is known as single-stage cluster sampling.

2. A random sample of clusters is selected, a list is made of all the individuals in each cluster, and a random sample of individuals is then selected independently within each cluster. This is known as two-stage cluster sampling with subsampling.

If a list of households is available and a random sample of individual persons is desired, a random sample of households may be selected and all individuals in the household may be interviewed or studied. This is an example of single-stage cluster sampling. If, after selecting the households, a roster of all individuals in each household is made and a random sample of one or more individuals is randomly selected from each roster, one has performed two-stage cluster sampling.

There may be more than two stages of sampling. For example, a list of blocks in a city may be available from the population census. A sample of blocks may be randomly selected. Each of the selected blocks may be canvassed to obtain a list of households. A sample of households may then be selected and for each household a roster of household members compiled. This procedure results in a three-stage sample with subsampling at all stages.

If not available, lists of such clusters can be constructed by the investigator. In addition, aerial photographs or maps can be used to divide a geographical area into smaller areas with definable boundaries and then samples of areas and sub-areas can be selected.

One form of cluster sampling is **random digit dialing** (RDD). In this technique, telephone numbers for households in a specific geographic area are selected at random from clusters of such telephone numbers. The investigator can then sample individuals in households with telephones (Hartge et al., 1984; Waksberg, 1978; Wacholder et al., 1992; Greenberg, 1990). There are many potential problems in random digit dialing, including the inability to include in the sample individuals in households lacking a telephone, the greater likelihood of sampling households with two telephone numbers than those with only one number, and the different numbers of individuals living in each household. Methods have been developed to circumvent these difficulties. The interested reader is referred to the reviews of Greenberg (1990) and Wacholder et al. (1992) for further information.

Cluster sampling is convenient not only when no population lists are available but also when the investigator wants to study people living in a small number of households or villages rather than individuals in more scattered populations.

Cluster multistage samples have larger sampling errors than simple random samples of the same size. A cluster is composed of individuals who are likely to be more similar to each other than those selected at random from the population. For example, individuals in the same household have similar dietary and smoking habits (generally known as ''intra-class correlation''). In addition, fewer large clusters will be available for sampling and the sample will be concentrated in a smaller number of clusters. It is therefore preferable to have a large number of small clusters than a small number of large clusters. It should be emphasized that biases can result if a cluster sample of individuals is analyzed as if it were a random sample of individuals. It should also be noted that clusters, like individuals, can be grouped into more homogeneous strata and a certain percentage of clusters selected from within each stratum. Thus, the methods used in analyzing stratified sampling can be applied. Again, the reader is referred to Cochran for a detailed discussion of these methods (1977).

ESTIMATING POPULATION CHARACTERISTICS AND THEIR SAMPLING VARIABILITY

Drawing a sample so that biases of selection are avoided does not guarantee that it will be completely representative of the population from which it was derived. The sampling procedure itself (unless it is a "sample" of 100 percent of the population) will eliminate individuals with certain characteristics. If many different samples are drawn from the same population by random sampling or by one of its variants, different values or estimates will be obtained of the same characteristic from each sample selected. If all the possible samples of a certain size drawn from a population vary considerably, the investigator has less assurance that his particular selection is representative of the population characteristic to be estimated. However, if there is little variation from sample to sample and no biases are present, either in the method of selecting the sample or in the way the population characteristic is estimated, the investigator has more assurance that a particular sample is a representative one.

Estimating Population Characteristics

The selection of the sample from a population allows for the characterization of various features of that population, e.g., serum cholesterol concentration, prevalence of cigarette smoking, etc. Three measures (the mean, the median, and the mode) are used to summarize the characteristics of interest. Each has its advantages and disadvantages in describing the features of a sample and the population from which the sample was drawn. In discussing these three summary measures, we will refer to the systolic blood pressures in a random sample of 63 nulliparous pregnant women measured at the start of their second trimester shown in Table A–2.

The mean

The *mean* is the most frequently used summary measure. Also known as the *arithmetic mean* or the *arithmetic average,* it is symbolized as $\bar{x}$ (termed "x-bar"). The mean is calculated by summing all of the observed values and dividing by the sample size. For the data in Table A–2, the mean is calculated as: (113 + 114 + 100 + 113 + 115 + ... + 102 + 109 + 128) mmHg/63, which is equal to 106.38 mmHg. Although there may be considerable variation in the individual

Table A–2. Measurements of Systolic Blood Pressure among 63 Nulliparous Pregnant
Women at the Beginning of the Second Trimester

113	114	100	113	115	84	115	119	99	95	113	111	114
128	96	107	88	93	99	103	92	108	122	107	104	99
95	122	97	112	120	105	100	105	111	113	110	121	106
107	114	102	103	99	96	93	103	107	102	105	116	95
118	114	105	111	92	113	97	103	102	109	128		

values of a characteristic in samples from the same population, the means for
those samples will tend to be similar in value. This consistency is one advantage
of the mean. Another is its use in many statistical tests (described below). However, the mean has one major disadvantage: depending on the simple size, it can
be greatly affected by an extreme value, i.e., an observation that differs greatly
from the other ones (sometimes referred to as "outliers"). For example, suppose
that in addition to the values in Table A–2, there were a 64th individual in the
sample, whose systolic blood pressure was 300 mmHg. Clearly, this value is quite
different from the other 63. If it were included in the calculation of the mean,
then $\bar{x}$ would be 109.4 mmHg. In order to reduce the effect of one or more outliers
on the characterization of a population, some investigators use a different summary measure, the median, which relies only on the ranking of observations in
the sample.

The median

The *median* is defined as the observation that corresponds to the 50th per-
centile of the sample, i.e., the midpoint of the data. One-half of all of the data
are greater than the median, and one-half are less than the median. To calculate
the median, the observations are ranked in ascending order. Table A–3 shows the
data in Table A–2 assembled in ascending order. The median observation is then
the 32nd observation (31 observations above the median, 31 observations below
the median), 106 mmHg. If there is an even number of observations, the median
is the mean of the middle two observations.

The main advantage of the median is the lack of effect of extreme values on
it. For instance, if there were a 64th observation of 300 mmHg for the data in
Table A–3, the median would be 106.5 (the average of the 32nd and 33rd observations). This benefit contrasts with the disadvantage that the median is not as
amenable to statistical testing as the mean. Hence, although the median is sometimes used as a summary measure, it is less often used than the mean.

Table A–3. Measurements of Systolic Blood Pressure among 63 Nulliparous Pregnant Women, Arranged in Ascending Order

RANK	OBSERVATION	RANK	OBSERVATION	RANK	OBSERVATION
1	84	23	103	45	113
2	88	24	103	46	113
3	92	25	103	47	113
4	92	26	103	48	113
5	93	27	104	49	114
6	93	28	105	50	114
7	95	29	105	51	114
8	95	30	105	52	114
9	95	31	105	53	115
10	96	32	106	54	115
11	96	33	107	55	116
12	97	34	107	56	118
13	97	35	107	57	119
14	99	36	107	58	120
15	99	37	108	59	121
16	99	38	109	60	122
17	99	39	110	61	122
18	100	40	111	62	128
19	100	41	111	63	128
20	102	42	111		
21	102	43	112		
22	102	44	113		

The mode

The third summary measure is the *mode,* which is the most frequently occurring value. For the data in Table A–2, the mode is 113; this is considerably different from both the mean and the median. Frequently, there is no particular value in a sample that occurs more often than all the other values; in this instance, the mode does not exist. Although the mode can summarize some information regarding a characteristic in a sample (and the population from which it was drawn), it does not provide as much information as the mean or the median. For this reason, it is not frequently used by investigators.

Assessing Sampling Variability

Random sampling provides the means of measuring the degree of assurance from the particular sample selected. It can be shown theoretically or by experimental sampling that the amount of variation in the frequency of a characteristic from one sample to another depends upon the amount of variation of the characteristic (whether quantitative or qualitative) in the population. Random sampling allows one to obtain from any selected sample an unbiased estimate of the population variation. This estimate is then used to set limits within which the population value being estimated will lie, with varying degrees of confidence. A numerical value for these degrees of confidence can be calculated by making some assumptions, or preferably by having some knowledge about the distribution of the estimated characteristic in the population.

As already mentioned, when random sampling is used, the variability of samples drawn from a population can be measured in terms of the variability found in the population itself, which can be estimated from the selected sample. For example, if the average age at menarche is estimated from a sample, the variation in the estimate from that sample reflects the variation in the age of menarche in the population, which can be estimated in a randomly selected sample.

Variation of individuals in a population can be measured in several ways. Most frequently it is measured by its variance or the square root of the variance, the standard deviation. The *variance* of a characteristic or measurement is defined as the mean of the sum of squared deviations of individuals from the population's arithmetic mean. The standard deviation of a characteristic is usually denoted by the Greek lowercase letter sigma (σ) and the variance as σ^2. Symbolically, the variance may be defined as:

$$\sigma^2 = \frac{1}{N} [(x_1 - \overline{X})^2 + (x_2 - \overline{X})^2 + \ldots + (x_N - \overline{X})^2]$$

where N is the size of the population, x is the particular characteristic being measured, x_i is the value of the characteristic for the ith individual in the population, and $\overline{X}$ is the arithmetic mean of the xth characteristic in the population.

An equivalent formula which makes the calculation of σ^2 easier is:

$$\sigma^2 = (\Sigma x_i^2 - N\overline{X}^2)/N.$$

If the characteristic being examined is dichotomous (i.e., present or absent) rather than a measurement, the variance reduces to $P(1 - P)$, where P is the proportion of individuals with the characteristic.

It is important to note that the sampling variation depends essentially on two quantities: the variance of the population (σ^2) and the sample size (n). Populations with more variable characteristics of interest require larger sample sizes to compensate for this fact. With a qualitative characteristic, the greatest amount of variation in the population occurs when P, the frequency of the characteristic in the population, equals 0.50. This decreases as P is higher or lower than 0.50. Thus, when sampling from a population where the characteristic occurs 50 percent of the time, much larger samples are necessary to provide the same degree of assurance one has in a population where the characteristic occurs only 10 percent of the time.

Study results are usually assessed in terms of the standard deviation. The formula used to determine the precision of the sample mean or proportion is:

$$\sigma_{\bar{x}} = \frac{\sigma}{\sqrt{n}}.$$

It should be noted that a change in the sample size affects the standard deviation. To reduce the standard deviation by one-half, for example, it is necessary to quadruple the sample size. Thus it is possible to achieve any desired reduction in the standard deviation, but the necessary increase in the sample size may be prohibitively costly.

Rarely does the investigator have knowledge of the variance or standard deviation of the population being studied. When the sample is a probability sample, an estimate of the sampling variation is obtained from the sample itself. For a simple random sample, the estimated variance of a sample mean is:

$$s_{\bar{x}}^2 = \frac{s^2}{n}$$

where s^2 is the sample estimate of the variance defined by:

$$s^2 = \frac{1}{n-1} [(x_1 - \bar{x})^2 + (x_2 - \bar{x})^2 + \ldots + (x_n - \bar{x})^2],$$

where $x_1, x_2, \ldots, x_n$ are the sample values of the xth characteristic and $\bar{x}$ is the arithmetic mean of the xth characteristic in the sample. An equivalent formula which makes the calculation of s^2 easier is:

$$s^2 = (\Sigma x_i^2 - N\bar{x}^2)/(N - 1).$$

An example of the calculation of s^2, using the data in Table A–2, is shown in Table A–4. The standard error, $S_{\bar{x}}$, is the square root of the variance of the mean.

Table A–4. Calculation of s^2 for Data in Table A–2

$n = 63$

$\Sigma x = 6,702$

$\Sigma x^2 = 718,700$

$\bar{x} = \Sigma x/n = 6,702/63 = 106.38$

$s^2 = (\Sigma x^2 - n\bar{x}^2)/(n - 1) = (718,700 - [63 \cdot (106.38)^2])/62 = 5747.65/62 = 92.70$

$s = \sqrt{s^2} = \sqrt{92.70} = 9.63$

$s_{\bar{x}} = s/\sqrt{n} = 9.63/\sqrt{63} = 1.21$

The estimate of the variance of the sample proportion is:

$$P(1 - P)/N,$$

where P is the proportion of individuals in a sample of size N with the characteristic being studied.

Thus, if a simple random sample of 100 individuals is selected from a large population, among whom 40 persons have a certain characteristic, the estimated proportion of people with this characteristic in the population is $p_0 = \dfrac{40}{100} = 0.40$ (p_0 will be used as the sample estimate of P). The estimated sampling variability is:

$$s = \sqrt{\frac{p_0(1 - p_0)}{n}} = \sqrt{\frac{(.40)(1 - .40)}{100}} = \sqrt{.0024} = .049$$

or approximately .05. This can be interpreted to mean that while the estimated frequency of the characteristic in the population as derived from this sample was 40 percent, other samples of the same size, drawn similarly from the same population, would vary from each other on the average by about 5 percent.

However, the value of .049 was also derived from sample values so that another sample would likely give a different estimate of the precision or standard deviation of the sample. The estimates of precision are not likely to vary as much as the estimated proportions themselves. If only ten (or even ninety) persons had been found to have the characteristic rather than forty, the estimated precision would have changed from 5 to 3 percent.

The formula:

$$s = \sqrt{\frac{P(1 - P)}{n}}$$

is known as the standard error of a proportion. It refers to the variability of a sample proportion p_0 from one sample to another. It is estimated from the sample itself by:

$$s = \sqrt{\frac{p_0(1 - p_0)}{n}} \; .$$

CONFIDENCE INTERVALS FOR PROPORTIONS

The estimation of variation represents the average amount of sampling variability. Under certain conditions, however, it can be shown that for reasonably large samples [large enough so that $n(1 - p) > 10$], the proportion estimated from approximately 95 percent of samples of a given size will lie within ± 1.96 standard errors of the true population proportion P.

    If the value of P is known, it can then be stated that 95 percent of the samples of size n selected from this population have a proportion that will fall in the interval

$$P - 1.96 \sqrt{\frac{P(1 - P)}{n}} , P + 1.96 \sqrt{\frac{P(1 - P)}{n}} \; .$$

If, for example, random samples of size 100 are selected from a population in which 50 percent of the persons have a certain characteristic, 95 percent of the samples will provide estimates of this percentage that will lie between

$$0.50 - 1.96 \sqrt{\frac{0.5(1 - 0.5)}{100}} \text{ and } 0.50 + 1.96 \sqrt{\frac{0.5(1 - 0.5)}{100}}$$

or between 40 and 60 percent (the multiplier 2.0 can be used rather than 1.96 for convenience). Thus, estimates that are less than 40 percent or greater than 60 percent will occur in only 5 percent of the samples of size 100 selected from such a population. It can be further shown that 99 percent of the samples will lie within the interval

$$P - 2.58 \sqrt{\frac{P(1 - P)}{n}} \text{ and } P + 2.58 \sqrt{\frac{P(1 - P)}{n}} \; .$$

Using data from the above example, 99 percent of the estimates from samples of size 100 will lie between 38 and 62.9 percent.

Then, what can be inferred from any particular random sample of size n that is selected from this population? From the sample, first compute p_0, and then the following expression:

$$p_0 \pm 1.96 \sqrt{\frac{P(1 - P)}{n}} ,$$

i.e., $\left(p_0 - 1.96 \sqrt{\frac{P(1 - P)}{n}} \right) - \left(p_0 + 1.96 \sqrt{\frac{P(1 - P)}{n}} \right).$

This interval will include P only if p_0 is one of the 95 percent of all possible estimates that fall within the interval

$$P \pm 1.96 \sqrt{\frac{P(1 - P)}{n}} .$$

In the numerical example above, if p_0 were one of the estimates between 0.40 and 0.60, the interval formed by adding and subtracting

$$2 \sqrt{\frac{0.5(1 - 0.5)}{100}} = 0.10$$

will contain the population proportion, 0.50. This interval will not contain 5 percent of the samples that have estimates of p_0 greater than 0.60 or less than 0.40, and therefore will not contain the population proportion, 0.50. Thus, 95 percent of the samples will provide intervals that contain the population percentage, while 5 percent will not. Before selecting a particular sample of size n, the investigator is thus assured in 95 times out of 100 that the interval calculated from his sample will contain the population proportion he is interested in estimating.

The investigator will not know before (or after) selecting the sample whether or not this particular estimate is one of the 95 percent lying within the two standard error range of the true proportion or if it is one of the 5 percent outside this range. If the investigator's sample is one of the latter 5 percent, then the statement that the interval

$$p_0 \pm 2 \sqrt{\frac{P(1 - P)}{n}}$$

contains the population proportion will be wrong; otherwise, it will be a correct statement. For these reasons the interval

$$p_0 \pm 2 \sqrt{\frac{P(1 - P)}{n}}$$

is called a 95 percent confidence interval, the word "confidence" referring to the investigator's assurance that the selected sample is one of 95 percent of all samples that will provide a correct statement based on the interval.

It should be noted that in order to calculate these confidence intervals the unknown population proportion P has been used in the standard error formula. Since the investigator is either attempting to estimate P or to test some hypothesis about it, its value is not known. The obvious solution is to substitute the sample value of p_0 in the formula for the standard error and calculate the interval

$$p_0 \pm 1.96 \sqrt{\frac{p_0(1 - p_0)}{n}}.$$

This increases the variation of the interval since the standard error will vary from sample to sample. Fortunately, as was pointed out earlier, the standard error changes little from sample to sample, even though the sample proportion p_0 might. Thus, the statements that were made using P in the standard error hold fairly well when the sample estimate p_0 is used in place of P.

In summary: If a simple random sample of size n is selected from a population and the sample proportion p_0 is calculated, a 95 percent confidence interval for P, the population proportion, is given by

$$p_0 \pm 1.96 \sqrt{\frac{p_0(1 - p_0)}{n}}.$$

If a 99 percent confidence interval is desired, the multiplier 1.96 is replaced by 2.58. (For most practical applications, 1.96 can be replaced by 2.0 and 2.58 by 2.6 with little loss of accuracy.)

For example, suppose in a simple random sample of 400 persons from a large population of smokers, 80 are found to be "heavy" smokers (smoking more than one pack of cigarettes a day). The proportion of "heavy" smokers in the population can be estimated by the 95 percent confidence interval

$$p_0 \pm 2 \sqrt{\frac{p_0(1 - p_0)}{n}} = \frac{80}{400} \pm 2 \sqrt{\frac{\frac{80}{400} \left(1 - \frac{80}{400}\right)}{400}} = 0.20 \pm .04,$$

or 16 percent to 24 percent. Thus, it can be stated that there is a 95 percent probability that the percentage of "heavy" smokers in the population lies between 16 and 24 percent.

The confidence interval can be made as small as desired by increasing the sample size, but the decrease is proportional to the square root of the increase rather than to the increase itself. In the example, in order to decrease the confidence interval from 16–24 percent to 18–22 percent, the sample size would have to be quadrupled from 400 to 1,600 persons. Thus, beyond a certain level, reductions in the confidence interval can only be achieved at higher cost.

NINETY-FIVE PERCENT CONFIDENCE INTERVAL FOR RARELY OCCURRING EVENTS

We have seen that for a percentage or rate, good approximations for 95 percent confidence intervals are easily computed when the condition $n(1 - p) > 10$ is satisfied. But many diseases, such as cancer, have annual incidence, prevalence, or mortality rates ranging from 1 to 100 per 100,000 population so that sample sizes of 10,000 to 1,000,000 would be necessary before the above calculations of confidence limits could be used safely. In practice, rates must often be estimated from smaller samples.

In calculating confidence intervals for rarely occurring events, different methods must be used. These are based on the Poisson rather than the normal (Gaussian) distribution used earlier. With these methods, unfortunately, it is not possible to use multipliers for the standard error that are analogous to 1.96 and 2.58, which are derived from the normal curve. To simplify matters, a table of 95 percent confidence interval factors* was prepared by Haenszel, Loveland, and Sirken (1962) and is reproduced as Table A–5. The authors tabulated factors necessary to calculate 95 percent confidence limits for standardized mortality ratios (SMRs). The following calculation of 95 percent confidence limits for low incidence rates exemplifies the method used.

If, in a simple random sample of 5,000 adult males, 2 new cases of stomach cancer had occurred during a year of observation, which projects to an incidence rate of 40 per 100,000 population. In order to calculate 95 percent confidence limits, enter Table A–5 at $n = 2$ (observed number of cases on which the estimate is based). A lower limit factor (L) of 0.121 and an upper limit factor (U) of 3.61 are found corresponding to $n = 2$. To convert these numbers to a rate per 100,000, multiply both lower and upper limits by the sample rate per 100,000 (i.e., by 40). Thus, $L = 40 \times 0.121 = 4.84$, and $U = 40 \times 3.61 = 144.40$. The 95 percent confidence interval for the incidence of stomach cancer is therefore 4.84–144.40 cases per 100,000 of population. This interval is wide, reflecting the uncertainties based on estimates involving only two cases.

If, in a sample of any size, no cases are found, an upper 95 percent confidence limit can be estimated by using $n = 3$ as the upper limit. Thus, if in a sample of

*These factors facilitate the calculation of a confidence interval for a Poisson-distributed variable.

Table A–5 Tabular Values of 95 Percent Confidence Limit Factors for Estimates of a Poisson-Distributed Variable

OBSERVED NUMBER ON WHICH ESTIMATE IS BASED (n)	LOWER LIMIT FACTOR (L)	UPPER LIMIT FACTOR (U)	OBSERVED NUMBER ON WHICH ESTIMATE IS BASED (n)	LOWER LIMIT FACTOR (L)	UPPER LIMIT FACTOR (U)	OBSERVED NUMBER ON WHICH ESTIMATE IS BASED (n)	LOWER LIMIT FACTOR (L)	UPPER LIMIT FACTOR (U)
1	0.0253	5.57	21	0.619	1.53	120	0.833	1.200
2	0.121	3.61	22	0.627	1.51	140	0.844	1.184
3	0.206	2.92	23	0.634	1.50	160	0.854	1.171
4	0.272	2.56	24	0.641	1.49	180	0.862	1.160
5	0.324	2.33	25	0.647	1.48	200	0.868	1.151
6	0.367	2.18	26	0.653	1.47	250	0.882	1.134
7	0.401	2.06	27	0.659	1.46	300	0.892	1.121
8	0.431	1.97	28	0.665	1.45	350	0.899	1.112
9	0.458	1.90	29	0.670	1.44	400	0.906	1.104
10	0.480	1.84	30	0.675	1.43	450	0.911	1.098
11	0.499	1.79	35	0.697	1.39	500	0.915	1.093
12	0.517	1.75	40	0.714	1.36	600	0.922	1.084
13	0.532	1.71	45	0.729	1.34	700	0.928	1.078
14	0.546	1.68	50	0.742	1.32	800	0.932	1.072
15	0.560	1.65	60	0.770	1.30	900	0.936	1.068
16	0.572	1.62	70	0.785	1.27	1000	0.939	1.064
17	0.583	1.60	80	0.798	1.25			
18	0.593	1.58	90	0.809	1.24			
19	0.602	1.56	100	0.818	1.22			
20	0.611	1.54						

Source: Haenszel et al. (1962).

10,000 persons, $n = 0$ cases of a disease were found, the upper 95 percent confidence limit would be calculated as 3 per 10,000 cases, or 30 per 100,000.

This method is also applicable to subclasses of the sample population. If simple random sampling is not used, or if the numerators and denominators of the rates are not derived from the same survey, then certain complications can arise from using Table A–5. Some of these complications are discussed by Haenszel et al. (1962).

TESTS OF HYPOTHESES FOR PROPORTIONS

Samples are often selected not only to estimate the frequencies or proportions but also to test certain hypotheses. It is often desirable to know if an incidence or prevalence rate for a certain group of the population has decreased or increased over a period of time. The new rate p_0 can be estimated from a simple random sample and the investigator wants to determine ("test the hypothesis") whether the sample with this rate may have come from a population with a certain hypothesized rate. Is the difference between the observed and hypothesized rate large enough to exclude sampling variation as an explanation? For example, it might be known that the yearly survival rate from a certain group of diseases is 30 percent. After a new method of treatment is introduced, it is observed in a random sample of 100 persons with the disease, that 50 have survived one year. Is this difference of 20 percent due to sampling variation or must one hypothesize another explanation of the difference? (This issue is hypothetical since, as discussed in Chapter 8, a randomized clinical trial is the best method for determining whether a new treatment has an effect.)

In the previous section, it was noted that for samples which are large enough $[n(1 - p) > 10]$, the 95 percent confidence interval is

$$p_0 - 2.0 \sqrt{\frac{P(1 - P)}{n}} \leq P \leq p_0 + 2.0 \sqrt{\frac{P(1 - P)}{n}}.$$

This relationship would be true for 95 percent of the samples selected from that population. This can be rewritten in the form:

$$|p_0 - P| \leq 2.0 \sqrt{\frac{P(1 - P)}{n}}.$$

The vertical strokes on either side of a quantity refer to the absolute value of the quantity regardless of algebraic sign.

Thus, if a sample with a proportion p_0 comes from a population with proportion P, the difference (either in a positive or negative sense) can be expected to exceed twice the standard error *only* 5 percent of the time. If the observed difference does, indeed, exceed twice the standard error, it can be concluded that this sample belongs to that group that occurs infrequently (less than 5 percent of the time), or that it has in fact been derived from some other population. If the latter explanation is accepted, then there is a 5 percent chance of being wrong.

In the hypothetical survival rate problem, $p_0 = \dfrac{50}{100} = .50$, $P = .30$, and

$$\sqrt{\frac{P(1 - P)}{n}} = \sqrt{\frac{(.30)(.70)}{100}} = .046;$$

$1.96(0.46) = .0902$ and $|p_0 - P| = |.50 - .30| = .20$. Since the difference of .20 is greater than .090, one can conclude that either there was no increase in survival and a rather rare event was observed, or that there really was an increase in survivorship, resulting in the observed difference.If the investigator is unwilling to accept the possibility that the study sample is one that occurs rarely, then the difference is said to be statistically significant at the 5 percent probability level. If one is reluctant to accept a sample that occurs less than 5 percent of the time as being rare, a higher level of statistical significance may be specified; for example, by classifying as rare those samples that occur less than 1 percent of the time. It is then necessary that the difference $|p_0 - P|$ exceed

$$2.6 \sqrt{\frac{P(1 - P)}{n}} \, .$$

This will occur less than 1 percent of the time if the hypothesis is true that p_0 was derived from a population with proportion P. If this hypothesis is rejected, there is a 1 percent chance of having rejected a true hypothesis.

The test appears in its simplest form if the following quantity is calculated:

$$\frac{|p_0 - P|}{\sqrt{\dfrac{P(1 - P)}{n}}} = \frac{\text{difference}}{\text{standard error (S.E.)}}$$

If this difference exceeds 2.0, the difference is said to be statistically significant at the 5 percent level; if it exceeds 2.60 the difference is said to be statistically significant at the 1 percent level. The 5 percent and 1 percent levels correspond to α, the chance of a Type I error occurring, that was discussed in Chapter 8 (p. 161).

CONFIDENCE INTERVALS AND TESTS OF HYPOTHESES FOR THE SAMPLE MEAN

There are also 95 percent confidence interval and statistical tests for the mean $(\bar{x})$ of sample data that are "continuous," i.e., not dichotomous. The maternal systolic blood pressure readings given in Table A–2 are examples of such data. The 95 percent confidence interval for the mean of such continuous data $(\bar{X})$ would be

$$\bar{x} - 1.96\sqrt{(\sigma^2/N)}, \bar{x} + 1.96\sqrt{(\sigma^2/N)}.$$

(This confidence interval should only be used if the population distribution from which the data were drawn is a normal one or if $N \geq 30$.) For the data given in Table A–2, the mean was 106.38 mmHg. Suppose that the variance (σ^2) were known from previous surveys to be 100.2 mmHg^2. Then the 95 percent confidence interval would be

$$106.38 - 1.96\sqrt{(100.2/63)}, 106.38 + 1.96\sqrt{(100.2/63)}$$

or 103.91 mmHg to 108.85 mmHg.

An alternative analysis of these data might use the investigator's knowledge that the average maternal systolic blood pressure in the general population is 110.1 mmHg. The investigator wishes to determine whether the difference between the population value and the mean for the sample is due to sampling variation or whether some other explanation must be sought. The 95 percent confidence interval for $\bar{X}$ is

$$\bar{x} - 1.96\sqrt{(\sigma^2/N)} \leq \bar{X} \leq \bar{x} + 1.96\sqrt{(\sigma^2/N)}.$$

This relationship may be rewritten as

$$|\bar{x} - \bar{X}| \leq 1.96\sqrt{(\sigma^2/N)}.$$

or

$$\frac{|\bar{x} - \bar{X}|}{\sqrt{(\sigma^2/N)}} \leq 1.96.$$

If the left side of this equation is found to be less than 1.96, then the investigator would conclude that there is at least a 5 percent chance that the difference between the sample mean and the known population value resulted from sampling variation; i.e., no other explanation is needed to explain the discrepancy. Alternatively, if the left side of the equation is greater than 1.96, then the probability that this difference results from sampling variation is less than 5 percent; i.e., there are other explanations for the discrepancy. Substituting the sample mean and the population values into this criterion, one finds that

$$\frac{|\bar{x} - \overline{X}|}{\sqrt{(\sigma^2/N)}} = \frac{|106.38 - 110.1| \text{ mmHg}}{\sqrt{(100.2 \text{ mmHg}^2/63)}}$$

$$= (3.72 \text{ mmHg})/(1.26 \text{ mmHg})$$
$$= 2.95.$$

Hence the investigator would conclude that the sample mean is statistically significantly different from the population mean at the 5 percent level.

Suppose that the variance for the data in Table A–2 were not known before the sample was selected. The investigator may still test the hypothesis that the difference between the sample mean and the population mean is attributable to sampling variation, but the formula used differs slightly from that presented above. In particular, since σ^2 must be estimated by s^2, the test criterion is:

$$\frac{|\bar{x} - \overline{X}|}{\sqrt{(s^2/N)}} \le t_{N-1}.$$

where t_{N-1} is the value of the t-distribution (a statistical frequency distribution) with $N - 1$ "degrees of freedom" (df) for the desired level of significance. Selected values of the t-distribution for various degrees of freedom are given in Table A–6. It is important to recognize that the degrees of freedom depend only on the sample size, not on the magnitude of $\bar{x}$, s, or $\overline{X}$.

Suppose that the investigator wishes to determine if the sample mean of 106.38 mmHg differs significantly from the population value of 110.1 mmHg and does not know the value of σ^2. Using the information in Table A–4, we can see that the test criterion is

$$\frac{|106.38 - 110.1|}{\sqrt{(s^2/63)}} \le t_{62},$$

$$\frac{3.72}{1.21} \le t_{62},$$

$$3.07 \le t_{62}.$$

Since the left side of the equation is greater than the right side, the investigator would conclude that the sample mean is statistically significantly different from the population mean at the 5 percent level; i.e., sampling variation alone cannot explain the difference. For more information on the t-distribution, the reader is referred to Colton (1974) and Snedecor and Cochran (1977).

Table A–6. Value of the *t*-
Distribution for 5 Percent Statistical
Significance Tests for Various Degrees
of Freedom

DEGREES OF FREEDOM (df)	t_{df}
1	25.45
2	6.21
3	4.18
4	3.50
5	3.16
6	2.97
7	2.84
8	2.75
9	2.69
10	2.63
15	2.49
20	2.42
25	2.39
30	2.36
35	2.34
40	2.33
45	2.32
50	2.31
55	2.30
60	2.30
70	2.29
80	2.28

TESTING HYPOTHESES ABOUT TWO SAMPLE PROPORTIONS

It can be shown that the standard error of the difference between two sample percentages p_1 and p_2 from the same population will have a standard error of

$$\sqrt{\frac{P(1 - P)}{n_1} + \frac{P(1 - P)}{n_2}}.$$

where P is the proportion of the population with the characteristic, $(1 - P)$ is the proportion of the population without the characteristic, n_1 is the size of one sample, and n_2 is the size of the other sample. If one wants to test the hypothesis that the two samples have been independently selected from a population having the common population proportion P, a ratio is calculated that is similar to the one given in previous sections, namely,

$$\frac{\text{difference between proportions}}{\text{standard error of difference}} = \frac{|p_1 - p_2|}{\sqrt{\dfrac{P(1 - P)}{n_1} + \dfrac{P(1 - P)}{n_2}}}.$$

This provides a satisfactory method of testing the hypothesis that there is no difference between p_1 and p_2 at the 5 percent or 1 percent significance level, if an estimate of P and $(1 - P)$ is available. Up to this point we have assumed that the values of P and $(1 - P)$ were provided or known. The hypothesis to be tested states that the two samples come from a population with a common population proportion without specifying the value of the proportion. Thus, it is necessary to estimate the value of P from the two samples by taking a weighted average of their proportions,

$$\hat{p} = \frac{n_1 p_1 + n_2 p_2}{n_1 + n_2} = \frac{\text{total number in both samples}}{\text{total number of observations}}$$

The test criterion then becomes:

$$\frac{\text{difference between proportions}}{\text{standard error of difference}} = \frac{|p_1 - p_2|}{\sqrt{\dfrac{\hat{p}(1 - p)}{n_1} + \dfrac{\hat{p}(1 - \hat{p})}{n_2}}}.$$

If this value exceeds 1.96 (or 2.0), then the hypothesis, that the observed difference is due to sampling alone, is rejected at the 5 percent level of statistical significance. If it exceeds 2.58 (or 2.6), the hypothesis is rejected at the 1 percent level.

For a simple example of the procedure, assume that an investigator has observations on the number of patients who have and have not been cured after receiving one of two treatments, A and B, as shown in Table A–7. The hypothesis to be tested is whether the observed cure rate of those who had received treatment A is significantly different from those who had received treatment B. This can be restated as follows: would one frequently observe a difference of .156 (or 15.6 percent) in these cure rates if these two samples being compared were derived from a population with the same cure rate? The estimate of the population cure rate is given by $\hat{p} = \dfrac{75}{200} = .375.$

The statistical test can now be calculated as

$$\frac{.156}{\sqrt{\dfrac{(.375)(.625)}{40} + \dfrac{(.375)(.625)}{160}}} = \frac{.156}{.0866} = 1.8.$$

Table A–7. Determination of Percentage Cured for
Patients Receiving Treatments A and B

| TREATMENT | NUMBER OF PATIENTS | | |
	CURED	NOT CURED	TOTAL
A	10	30	40
B	65	95	160
Total	75	125	200

The cure rate for those receiving treatments A and B are
$p_a = 10/40 = .25, p_b = 65/160 = .406$, respectively. The
difference in cure rates is $p_a - p_b = .156$.

Since this value is less than 1.96, it is concluded that either the difference observed is due to sampling (or chance) variation in the two groups or that the sample sizes used in this comparison are not large enough to detect differences of this size.

The test can be put into another form that allows simpler computations. If the observations in the fourfold table (Table A–7) are expressed in a more general form, as in Table A–8, it is possible to obtain, after some algebraic manipulation, the following:

$$(\text{test criterion})^2 = \frac{N(ad - bc)}{(a + c)(b + d)(a + b)(c + d)} = X^2 \text{ (chi square)}.$$

This last quantity is often given as the computational form when data are expressed in a fourfold table such as A–7 or A–8. Rather than comparing the observed value with 1.96 to determine the significance, X^2 is compared with $(1.96)^2 = 3.84$. If X^2 is greater than 3.84, the difference of the observed proportions is said to be significantly different at a probability level of 0.05. Equivalently, there is said to be a significant association between the method of treatment

Table A–8. Symbolic Representation for Determining Cure
Rates for Receiving Treatments A and B

| TREATMENT | NUMBER OF PATIENTS | | |
	CURED	NOT CURED	TOTAL
A	a	b	a + b
B	c	d	c + d

Total $a + c = n_1; b + d = n_2$ $N = a + b + c + d = n_1 + n_2$

and cure of the disease. For a further explanation of X^2 tests and examples of their extension to other situations involving qualitative data, the reader is referred to Hill (1967), Snedecor and Cochran (1977), and Fleiss (1981).

TESTING HYPOTHESES ABOUT TWO SAMPLE MEANS

As was the case with the difference in two sample percentages from the same population, the standard error for the difference in two sample means from the same population is

$$\sqrt{[(n_1 - 1)s_1^2 + (n_2 - 1)s_2^2]/(n_1 + n_2 - 2)},$$

where s_1^2 is the estimated variance for one sample of size n_1 and s_2^2 is the estimated variance of the other sample of size n_2. If one wants to test the hypothesis that the two samples have been selected from the same population, a ratio is calculated similar to the one given in previous sections, namely,

$$\frac{\text{difference between means}}{\text{standard error of difference}} = \frac{|\bar{x}_1 - \bar{x}_2|}{\sqrt{[(n_1 - 1)s_1^2 + (n_2 - 1)s_2^2]/(n_1 + n_2 - 2)}}.$$

The degree of freedom for this ratio is given by $n_1 + n_2 - 2$. If the ratio exceeds the t-statistic in Table A–6 with the corresponding degrees of freedom, then the hypothesis, that the observed difference is due to sampling alone, is rejected at the 5 percent level of statistical significance.

For a simple example of the procedure, assume that an investigator has made observations on the total serum cholesterol levels in 41 men and 41 women. The average total serum cholesterol level for the men is 220 mg/dL (with a standard deviation of 10 mg/dL) and for the women, 198 mg/dL (with a standard deviation of 8 mg/dL). The investigator wishes to determine if the difference in the means of 22 mg/dL can be attributed to random sampling variation alone. This question can be restated as follows: Would one frequently observe a difference of 22 mg/dL in average total serum cholesterol if the two samples being compared were derived from the same population? The standard error of the difference would be

$$
\begin{aligned}
\text{S.E.} &= \sqrt{[(n_1 - 1)s_1^2 + (n_2 - 1)s_2^2]/(n_1 + n_2 - 2)} \\
&= \sqrt{[(41 - 1)(10)^2 + (41 - 1)(8)^2]/(41 + 41 - 2)} \\
&= \sqrt{[40(100) + 40(64)]/(80)} \\
&= \sqrt{6560/80} \\
&= 9.1 \text{ mg/dL.}
\end{aligned}
$$

The investigator would then calculate the ratio of the difference in the sample means to the standard error of the difference:

$$\frac{\text{difference in sample means}}{\text{standard error of difference}} = \frac{22 \text{ mg/dL}}{9.1 \text{ mg/dL}} = 2.42$$

This ratio is then compared with the t-statistic given in Table A–6 for $(n_1 + n_2 - 2) = 80$ degrees of freedom. Since this ratio is greater than the t-statistic (2.28), the investigator would conclude that random sampling alone cannot explain this large a difference in the sample means if the samples were derived from the same population. Hence, other explanations for the difference in the means must be sought.

CORRELATION AND REGRESSION

The statistical analysis of the relationship between two continuous variables may be considered by either of two approaches: (1) correlation and (2) regression. Although these two methods are related, they remain separate in their range of applications.

Correlation

The assessment of the linear association between two continuous variables is called *correlation*. The degree of such association is measured by the *correlation coefficient, r*, also known as *Pearson's correlation coefficient* or the *product-moment correlation coefficient*. If the ranks of the observations are substituted for the observations themselves, the correlation coefficient is then known as *Spearman's rank correlation coefficient*. For further information about rank correlation, see Colton (1974). For n pairs of observations of the two variables of interest, x and y, the correlation coefficient is

$$r = \frac{\Sigma(x_i - \bar{x})(y_i - \bar{y})}{\sqrt{[\Sigma(x_i - \bar{x})^2][\Sigma(y_i - \bar{y})^2]}} .$$

Computationally, the numerator of r may be calculated as $\Sigma(x_1 y_1) - n\bar{x}\bar{y}$, and the denominator as $\sqrt{[\Sigma(x_i^2 - n\bar{x}^2)\Sigma(y_i^2 - n\bar{y}^2)]}$. An example of the calculation of the correlation coefficient for hypothetical observations of annual per capita tobacco consumption and lung cancer incidence twenty years later is shown in Table A–9.

The correlation coefficient can range from -1 to 1. A value of 1 means that there is a strong positive linear association between the two variables; i.e., when the value of one variable is small, the other variable is small, and when the value of one variable is large, the other variable is large. If r is equal to -1, then there is a strong inverse linear association between the two variables; i.e., when the value of one variable is large, the value of the other variable is small, and vice versa. The closer the value of r is to either 1 or -1, the greater the degree of linear association present between the two variables, with values of .5 or $-.5$

Table A–9.   Example of the Calculation of the Correlation Coefficient

ANNUAL PER CAPITA TOBACCO CONSUMPTION (lbs) (x)	AVERAGE AGE-ADJUSTED LUNG CANCER RATE PER 100,000 PERSONS TWENTY YEARS LATER (y)
98	65.2
96	68.7
100	69.5
106	75.2
109	77.3
115	82.4
140	95.4
141	96.7
137	93.6
146	98.9
151	99.3
165	103.3
171	104.4
174	104.7
180	105.3
169	99.4
175	104.3
$n = 17$	$\Sigma x_i y_i = 222{,}175.1$
$\Sigma x = 2{,}373; \bar{x} = 139.6$	$\Sigma y = 1543.6; \bar{y} = 90.8$
$\Sigma x^2 = 345{,}857$	$\Sigma y^2 = 143{,}455.06$

$$r = \frac{\Sigma(x_i - \bar{x})(y_i - \bar{y})}{\sqrt{[\Sigma(x_i - \bar{x})^2][\Sigma(y_i - \bar{y})^2]}} = \frac{\Sigma(x_i y_i) - n\bar{x}\bar{y}}{\sqrt{[\Sigma(x_i^2 - n\bar{x}^2)][\Sigma(y_i^2 - n\bar{y}^2)]}}$$

$$= \frac{222{,}175.1 - (17 \times 139.6 \times 90.8)}{\sqrt{[(345{,}857 - (17 \times 139.6^2)][(143{,}455.06 - (17 \times 90.8^2)]}}$$

$$= \frac{6706.7}{6940.3} = 0.97$$

indicating moderate association. A value for r of 0 means that there is no linear association between the two variables.

An investigator may want to determine if the value of r observed in a sample can be attributed to sampling variation, i.e., is the value of the correlation coefficient in the population equal to 0? A test statistic for this purpose has been developed and is:

$$r\sqrt{\frac{(n-2)}{1-r^2}},$$

where r is the observed correlation coefficient and n is the number of pairs of the variables of interest. This statistic can then be compared to the entries in Table A–6, using $n - 2$ degrees of freedom. For the example in Table A–9, the test statistic is 15.4, which is greater than the corresponding entry in Table A–6 for 15 degrees of freedom. This suggests that the difference between the observed correlation coefficient and zero (indicating no linear association) is not accounted for by sampling variation alone, i.e., the investigator must seek other explanations for this degree of correlation. One explanation is that tobacco use is involved in the etiology of lung cancer and that two decades is necessary for the disease to become clinically apparent.

Correlation is useful for analyzing associations, but it does not provide the investigator with a method to mathematically relate the value of one variable to the value of the other variable. To obtain such a mathematical relationship, the investigator must use regression analysis.

Regression

In *regression analysis,* the mathematical relationship between two variables is examined. One variable, designated x, is known as the *independent variable,* and the other one, designed y, is the *dependent variable.* Using the example of annual per capita tobacco consumption and lung cancer incidence twenty years later, the annual per capita tobacco consumption would be the independent variable and lung cancer incidence twenty years later would be the dependent one.

The relationship between x and y is known as a *model.* It is possible for the model to assume different mathematical forms. In this section, we will discuss the linear model, in which $y = ax + b$; the investigator then must estimate a and b with the sample data. (Another regression model, the *logistic,* is discussed later in the Appendix, p. 324.) There are different statistical methods for estimating a and b. One of the most frequently used techniques is known as *least squares linear regression.* In this method, the distance between the observed value of y and the estimated value of y based upon the estimates of a and b is minimized.

In least squares linear regression, the estimate of a is

$$a = \frac{\Sigma(x_i - \bar{x})(y_i - \bar{y})}{\Sigma(x_i - \bar{x})^2}.$$

and for b, it is

$$b = \bar{y} - a\bar{x},$$

where $\bar{y}$ is the average of the observations of y and $\bar{x}$ is the mean of the observations of x. An example of the calculation of these two estimates is shown in Table A–10.

Although regression analysis and correlation are two distinct approaches to data analysis, there are certain relationships between the two areas. For example, the correlation coefficient and the least squares estimate of a in the linear model are related:

$$r = a\frac{s_x}{s_y},$$

where s_x is the standard deviation of the x observations and s_y is the standard deviation of the y observations. Accordingly, the statistical test described above

Table A–10.   Example of the Calculation of Linear Regression
Coefficients (a and b) Using Data from Table A–9

$n = 17\ \Sigma x_i y_i = 222{,}175.1$

$\Sigma x = 2{,}373;\ \bar{x} = 139.6\ \Sigma y = 1543.6;\ \bar{y} = 90.8$

$\Sigma x^2 = 345{,}857\ \Sigma y^2 = 143{,}455.06$

$$a = \frac{\Sigma(x_i - \bar{x})(y_i - \bar{y})}{\Sigma(x_i - \bar{x})^2} = \frac{\Sigma(x_i y_i) - n\bar{x}\bar{y}}{\Sigma x_i^2 - n\bar{x}^2}$$

$$= \frac{222{,}175.1 - (17 \times 139.6 \times 90.8)}{345{,}857 - (17 \times 139.6^2)}$$

$$= \frac{6{,}706.7}{14{,}556.3} = 0.46$$

$b = \bar{y} - a\bar{x}$
  $= 90.8 - 0.46(139.6)$
  $= 90.8 - 64.2$
  $= 26.6$

Hence, the least squares linear regression model would be:
$y = 0.46x + 26.6.$

---

for assessing whether r is statistically significantly different from 0 (suggesting that no linear association exists between x and y) is equivalent to the statistical test that a is 0.

THE RELATIVE RISK, THE ODDS RATIO, AND THE ATTRIBUTABLE FRACTION: DERIVATION, STATISTICAL TESTS, VARIANCE, AND CONFIDENCE INTERVALS

Relative Risk

In Chapter 10, the method of calculating the relative risk as a measure of association in cohort studies was presented, and the estimation of the relative risk by the odds ratio in the analysis of data collected in case-control studies was noted in Chapter 11. The reasons for the use of the odds ratio as an approximation of the relative risk may be seen in the derivation of the formula for the relative risk. Using the relationship of cigarette smoking to lung cancer as an example:

Let P = Frequency of lung cancer in population
p_1 = Frequency of smokers among lung cancer patients
$(1 - p_1)$ = Frequency of nonsmokers among lung cancer patients
p_2 = Frequency of smokers among non-lung cancer cases (controls)
$(1 - p_2)$ = Frequency of nonsmokers among non-lung cancer cases (controls).

In a population, the lung cancer cases and controls are distributed by smoking habits according to Table A–11. Therefore:

$$\text{The lung cancer rate among smokers} = \frac{p_1 P}{p_1 P + p_2(1 - P)}$$

$$\text{The lung cancer rate among nonsmokers} = \frac{(1 - p_1)P}{(1 - p_1)P + (1 - p_2)(1 - P)}$$

Table A–11. Distribution of Lung Cancer Patients and Controls by Smoking Habits

	LUNG CANCER PATIENTS	CONTROLS	TOTAL
Smokers	$p_1 P$	$p_2(1 - P)$	$p_1 P + p_2(1 - P)$
Nonsmokers	$(1 - p_1)P$	$(1 - p_2)(1 - P)$	$(1 - p_1)P + (1 - p_2)(1 - P)$
Total	P	$(1 - P)$	1

The Relative Risk is

$$RR = \frac{\text{Lung cancer rate among smokers}}{\text{Lung cancer rate among nonsmokers}} = \frac{\dfrac{p_1 P}{p_1 P + p_2(1 - P)}}{\dfrac{(1 - p_1)P}{(1 - p_1)P + (1 - p_2)(1 - P)}}$$

$$= \frac{p_1 P}{p_1 P + p_2(1 - P)} \times \frac{(1 - p_1)P + (1 - p_2)(1 - P)}{(1 - p_1)P}$$

and, *if P is small,* this reduces to $\dfrac{p_1(1 - p_2)}{p_2(1 - p_1)}$, which is an estimate of the relative risk. In terms of the symbols used in Table 10–1, this expression is equivalent to ad/bc.

Test of Significance, Variance and Confidence Intervals

When the relative risk equals one, then ad/bc as an approximation of the relative risk (RR) is exact. This is the case when the risk of disease for those with and without the characteristic under study is the same (ad/bc = 1 or ad = bc); one can therefore say that the disease and the characteristic are unrelated.

A test of whether or not the observed difference between ad and bc is due to sampling variation is provided by the χ^2 test for fourfold tables:

$$\chi^2 = \frac{\left(|ad - bc| - \dfrac{N}{2}\right)^2 N}{N_1 N_2 M_1 M_2}$$

where N = a + b + c + d; N_1 = a + c; N_2 = b + d; M_1 = a + b; M_2 = c + d, as shown in Table 10–1, with one degree of freedom. The term N/2, which is subtracted from the difference, is the correction factor that is needed to make the test valid for small sample sizes. If the value of χ^2 is greater than 3.84, one may conclude that it is unlikely that the difference in risk between the group with and the group without the characteristic is a result of chance, at a probability level of 0.05.

A more useful method of testing the hypothesis of equal realtive risks, which at the same time provides an estimate of the confidence limits of the relative risk, is that recommended by Haldane (1956). Confidence limits of the logarithm (to the base *e*) of a corrected relative risk are computed and the logarithmic confidence intervals are then reconverted to the original scale. The addition of 0.50 to each of the values a, b, c, and d corrects for a bias that can occur with small numbers of observations.

Using the log-relative risk rather than the relative risk itself simplifies calculations of standard errors necessary for computing confidence intervals. If the reconverted confidence interval does not contain the value 1.0, the hypothesis that there is no difference in risk between the two groups (cases and controls) is rejected. The risk of falsely rejecting the hypothesis depends upon the level of confidence interval selected. If, for example, a 95 percent confidence interval is selected, there will be a 5 percent chance of falsely rejecting the hypothesis of equal relative risk. If the hypothesis is rejected, an interval within which the investigator is confident the ''true'' relative risk lies is then provided.

For an example of the above procedure, consider the data of Breslow et al. (1954) presented in Table A–12.

$$\text{The relative risk of lung cancer} \atop \text{of smokers to nonsmokers} = \frac{ad}{bc} = \frac{(499)(56)}{(462)(19)} = 3.18.$$

The χ^2 test of equal risk is:

$$\chi^2 = \frac{\left(|ad - bc| - \frac{N}{2}\right)^2 N}{N_1 N_2 M_1 M_2}$$

$$= \frac{\left(|(499)(56) - (462)(19)| - \frac{1036}{2}\right)^2 1036}{(518)(518)(961)(75)} = 18.63$$

with one degree of freedom. The value of χ^2 is statistically significant at the 1 percent level, indicating that there is less than one chance in one hundred that such a relative risk could occur by chance alone if the two risks were equal.

While the χ^2 test shows that the risks are significantly different at the 1 percent level of significance, no indication is given of the limits within which the ''true'' relative risk might lie in the population from which these two sam-

Table A–12.   Distribution of Smokers and Nonsmokers Among Lung Cancer Patients and Controls

	LUNG CANCER PATIENTS	CONTROLS	TOTALS
Smokers	a = 499	b = 462	M_1 = 961
Nonsmokers	c = 19	d = 56	M_2 = 75
Total	N_1 = 518	N_2 = 518	N = 1036

Source: Breslow et al. (1954).

ples have been selected. The first step is to calculate $\log_e$ (corrected relative risk):

$$\log_e \frac{(a + 0.50)(d + 0.50)}{(b + 0.50)(c + 0.50)} = \log_e \frac{(499.5)(56.5)}{(462.5)(19.5)}$$

$$= \log_e(3.129)$$
$$= 1.1408.$$

One should note that the correction of 0.50 added to each cell made little difference in the relative risk calculated in this example (3.13 versus 3.18). When the sample size is of the order of 50 rather than 500 in each of the disease groups, the correction will be more important.

The formula given by Haldane for the variance of the $\log_e$ (RR) is

$$\text{Var}(\log_e \text{ RR}) = \frac{1}{(a + \frac{1}{2})} + \frac{1}{(b + \frac{1}{2})} + \frac{1}{(c + \frac{1}{2})} + \frac{1}{(d + \frac{1}{2})}.$$

Using the data in Table A–12:

$$\text{Var}(\log_e \text{ RR}) = \frac{1}{499.5} + \frac{1}{462.5} + \frac{1}{19.5} + \frac{1}{56.5} = .073145.$$

The standard error is the square root of this quantity, 0.2705. A 95 percent confidence interval for the $\log_e$ of the corrected relative risk is calculated as

$$\log_e(\text{corrected RR}) \pm 1.96 \text{ S.E.}(\log_e \text{ RR}) = 1.1408 \pm 1.96(0.2705)$$
$$= 0.6101 \text{ to } 1.6705.$$

Upon reconverting to the original measurement scale by taking antilogs of the upper and lower limits, one finds that the 95 percent confidence interval for the relative risk is 1.8406 to 5.3148, which means that one is approximately 95 percent confident that the risk of developing lung cancer is between 1.84 and 5.31 times as great in smokers as in nonsmokers.

Additional statistical methods for the use of the relative risk in both retrospective and prospective studies may be found in Fleiss (1981), Schlesselman (1982), and Kahn and Sempos (1989).

Attributable Fraction

The calculation of attributable fraction was presented in Chapter 10. It was derived in the following manner by Levin (1953):

Let X = Incidence of a disease in those without the
characteristic

RR = Relative risk

(RR)X = Incidence of disease in those with the
characteristic

P = Proportion of total population with the
characteristic

$1 - P$ = Proportion of total population without the
characteristic.

Then:

1. $P(RR)X + X(1 - P)$ = The incidence of disease in the total population and

2. $\dfrac{(RR)X - X}{(RR)X} = \dfrac{X(RR - 1)}{X(RR)} = \dfrac{RR - 1}{RR} =$ The proportion of disease attributable to the characteristic among those with the characteristic

3. $\dfrac{P(RR)X \left(\dfrac{RR - 1}{RR}\right)}{P(RR)X + X(1 - P)} = \dfrac{P(RR - 1)}{P(RR - 1) + 1} =$ The proportion of disease in the population that is attributable to the characteristic, that is, the attributable fraction (AF).

Walter (1975) has derived a formula from which the variance of the attributable fraction can be estimated from a retrospective study. Using the symbols of Table 10–1, the variance of $\log_e(1 - AF)$ is

$$\frac{a}{c(a + c)} + \frac{b}{d(b + d)}.$$

Walter showed that $\log_e(1 - AF)$ is normally distributed, and tests of significance and approximate confidence intervals can therefore be calculated using the normal distribution. Whittemore (1983) extended this work to include situations in which confounding is present.

CONTROLLING EXTRANEOUS FACTORS

We have been assuming that the groups being compared were homogeneous with respect to all characteristics other than the specific ones for which the strength of association was being measured. Thus, when measuring the association between stroke and elevated blood pressure, we assumed that the individuals with stroke and those without the disease were similar in all respects (age, gender, socioeconomic status) except for the factor being studied, namely, their blood pressure levels.

If the samples of diseased and nondiseased persons are randomly selected from the populations of diseased or nondiseased persons, they may be similar with regard to the distribution of some extraneous factors if the populations from which they were derived are similar with respect to these factors. However, any population differences would be reflected in these samples. If, for example, lung cancer patients differ in age and gender from the population from which the controls are selected, the samples will also differ in these characteristics. To avoid biases that can arise from such differences, various methods of selection or analysis are available to the investigator. The adjustment procedure described in Chapter 4 is useful when comparing incidence or mortality rates as well as other sets of data.

It is also possible to make a series of specific comparisons for each level of the extraneous factor; for example, age- and sex-specific comparisons of the frequency of stroke in persons with normal blood pressure and persons with elevated blood pressure. One disadvantage with factor-specific comparisons is that they separate the total sample into many segments, and some of these may contain too few observations (or none at all) to make a factor-specific comparison within these segments. Even when a particular segment contains both cases and controls, there may be a large number of cases but only a small number of controls, or vice versa. Generally speaking, the precision of the comparison varies with the factor,

$$\frac{1}{\sqrt{\dfrac{1}{n_1} + \dfrac{1}{n_2}}}$$

where n_1 is the number of cases in a particular segment and n_2 is the number of controls. For a fixed total $n = n_1 + n_2$, the precision will be greater when $n_1 = n_2$. If n_1 happens to be small, an increase in the size of n_2 will not necessarily compensate for this. If a random sample is drawn from both the case and control populations, the factor-specific comparisons will vary in their degrees of precision and the comparisons that have the lowest precision may be in those segments where the greatest interest lies.

Group Matching

One means of assuring equal numbers of disease and control samples for each factor level is to "group match" the samples by stratification of one of the groups, using each factor level as a stratum. Usually the cases are self-selected in terms of the disease, with the investigator having no control over the number of cases at each factor level. The investigator then attempts to select controls that have the same characteristics as the cases. If the characteristics of the cases are known in advance, the best method of group matching is to stratify the control population on the levels of the factor to be controlled. Simple random samples of the same size as found in the disease sample at each factor level are then selected independently from the corresponding stratum of the population controls.

If the comparisons are to be made on a factor-specific basis, the percentage with and without the characteristic can be compared at each factor level by the simple binomial test described earlier. However, a useful method of combining the comparisons for each factor level has been developed by Cochran (1954) and modified by Mantel and Haenszel (1959). It takes into account the variation in the number of observations in both cases and controls at each factor level and the variation in the proportion of individuals (cases and controls combined) having the characteristic of interest at each level. The method and its limitations are reviewed by Snedecor and Cochran (1967), Fleiss (1981), Kahn and Sempos (1989), and Schlesselman (1982).

For the ith factor level, let

$$n_{i1}, n_{i2} = \text{sample sizes of cases and controls, respectively}$$
$$p_{i1}, p_{i2} = \text{observed proportion with the characteristics of interest}$$
$$\text{in the two groups}$$
$$\hat{p}_i = \text{combined proportion} = \frac{n_{i1}p_{i1} + n_{i2}p_{i2}}{n_{i1} + n_{i2}}$$
$$\hat{q}_i = 1 - \hat{p}_i$$
$$d_i = p_{i1} - p_{i2} = \text{observed difference in proportions}$$
$$w_i = \frac{n_{i1}n_{i2}}{n_{i1} + n_{i2}} \; ; w = \Sigma w_i.$$

The weighted mean difference is first computed:

$$\bar{d} = \frac{\Sigma w_i d_i}{w}$$

which has a standard error of

$$S.E. = \frac{\sqrt{\Sigma w_i \hat{p}_i \hat{q}_i}}{w} .$$

As in the binomial test, the criterion for testing the hypothesis of no difference in proportions is:

$$\frac{\overline{d}}{S.E.} = \frac{\Sigma w_i d_i}{\sqrt{\Sigma w_i \hat{p}_i \hat{q}_i}} .$$

(This is referred to in the tables of normal distribution.) If it is greater than 1.96, it is concluded that the overall difference is statistically significant at a probability of 5 percent.

An example of the computations is presented in Tables A–13 and A–14. These are derived from a study of the possible relationship between prenatal and perinatal factors and childhood behavior disorders by Rogers et al. (1959). The cases were those children referred by their teachers as behavior problems and the controls were those not so referred. A factor of interest was the history of previous infant loss prior to the birth of the study children as reported on the birth certificates of the study children among the mothers of case and control children. Since this is influenced by the birth order of the child, and its distribution may vary in the cases and controls, it was necessary to take the birth order into account in comparing the cases and controls. The criterion for the significance test in the

Table A–13. Number and Percent of Mothers with History of Previous Infant Loss among Cases and Controls by Birth Order (Birth Certificate Data)

BIRTH ORDER	CHILDREN'S STATUS	NO. OF MOTHERS WITH HISTORY OF		TOTAL	PERCENT WITH HISTORY OF LOSS
		LOSSES	NO LOSSES		
2	Cases	14	86	$100 = n_{11}$	$14.0 = p_{11}$
	Controls	7	67	$74 = n_{12}$	$9.5 = p_{21}$
	Total	21	153	$174 = n_1$	$12.1 = p_1$
3–4	Cases	22	44	$66 = n_{21}$	$33.3 = p_{21}$
	Controls	7	35	$42 = n_{22}$	$16.7 = p_{22}$
	Total	29	79	$108 = n_2$	$26.9 = p_2$
5+	Cases	22	14	$36 = n_{31}$	$61.1 = p_{31}$
	Controls	10	7	$17 = n_{32}$	$58.8 = p_{32}$
	Total	32	21	$53 = n_3$	$60.3 = p_3$

Source: Rogers et al. (1959).

Table A–14. Computations for the Combined Test

BIRTH ORDER	d_i	p_i	$p_i q_i$	w_i^*	$w_i d_i$	$w_i p_i q_i$
2	+ 4.5	12.1	1,063.6	42.5	+191.3	45,203.0
3–4	+16.6	26.9	1,996.4	25.7	+426.6	51,307.5
5+	+ 2.3	60.3	2,393.5	11.6	+ 26.68	27,769.2

$$*w_i = \frac{n_{i1} n_{i2}}{n_{i1} + n_{i2}}$$

$\Sigma w_i d_i = 644.6$

$\Sigma w_i p_i q_i = 124,279.7$

$$\text{Test Criterion} = \frac{\Sigma w_i d_i}{\sqrt{\Sigma w_i \hat{p}_i \hat{q}_i}} = \frac{644.6}{\sqrt{124,279.7}} = 1.83$$

example is 1.83, which is referred to the table of the normal distribution. This indicates a P value of 0.07, which is slightly higher than the usually accepted value of 0.05 for statistical significance. However, one can regard the difference as having borderline significance.

Relative risks can also be calculated for group matching with the method developed by Mantel and Haenszel (1959), and for this reason, the statistical test is generally referred to as the "Mantel-Haenszel test." This and other methods are more fully discussed in Fleiss (1981), Kahn and Sempos (1989), and Schlesselman (1982).

Logistic Regression

Another approach to the calculation of a relative risk adjusted for the effect of extraneous factors uses *logistic regression*. In this technique, a logistic model is fitted by statistical regression to the sample data. For one variable x, the logistic model is

$$\text{Pr(disease)} = \frac{1}{1 + e^{-(a + bx_i)}},$$

where Pr(disease) is the probability of the disease in the ith individual, and the value of variable x in that individual is x_i. The values of a and b are estimated from the sample data. If the relative risk associated with exposure to x is one, then the value of b will be zero; conversely, if the value of b is greater than zero, then the relative risk for x will be greater than one; for negative values of b, the corresponding relative risk is less than one. For further information on logistic regression, see Kahn and Sempos (1989), Schlesselman (1982), and Breslow and Day (1983, 1987).

Individual Case-Control Matching

As an alternative to group matching, individual cases and controls can be matched for various factors so that each case in the study has its own pairmate. Ideally, pairmates should be as much alike as possible in all characteristics except the one being studied. If many factors are selected for matching, it becomes difficult to find matches for each of the cases. In epidemiologic studies there is usually a limited number of cases and a large number of controls. Each case is then classified according to the factor to be controlled, and a search is made for a control with the same characteristics. If the number of factors and their levels are not too great and there is a large enough number of controls from which to select, matching may be carried out with little effort. Matching becomes difficult and time-consuming if a large number of factors and levels are considered and the number of potential controls is of a magnitude similar to the number of cases. It is likely that there will be many cases for which no control can be found. Therefore, it becomes necessary either to eliminate some of the factors or to reduce the number of levels of some factors. If age is a factor, for example, it is unlikely that pairs can be formed readily using six-month or one-year age intervals; but with five- or ten-year age intervals, matching becomes feasible.

While matching is probably desired to reduce biases, the number of factors or levels on which it is practical is rather small. There should be good reasons for including a factor as a matching variable in any study. Matching should usually be limited to a small number of factors, rarely more than four, each consisting of a small number of levels or categories (Ury, 1975).

In addition to eliminating bias, matching also increases the precision of the comparisons by providing more homogeneous groups within which the comparisons are made. The increased precision is largely dependent on the degree of association of the matching factor with the variable of interest. Rather strong associations must exist before substantial increases in precision can be expected. Therefore, the major aim of matching in case-control studies should be to provide comparisons that are relatively free from bias that might arise from the dissimilarities of the case and control populations.

When cases and controls are individually matched, the fourfold table assumes the form presented in Table 11–12. For matched pairs where RR = s/t (Kraus, 1958), (using the symbols in Table 11–12), Fleiss (1981) shows that the estimated variance $= (1 + RR)^2 \left(\dfrac{RR}{s + t} \right)$ and the estimated standard error $=$

$(1 + RR) \sqrt{\dfrac{RR}{(s + t)}}$.

A useful test of significance for matched pairs, when s and t are not small (>3), is the McNemar test:

$$\chi^2 = \frac{(|t - s| - 1)^2}{t + s},$$

with one degree of freedom.

In this section we have dealt only with factors that are qualitative and dichotomous. The reader is referred to Fleiss (1981) for a more detailed discussion of these issues, including the use of multiple controls in such studies. When the study characteristics are quantitative, other methods of controlling for extraneous factors are available. Extraneous effects often can be eliminated more efficiently in the analysis of the data by the method of analysis of covariance. This allows the investigator to select simple random samples of case and control groups without first matching pairs for the factors to be controlled. The reader is referred to Snedecor and Cochran (1967) for details of this technique.

LIFE TABLES AND SURVIVORSHIP ANALYSIS

In the previous sections, we discussed analyses of epidemiologic study data in which the time until the occurrence of the event of interest was not a focus of the investigation. However, the time to occurrence of an outcome (whether mortality or a form of morbidity) is often of interest. The statistical analysis of these time periods and their relationship to various factors is known as *survivorship analysis*. The techniques used in survivorship analysis derive from the *life table*.

The Life Table

The life table provides a simple, systematic way of organizing and analyzing survivorship data. Suppose that an investigator has identified 500 Parkinson's disease patients who have started to use a new treatment that stabilizes their condition and wishes to know the probability of these patients having no progression of their disease. Each year, the investigator evaluates each patient to determine if the condition has progressed. The hypothetical data collected after five years of follow-up for each patient are given in Table A–15.

Table A–15.   Example of a Life Table for 500 Persons Using a New Therapy for Parkinson's Disease

YEAR (x)	NUMBER OF PERSONS WITH STABLE DISEASE STATUS AT START OF YEAR (Q_x)	NUMBER OF PERSONS WHOSE DISEASE STATUS DECLINED DURING YEAR ($_nd_x$)	PROBABILITY OF DISEASE STATUS DECLINING ($_nq_x$)	PROBABILITY OF DISEASE STATUS REMAINING STABLE ($_np_x$)
1	500	100	0.22	0.78
2	400	100	0.29	0.71
3	300	150	0.67	0.33
4	150	90	0.86	0.14
5	60	38	0.93	0.07

There are two measures of interest for the investigator: the probability of progression in a given year and the probability of an individual's disease remaining stable throughout the five years of follow-up. The probability of declining disease status can be estimated for each year of follow-up using the data in Table A–15. For the time period from x to $x + n$, this probability ($_nq_x$) is equal to,

$$\frac{\text{the number of persons whose disease status declined during the year}}{\text{the mid-year number of persons at risk of declining disease status}}$$

or

$$_nq_x = \frac{_nd_x}{O_x - (_nd_x/2)},$$

where O_x is the number of persons who began the xth year with stable disease status and $_nd_x$ is the number of those persons who began the xth year with stable disease status but whose disease status declined by the end of the $(n + x)$th year. This estimate assumes that the number of persons whose disease status declines is equal in both the first half of the year and in the latter half; if this assumption is incorrect, the number used to divide $_nd_x$ in the denominator would need to be adjusted accordingly.

A second estimate shown in Table A–15, $_np_x$, is the probability of an individual finishing the $(n + x)$th year with stable disease status given that the individual's disease status was stable at the start of the year. The probability of an individual completing the five years with stable disease status can be estimated by multiplying the $_np_x$ for each of the years, i.e.,

$$(0.78)(0.71)(0.33)(0.14)(0.07) = 0.0016.$$

Hence, the probability of completing all five years with stable disease status is 0.00106, or about 1.5 in 1,000 persons using the new therapy for five years.

Further information on life tables and their calculation, including the standard error of the various probabilities estimated in them, may be found in Chiang (1968) and Kahn and Sempos (1989).

The Logrank Test

The logrank test was suggested by Mantel (1966) as a method for comparing two groups with regard to the time until the occurrence of the outcome of interest. In the logrank test, these times are ranked and the ranks are compared using a χ^2 test. For computational details of the logrank test, the reader is referred to Peto et al. (1977) or Kahn and Sempos (1989).

AGE-ADJUSTED MORTALITY RATES: VARIANCE AND STANDARD ERRORS

The direct method of age adjustment of death rates and the standardized mortality ratio (SMR) were described in Chapter 4. It is often useful to calculate the variance and standard error of these rates, and therefore the formulas for these statistics will be presented. For a more detailed discussion, the reader may consult Kahn and Sempos (1989) and Fleiss (1981).

Age Adjustment by the Direct Method

Let r = the age specific death rate in the ith age group
N_i = the number of people in the ith age group of the standard population
n_i = the number of people in the ith age group of the population that is being age-adjusted

The age-adjusted death rate is then $R = \Sigma \left(\dfrac{N_i}{\Sigma N_i} \right) r_i$, the

$$\text{Variance of } R = \Sigma \left(\frac{N_i}{\Sigma N_i}\right)^2 \frac{r_i(1 - r_i)}{n_i} \text{ and the}$$

$$\text{Standard Error } = \sqrt{\Sigma \left(\frac{N_i}{\Sigma N_i}\right)^2 \frac{r_i(1 - r_i)}{n_i}} .$$

Standardized Mortality Ratio (SMR)

The SMR $= \dfrac{\text{O (Observed number of deaths per year)}}{\text{E (Expected number of deaths per year)}} \times 100$, and is usually expressed as a percentage.

Assuming that the standard population from which the expected numbers are calculated is much larger than the population being studied, and that the age-specific death rates in the standard population are small, which is usually the case, the variance of SMR (or O/E) is approximately O/E^2, and the standard error $= \sqrt{O}/E$.

KAPPA AND THE ASSESSMENT OF INTER- AND INTRA- OBSERVER VARIABILITY

The use of the κ (kappa) statistic for an assessment of inter- and intra-observer variability was presented in Chapter 6 (p. 124). Two situations may occur: an individual classifies a set of data twice and the disagreements in classification are analyzed, or two individuals classify the same data and their disagreements are analyzed. In either case, the analysis of the data is the same. κ, developed by Cohen (1960), adjusts for agreement in classification that would occur by chance. Formally stated,

$$\kappa = \frac{\text{Observed frequency of agreement } - \text{ Expected frequency of agreement}}{\text{Total observed } - \text{ Expected frequency of agreement}} .$$

If there is only chance agreement between two classifications, then the value of κ is zero. If there is perfect agreement, then the value of κ is one. It is possible to use κ for situations involving many different classification categories. In this example, however, we will restrict our consideration to the case of two classification categories.

An example of the calculation of κ may provide insight into its use. The data in Table A–16 from Paganini-Hill and Ross (1982) were cited by Kelsey et al. (1986) in such a description. These data compare a patient's recall of reserpine use with the history of use on the patient's medical chart. The expected frequency

Table A–16. Example of the Calculation of Kappa: Agreement Between Personal Interview and Medical Chart Concerning Use of Reserpine Among Control Subjects from a Case-Control Study of Breast Cancer in Two Retirement Communities

| | | HISTORY OF USE OF RESERPINE ACCORDING TO MEDICAL CHART | | |
		YES	NO	TOTAL
History of use of reserpine according to patient's report	Yes	14	7	21
	No	25	171	196
Total		39	178	217

Source: Paganini-Hill and Ross (1982).

of agreement between the patient's recall of reserpine use and that which was indicated on the medical chart is the expected frequency of both indicating such use ((21)(39)/217) and the expected frequency of both indicating no such use ((196)(178)/217), i.e., 164.5. The observed frequency of agreement is 14 + 171, i.e., 185. Hence,

$$\kappa = \frac{\text{Observed frequency of agreement } - \text{ Expected frequency of agreement}}{\text{Total observed } - \text{ Expected frequency of agreement}}$$

$$= \frac{185 - 164.5}{217 - 164.5} = \frac{20.5}{52.5} = 0.39.$$

This result suggests that there is only fair agreement between the two sources of information about a patient's past use of reserpine.

For further information about κ, the reader is referred to Fleiss (1981) and Kelsey et al. (1986).

REFERENCES

Breslow, L., Hoaglin, L., Rasmussen, G., and Abrams, H. K. 1954. "Occupations and cigarette smoking as factors in lung cancer." *Amer. J. Public Health* 44:171–181.
Breslow, N. E., and Day, N. E. 1983. *Statistical Methods in Cancer Research, Vol. 1. The Design and Analysis of Case-Control Studies.* Lyon: International Agency for Research on Cancer.
———. 1987. *Statistical Methods in Cancer Research, Vol. 2. The Design and Analysis of Cohort Studies.* Lyon: International Agency for Research on Cancer.

Chiang, C. L. 1968. *Introduction to Stochastic Processes in Biostatistics,* New York: John Wiley and Sons.

Cochran, W. G. 1954. "Some methods of strengthening the common χ^2 tests." *Biometrics* 10:417–451.

———. 1977. *Sampling Techniques.* 3rd ed. New York: John Wiley and Sons.

Cohen, J. 1960. "A coefficient of agreement for nominal scales." *Educ. Psych. Meas.* 20: 37–46.

Colton, T. 1974. *Statistics in Medicine.* Boston: Little, Brown and Company.

Fleiss, J. L. 1981. *Statistical Methods for Rates and Proportions,* 2nd ed. New York: J. Wiley and Sons.

Greenberg, E. R. 1990. "Random digit dialing for control selection. A review and a caution on its use in studies of childhood cancer." *Am. J. Epidemiol.* 131:1–5.

Haenszel, W., Loveland, D., and Sirken, M. G. 1962. "Lung-cancer mortality as related to residence and smoking histories." *J. Natl. Cancer Instit.* 28:947–1001.

Haldane, J.B.S. 1956. "The estimation and significance of the logarithm of a ratio of frequencies." *Ann. Hum. Genet.* 2:309–311.

Hartge, P., Brinton, L. A., Rosenthal, J. F., Cahill, J. I., Hoover, R. N., and Waksberg, J. 1984. "Random digit dialing in selecting a population-based control group." *Am. J. Epidemiol.* 120:825–833.

Hill, A. B. 1977. *A Short Textbook of Medical Statistics.* 10th ed. Philadelphia: J. B. Lippincott.

Kahn, H. A., and Sempos, C. T. 1989. *Statistical Methods in Epidemiology.* NewYork: Oxford University Press.

Kelsey, J. L., Thompson, W. D., and Evans, A. S. 1986. *Methods in Observational Epidemiology.* New York: Oxford University Press.

Kendall, M. G. and Smith, B. B. 1938. "Randomness and random sampling numbers." *J. Roy. Stat. Soc.* 101:147–166.

Kraus, A. S. 1958. "The use of family members as controls in the study of the possible etiologic factors of a disease." Sc.D. Thesis. Graduate School of Public Health, University of Pittsburgh.

Levin, M. L. 1953. "The occurrence of lung cancer in man." *Acta Unio. Internat. Contra Cancrum* 9:531–541.

Mantel, N. 1966. "Evaluation of survival data and two new rank order statistics arising in its consideration." *Cancer Chemother. Reports* 60:163–170.

Mantel, N., and Haenszel, W. 1959. "Statistical aspects of the analysis of data from retrospective studies of disease." *J. Natl. Cancer Inst.* 22:719–748.

Paganini-Hill, A., and Ross, R. K. 1982. "Reliability of recall of drug usage and other health-related information." *Am. J. Epidemiol.* 116:114–122.

Peto, R., Pike, M. C., Armitage, P., Breslow, N. E., Cox, D. R., Howard, S. V., Mantel, N., McPherson, K., Peto, J., and Smith, P. G. 1977. "Design and analysis of randomized clinical trials requiring prolonged observation of each patient: II. Analysis and examples." *Brit. J. Cancer* 35:1–39.

Rand Corporation. 1955. *A Million Random Digits.* Glencoe, Ill.: Free Press.

Rogers, M. E., Lilienfeld, A. M., and Pasamanick, B. 1959. *Prenatal and Paranatal Factors in the Development of Childhood Behavior Disorders.* Baltimore, Md.: The Johns Hopkins University School of Hygiene and Public Health.

Schlesselman, J. J. 1982. *Case-Control Studies.* New York: Oxford University Press.

Snedecor, G. W., and Cochran, W. G. 1967. *Statistical Methods.* 6th ed. Ames, Iowa: Iowa State University Press.

Ury, H. K. 1975. "Efficiency of case-control studies with multiple controls per case: continuous or dichotomous data." *Biometrics* 31:643–649.

Wacholder, A., McLaughlin, J. K., Silverman, D. T., and Mandel, J. S. 1992. "Selection of controls in case-control studies. II. types of controls." *Am. J. Epidemiol.* 135: 1029–1041.

Waksberg, J. 1978. "Sampling methods for random digit dialing." *J. Am. Stat. Assn.* 73: 40–46.

Walter, S. D. 1975. "The distribution of Levin's measure of attributable risk." *Biometrika* 62:371–374.

Whittemore, A. S. 1983. "Estimating attributable risk from case-control studies." *Am. J. Epidemiol.* 117:76–85.

ANSWERS TO PROBLEMS

Chapter 1

1. The epidemiologist views disease from the perspective of its occurrence among persons, in places, and at varying times. Essentially, it is the intersection of time, place, and persons that defines the development of disease in a given population.

2. An ecological fallacy may be operating when an association between a characteristic and a disease is based on the study of group characteristics rather than of characteristics among individuals in the group. For example, an investigation into the relationship between religion and suicide might find that regions of Europe in which Protestants are more prevalent than Catholics have higher suicide rates compared with rates in those areas in which Catholics are more prevalent. The conclusion that Protestantism is associated with suicide would be an ecological fallacy if, in an epidemiologic study, the risk of suicide among Catholics was the same as or higher than that for Protestants.

3. Population-based data, such as mortality rates, provide an initial means by which the epidemiologist can compare populations. Such comparisons seek to develop hypotheses for the pattern of diseases observed among the populations. Caution is needed in using such data since the possibility of an ecological fallacy exists.

4. The major steps in the investigation of a food-borne outbreak are:
   (a) to identify the disease being investigated,
   (b) to define what a case is,

(c) to ascertain cases,

(d) to determine a common event among cases,

(e) to define the population present at the common event,

(f) to develop a questionnaire to assess consumption of food items at the common event,

(g) to administer the questionnaire to all those present at the common event,

(h) to calculate food-specific attack rates to determine which food item was contaminated,

(i) to investigate the preparation of the contaminated food item, including medical examinations of all food handlers involved in such preparation,

(j) to take appropriate public health action to stop the possibility of such outbreaks in the future (e.g., slaughtering of infected flocks producing contaminated eggs).

5. (a)

	CONSUMED FOOD			DID NOT CONSUME FOOD		
TYPE OF FOOD	NUMBER OF INDIVIDUALS	NUMBER III	ATTACK RATE (%)	NUMBER OF INDIVIDUALS	NUMBER III	ATTACK RATE (%)
Tomato Juice	204	47	23	263	21	8
Cantaloupe	290	53	18	177	15	3
Chipped beef with sauce	147	60	41	320	8	3
Potatoes	161	44	27	306	24	8
Eggs	169	39	23	298	29	10
Pastry	204	34	17	263	34	13
Toast	238	46	19	229	22	10
Milk	301	50	17	166	8	1

(b) The chipped beef is the likely culprit since it produced the highest attack rate of all consumed foods (41%). Those who did not consume the chipped beef had a low attack rate (3%).

(c) Additional investigations that could be conducted to determine the source and the likely microorganism include:

1. Using microbiological laboratory methods to culture a pathogen from leftover food.

2. Attempting to isolate and culture pathogens from the stools of victims.

3. Examining food handlers in search of skin lesions that may lead to food contamination, including bacterial culture studies of stools of food handlers. In this epidemic, the disease was caused

by enterotoxin-producing staphylococcal organisms that were
found in the food, in the stools of victims, and in a skin lesion
("boil") on the thumb of the cook. The salty and fatty sauce
provided a good growth medium for this microorganism.

(d) Proper storage (refrigeration) and cooking (heating) of food has
proven more effective than physical examination of food handlers in
preventing food-borne disease outbreaks due to bacterial contamination.

Chapter 3

1. The latency period for noninfectious diseases is the time between exposure to a disease-causing agent and the appearance of manifestations of
the disease. It varies with the specific disease. In some instances in which
the time of exposure to the disease-causing agent is known, the latency
period for disorders has been quantified. For example, the latency period
for leukemias following the radiation exposure from the explosion of the
atomic bomb at Hiroshima is five to six years, while that for female breast
cancer from the same exposure is about twenty years.

2. (a) In a common-vehicle, single-exposure outbreak, the epidemic curve
is skewed to the right, with a sharp initial rise and a gradual tapering, as
in Figure 3–4. (b) In a common-vehicle, continuous-exposure outbreak,
the epidemic curve also shows a sharp initial rise with a gradual tapering,
but the curve does not taper as fast as the single-exposure curve would
and it does not decrease to zero cases. Rather, it becomes a series of peaks
and troughs as new cases occur. (c) The curve for an outbreak propagated
by serial transfer is a flat line with occasional bumps in the curve as
exposures and subsequent cases occur. (d) In an epidemic due to a slow
virus, the epidemic curve will be the same as for a common-vehicle,
continuous-exposure epidemic, which is, after all, what it is.

3. Herd immunity is important to the public health administrator because it
implies that in order to contain or prevent an outbreak of disease, immunization of the entire population is not mandated. Only as large a proportion as required for herd immunity to develop in the population need
be immunized to prevent an outbreak of disease.

4. Subclinical cases of both infectious and noninfectious diseases pose several problems for the epidemiologist: (a) the identification of all factors
relating to the occurrence of the disease will be limited to those that
characterize the clinical cases; (b) the testing of a biological hypothesis
will be limited to the clinical cases; and (c) the characteristics of the
subclinical cases (particularly those which prevent the clinical manifestation of the disease) cannot be elucidated.

The applicability of these problems to both infectious and noninfectious diseases should underscore the importance of the "spectrum of disease" concept in any epidemiologic investigation. The major impact of subclinical cases concerns the prognosis of a given clinical case. It is only with information about the "spectrum of disease," including both clinical and subclinical cases, that an accurate assessment of prognosis can be made.

5. This observation suggests that the etiologic event was either prenatal or perinatal. It suggests that studies focused on prenatal or perinatal factors would be useful in determining the etiologic agent of Legg-Perthes disease.

6. The sexually transmitted disease epidemic in the United States today is a combination of epidemiologic categories of outbreaks. If a single instance of infection is not treated, it will serve as a continuous source of the agent. Since that individual infection can also serve as a common exposure for others, it would also be a common vehicle.

7. (a)

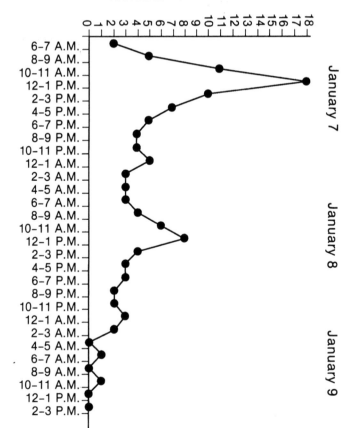

NUMBER OF ILL PERSONS

(b) This was a common-vehicle, single-exposure outbreak. Secondary cases occurred as a result of serial transfer from the primary case. The epidemic curve for the secondary cases can be seen as being imposed on that of the primary cases around noon, January 8.

(c) The bimodality is the result of the occurrence of both primary and secondary cases.

(d) The health officer should define the disease that is being investigated. After he or she has defined the disease, the common exposure of the primary cases can be determined. This part of the investigation would be similar to that described in Chapter 1 (pp. 13–18). The health officer should then determine if the secondary cases were the result of serial transfer from the primary ones.

8. The correlations found by Rose suggest that the latency period of coronary heart disease is at least 10 years. Similar correlations should be sought in other population groups.

Chapter 4

1. The numerators are the number of deaths from all accidents occurring in those 5–44 years old in the United States, Alaska, and Florida in 1987. The denominators are the numbers of those 5–44 years old living in the United States, Alaska, and Florida in 1987. The death rates for accidents among those 5–44 years old are:

$$\text{United States} = \frac{50,377}{150,020,000} \times 100,000 = 33.6 \text{ per } 100,000 \text{ per year}$$

$$\text{Alaska} = \frac{242}{368,000} \times 100,000 = 65.8 \text{ per } 100,000 \text{ per year}$$

$$\text{Florida} = \frac{2,584}{6,543,000} \times 100,000 = 39.5 \text{ per } 100,000 \text{ per year}$$

2. The numerators are the number of deaths from all malignant neoplasms occurring in those 65 and over in the United States, Alaska, and Florida in 1987. The denominators are the numbers of people 65 and older living in the United States, Alaska, and Florida in 1987. The death rates for malignant neoplasms among those 65 and older are:

$$\text{United States} = \frac{242,617}{29,840,000} = 100,000 = 813.1 \text{ per } 100,000 \text{ per year}$$

$$\text{Alaska} = \frac{210}{19,000} \times 100,000 = 1105.3 \text{ per } 100,000 \text{ per year}$$

$$\text{Florida} = \frac{21,599}{2,140,000} \times 100,000 = 1009.3 \text{ per } 100,000 \text{ per year}$$

3. The numerators are the total deaths from malignant neoplasms and from accidents in the United States, Alaska, and Florida in 1987. The denominators are the total populations of the United States, Alaska, and Florida in 1987. The overall death rates from malignant neoplasms are:

$$\text{United States} = \frac{363,656}{243,400,000} \times 100,000$$
$$= 149.4 \text{ per } 100,000 \text{ per year}$$

$$\text{Alaska} = \frac{442}{525,000} \times 100,000 = 84.2 \text{ per } 100,000 \text{ per year}$$

$$\text{Florida} = \frac{30,164}{12,023,000} \times 100,000 = 250.9 \text{ per } 100,000 \text{ per year}$$

The overall death rates from all accidents are:

$$\text{United States} = \frac{94,893}{243,400,000} \times 100,000 = 39.0 \text{ per } 100,000 \text{ per year}$$

$$\text{Alaska} = \frac{320}{525,000} \times 100,000 = 61.0 \text{ per } 100,000 \text{ per year}$$

$$\text{Florida} = \frac{5,120}{12,023,000} \times 100,000 = 42.6 \text{ per } 100,000 \text{ per year}$$

4. The expected number of deaths from malignant neoplasms for Alaska and Florida's age distribution are calculated by multiplying the age-specific death rates for each state by the U.S. population in each age group. The expected number of deaths are divided by the total U.S. population (check table in problem 3 to see what the death rate would be if the U.S. had the age structure of Alaska or Florida.

| AGE GROUP | EXPECTED NUMBER OF DEATHS | |
	ALASKA	FLORIDA
<5	0	548
5–44	24,753	21,153
45–64	124,912	97,628
65+	301,175	329,822
Total	450,840	449,151

$$\text{Mortality rate for Alaska} = \frac{450,840}{243,400,000} \times 100,000$$
$$= 185.2 \text{ deaths per } 100,000$$

$$\text{Mortality rate for Florida} = \frac{449,151}{243,400,000} \times 100,000$$
$$= 184.5 \text{ deaths per } 100,000$$

5. In the indirect method (SMR) the expected number of deaths from accidents for Alaska and Florida is calculated by multiplying the U.S. age- and cause-specific death rates by the populations in each age group for Alaska and Florida. The expected number of deaths is divided by the actual number of deaths and multiplied by 100 to produce the standardized mortality ratio.

| AGE GROUP | EXPECTED NUMBER OF DEATHS | |
	ALASKA	FLORIDA
<5	13	172
5–44	124	2,198
45–64	27	885
65+	16	1,853
Total	180	5,108
Total observed number of deaths (from table in problem 1)	320	5,120

$$\text{SMR Alaska} = \frac{180}{320} \times 100 = 56.3$$

$$\text{SMR Florida} = \frac{5{,}108}{5{,}120} \times 100 = 99.8$$

6. The crude rates show Florida's death rate from malignancies to be three times higher than Alaska's, but age adjustment shows the rates to be more similar (185.2 and 184.5 for Alaska and Florida, respectively).
7. The crude rates show Florida as having a lower rate of deaths from accidents than Alaska. The age-adjusted rates show Alaska's death rate from accidents to be lower than Florida's.
8. Age adjustment is especially useful in these examples because we are comparing two populations with different age structures, because the two populations are of different sizes, and because the diseases are associated with age (death from accidents occurs most frequently in younger people, deaths from malignancies occur mostly in older people).

Chapter 5

1. These are some of the possible explanations of why motor vehicle deaths vary with the day of the week:
   (a) The variation is a result of chance and has no other meaning.
   (b) People do more driving on Fridays, Saturdays, or Sundays.
   (c) Different people (worse drivers) drive on Fridays, Saturdays, or Sundays.
   (d) People are more likely to drink and drive on weekends.
   (e) Hospital care is worse on the weekend and accident victims are more likely to die.
   (f) Day of death is not filled out correctly for accident deaths.
2. (a) Some hypotheses to explain high HIV death rates are:
   • Urban areas are associated with behaviors such as intravenous drug use and needle sharing or unprotected sex with multiple partners that can lead to HIV infection.
   • Urban areas have hospitals that will care for dying HIV patients.
   • Washington, D.C., New Jersey, New York, California, and Florida all have large proportions of age groups that are more likely to engage in behaviors leading to death from HIV.
   • The disease spreads from the two coasts to the rest of the country.
   Some hypotheses to explain low HIV death rates are:
   • Deaths from HIV in South Dakota, North Dakota, Montana, Wyoming, Idaho, and Iowa are coded under another cause.
   • Westerners are resistant to HIV.
   • Persons in the West who are diagnosed with HIV move to another

part of the country to receive care and die where they receive treatment.

- Residents of these states do not engage in behaviors that lead to HIV infection.

(b) Washington, D.C., is a city, entirely urban, but New York is a state and mixes urban and rural populations, areas with a high and low HIV mortality. A comparison of Washington, D.C., to New York City would probably show more similar rates. Data for Washington, D.C., are summarized separately from other states for political rather than scientific reasons. From an epidemiologic point of view it would be preferable to compare similar geographic units.

3. (a) The trend is steadily downwards over 70 years. The decline in mortality is dramatic; in 1987 it is less than one-tenth of what it was in 1915–1919 for whites, and slightly above one-tenth for blacks. The decline occurred in both whites and blacks.

   (b) Improved birth registration would increase the denominator (live births) and decrease the infant mortality rate.

   (c) Improved death registration would increase the numerator (deaths for infants under 1 year of age) and increase the infant mortality rate.

4. The elimination of many infectious diseases through improved sanitation, sterile techniques, vaccinations, and antibiotics could explain the decline in infant mortality between 1915 and 1960.

5. Between 1960 and 1987 hospital-based technology reduced the mortality for many high-risk infants including those born at low or very low birth weight and those with congenital malformations.

6. Some hypotheses are:

   (a) Black infants have genetically determined lower survival rates.

   (b) Black mothers are less likely to have access to medical care during pregnancy.

   (c) Black mothers are more likely to be of lower socioeconomic class than are white mothers.

   (d) Black infants are more likely to be low birth weight than are white infants.

   (e) Deaths of white infants are less likely to be recorded than deaths of black infants.

   (f) Births of black infants are less likely to be recorded than are births of white infants.

Chapter 6

1. Positive predictive value is the probability of the disease being present given a test result. For the clinical health care provider, this probability

provides a basis for interpreting a positive test result, one which the patient might also understand. The same is true for negative predictive values, negative test results, and the absence of disease. However, neither positive nor negative predictive values provide a basis for evaluating the performance of a test.

2. The number of individuals likely to be identified with the virus in the early 1980s was low, but even with a very specific test, the number of false-positive persons would likely be high (perhaps even greater than the number of true positives identified). The other problem with the proposed policy in the early 1980s was that there were no treatments for HIV infection at that time.

3. The major strength of a registry is that it provides a central place where all cases of a disease in a community can be ascertained. Such data are useful for epidemiologic observational studies (discussed in Chapters 10 and 11) and also for enrolling those with the disease in therapeutic randomized clinical trials (discussed in Chapter 8). Registries provide unique information for characterizing secular trends of a disease. The weakness of registries is their cost. They are generally expensive to operate.

4. The sensitivity and specificity of the test may be characterized and compared with those for other early lung cancer screening tests. Also, a study could be initiated to determine if those who have been screened with the test have greater survivorship than those not screened.

5. Major problems will include different standards used to diagnose cardiovascular disease, different patterns of access to medical care for diagnosis of the disease, and different patterns of migration to and from the communities being monitored. An additional problem is obtaining the support of health care providers in each community where a registry is to be established.

6. Such data provide a basis for assessing diagnostic criteria, survivorship, and referral patterns. A given tumor registry, however, will often lack a defined population. This makes it difficult to calculate rates of disease. Also, since there may be many factors that influence which patients with which diseases present to which hospitals, there may be selection bias.

7. The prevalence of osteoarthritis is 2,500 cases per 100,000 population.

8. The observation may be artifactual, resulting from increased accessibility of health care. It may represent a genetic etiology of the condition. It may result from the common environment of the family, with consequent exposure to the environmental agent of the disease. Or it may result from a combination of genetic and environmental factors (i.e., a genetic susceptibility coupled with exposure to the environmental agent of the disease).

9. It is desirable to minimize the percentage of individuals with false-negative test results if the disease is very serious or fatal and a treatment exists that affects the prognosis of the disease. It is desirable to minimize the percentage of individuals with false-positive results if such a finding has adverse social or economic consequences or if the treatment itself has adverse side effects.

Chapter 7

1. The development of cases in the summer and early autumn reflects the availability of the insect agents responsible for the transmission of the agent to humans, i.e., the mosquito. This means of transmission is much less available during other times of the year, hence the fewer cases observed at other times.

2. Three possible explanations for these changes are (1) changes in the pathogenicity of the different types of bacteria, with staphlococcus and streptococcus bacteria becoming much less pathogenic by the 1960s and 1970s compared with the 1930s, 1940s, and 1950s; (2) the increased use of antibiotics, with consequent change in the availability of pathogenic bacteria to infect a given host; and (3) the increased use of immunosuppressive agents (including those used in cancer chemotherapy), which allows agents such as gram negative bacteria, from which a host is normally protected by a fully functioning immune system, to thrive.

3. The large number of immigrants to the United States from areas of world in which tuberculosis is much more common than the United States (the 1980s saw more immigrants to the United States than in any decade since the 1920s) and the increasing number of AIDS cases (first reported in 1980) in the United States have together resulted in the increasing number of tuberculosis cases observed in the United States.

4. (a) These data indicate that the prevalence rates were higher in 1973 than in 1964–1965 for all age groups among both men and women. The rates among women were greater than among men. From these data, one may conclude that women have a greater prevalence of diabetes than men, that the prevalence increases with ascending age, and that the prevalence of disease may have increased from 1964–1965 to 1973.

   (b) It would be desirable to have validation of the data, including diagnostic criteria, further information on case ascertainment, confirmation of the diagnoses, and information on changes in survivorship of those with the disease.

   (c) The data suggest the need for studies to validate diagnoses in both time periods and for further analysis of secular trends.

5. The differences in rates among whites and blacks may be artifactual, reflecting underascertainment of the black population. Assuming that errors in the population data could not account for the differences, the possibility of different definitions of disease being used by health care providers for blacks and whites must be considered. Lastly, it is possible that these differences result from differences in the incidence of esophageal cancer in both populations. Such differences could be due to genetic or environmental etiological factors being more common in the black population.

6. These differences could be the result of inconsistencies in data collection and analysis between the two areas or of differences in population enumeration. Assuming that such inconsistencies do not exist, it is possible that a herd immunity effect was present among the older population of Baltimore, accounting for the marked decrease in older age groups compared with St. Lawrence Island.

Chapter 8

1. Randomization is the process by which subjects are assigned to groups in an investigation such that each subject has the same chance of being assigned to each of the groups. Randomization performs three functions in a randomized clinical trial. First, it eliminates bias resulting from assignment to either treatment or placebo (or comparison) groups. Second, it assures the comparability of the two groups. Third, randomization facilitates the use of statistical tests of significance (or the calculation of confidence intervals).

2. Before using a new agent in a randomized clinical trial, one would need to determine its toxicology, both in animals and, to the degree possible in a small clinical study, in humans. This knowledge is essential if the clinical trial is to be conducted without bringing avoidable harm to individuals using the agent. Also, pharmacokinetic information is needed for adequate dosing of individuals using the agent.

3. The limitations of the randomized clinical trial are that it is relatively expensive, it is ethically difficult or impossible to conduct for some questions, it is only useful for beneficial outcomes, and poor compliance in either the experimental or the comparison groups is possible.

4. (a) Tabulations that will be needed include center-specific comparisons of the characteristics of the experimental and control groups, center-specific comparisons of the outcomes, and center-specific comparisons of adverse reactions. Aggregate tabulations of these comparisons would also be required to assess the drug's effectiveness.

    (b) The inference that could be derived from this trial is that the drug is effective at a certain dose in treating a certain disease in a specific population.

(c) The problems that may occur during the course of such a study are manifold. An important one is withdrawals, which can be handled by having a sufficiently large sample size to allow for the withdrawals and by following the withdrawals to determine if they are different from those who continue in the study. Other problems are adverse reactions, which may require that the trial be halted, and a treatment that is so efficacious that the continuance of the trial would be unethical.

(d) Physicians must consider several issues before prescribing the drug. Is the patient population studied in the trial comparable to those for whom the drug would be prescribed? What dosages of the drug were used? What adverse reactions accompanied the use of the drug at that dose? What were the definitions of disease used in the trial? Was the trial properly designed? Were the results analyzed properly? These questions would serve as a guide for physicians considering whether or not to prescribe the drug.

5. A randomized clinical trial would be unethical if no alternative treatment existed for the disease and the treatment had some effectiveness, or if the treatment was known to cause major disease or to have some toxicity with an unclear benefit to patients using it. If a randomized clinical trial can not be conducted, observational data could be collected in an epidemiologic study to provide additional insight into the issue. The limitation of the nonrandomized studies are due to the possibility that strong selection biases may be present.

6. The power of the trial may be inadequate to detect the small beneficial effect.

7. The randomized clinical trial can detect adverse reactions, but only if they are common enough to occur in the relatively small sample sizes used in such studies. It is for this reason that so-called postmarketing surveillance studies are conducted after a new drug has been approved by the federal government. It is also for this reason that morbidity and mortality surveys are needed to detect the less common adverse reactions.

8. The problem with this approach is that there is no comparison group against which the treatment's true efficacy can be assessed.

9. Three (60 × 0.05) statistical tests would be expected to be statistically significant even if there were no true difference. The best way to protect against this phenomenon (commonly referred to as ''multiple comparisons'') is to use statistical tests wisely and not to use them when they are not needed. Statisticians have developed techniques to deal with such

situations; consulting a statistician before using such tests (and during the design of the trial) should protect against this problem.

Chapter 9

1. The major difference between randomized clinical trials and community trials is that in randomized clinical trials the efficacy of a preventive or therapeutic agent or technique is tested in individual subjects, while in community trials it is tested in a group of subjects as a whole. Natural experiments and community trials are quite similar, the major difference being the control that the investigator has over the populations studied.

2. The main reason for conducting a community trial is to test an etiologic hypothesis or preventive procedure in an experimental setting comparable to that which might be used by a local or federal public health department in developing programs to prevent or reduce the incidence of disease in a population. Community trials facilitate the evaluation of such programs, specifically evaluation of their efficacy. If the activity to reduce disease incidence or to prevent disease is community-based, then it must be evaluated in a community trial, not in a randomized clinical trial.

3. These inferences are limited insofar as there may have been considerable differences among the communities studied. There was no randomized assignment of treatment, hence such differences might affect the results of the study. Another limitation was that the follow-up focused on the risk factors for cardiovascular diseases, not the incidence of cardiovascular disease. Although it is reasonable to expect that intervention aimed at the risk factors will result in a decline in cardiovascular disease, without such data from the trial, one cannot assume that such a decline will indeed take place.

4. Community trials are subject to ecological fallacy. The lack of specific information on individuals in community trials provides an opportunity for an ecological fallacy to occur.

5. When using historical controls, the investigator loses some control over the conditions within which the trial is conducted. Since there may be a loss of comparability in the communities studied and there may also be a lack of comparability in the methods used for disease diagnosis or risk factor assessment at different times, the use of historical controls greatly reduces the validity of the study findings.

6. The design of a randomized clinical trial is more important than its analysis because the quality of the data being analyzed is determined by the design of the trial. If the design of the trial is faulty, it is doubtful that the analysis will provide much meaningful information. The same reasoning applies to a community trial. Good study design facilitates proper analysis of the data, regardless of the type of study being discussed.

7. Community trials are conducted in those situations in which an intervention is best undertaken for an entire community, such as health education.

8. (a) These data suggest that making the privies flyproof reduced the occurrence of typhoid fever, presumably by reducing its transmission. However, it is important to note that the comparison data were not collected concurrent with the data on the intervention.

   (b) It would be very important to know what other changes took place in the city. Specifically, did the water supply change? Also of importance would be knowledge of changes in any other risk factor for typhoid fever.

Chapter 10

1. The SMR and the relative risk are not necessarily the same. The relative risk compares the frequency of disease in a given population that was exposed to a factor and the frequency of that disease in a similar population that was not exposed to that factor. In contrast, the numerator of an SMR is the number of cases in a group exposed to a factor. The denominator includes the number of cases that would have occurred in that group if their mortality experience had been the same as that of some comparison population. The comparison population may or may not have been exposed to the factor; alternatively, it might include some individuals who have been exposed to the factor. If no such persons are present in that population, then the SMR is indeed equivalent to the relative risk.

2. The attributable fraction is useful to the epidemiologist as a guide to how many risk factors it is worthwhile to investigate. For example, if a factor F has an attributable fraction of 95 percent for disease D, further investigations into those factors responsible for the other 5 percent of the disease are likely to be very difficult to conduct and unproductive in finding a relationship.

3. The basic design of this study would be:
   (a) Identify a high-risk group for D (such as college students for infectious mononucleosis or homosexual men for AIDS).
   (b) Recruit members of the high-risk group into the study.
   (c) Eliminate from the study any individuals with D.
   (d) Obtain blood or sera from study participants.
   (e) Determine, from the sera, which individuals have been exposed to V.
   (f) Follow all study participants for the development of D.
   (g) Compare the incidence rate of D for those individuals with V in their sera (or a marker for V, such as antibodies) to that for individuals without the virus or the marker in their sera.

This design is unchanged if V is a slow virus. It is also unchanged if D is thought to be noninfectious.

4. These databases may be used to determine exposures in the past, such as operations or pharmaceutical use, and relate it on an individual-by-individual basis to the subsequent development of a disease (which would be noted in the HMO's records for that patient.) Such a study would be nonconcurrent. If the exposure is determined at present with follow-up occurring from the present into the future, then the study would be concurrent.

5. The question that the surgeons have posed is one of exposure (What is the effect of tonsillectomy?). The surgeons could either identify a group of patients at some time in the past and a similar group of surgical patients (perhaps having hernia repairs or appendectomies), and in a nonconcurrent manner, follow up those patients through the National Death Index or some similar means. An alternative approach would be for the surgeons to identify a group of patients currently undergoing tonsillectomies and a similar group not having that operation and following both groups for subsequent mortality. This would be the concurrent approach.

Chapter 11

1. The choice of an appropriate control group may vary with the hypothesis to be tested. Often one chooses more than one type of control. Some possible answers are:

   (a) Babies born at normal birth weight (over 2500 gms), babies born over 1500 gms, or babies with birth defects. Exclude twins since low birth weight is related to twinness.

   (b) Infants with strep throat, infants coming to pediatrician for well baby visits, or infants coming to pediatricians for all causes except ear infections or well baby visits. Exclude infants with tubes in ears since they have a lower likelihood of becoming cases.

   (c) Transplant patients who do not reject transplant.

   (d) All other suicide victims, all other handgun victims (suicide or not), handgun owners, handgun suicide victims, or handgun suicide victims where witnesses were present.

2. (a) The odds ratio is $\dfrac{(11)(21)}{(33)(3)} = 2.33$, suggesting that drug and alcohol use increases the risk of death by Russian roulette compared to handgun suicide.

   (b) The odds ratio is $\dfrac{(9)(35)}{(19)(5)} = 3.31$. Cocaine use may increase by about three-fold the probability of suicide from Russian roulette compared to suicide by handgun.

3. Some advantages of the case-control design in studying this question are:

- Suicide by Russian roulette is a rare event that is most easily studied by the case-control method.
- The study used small sample sizes ($N = 68$) and was relatively inexpensive to conduct.
- The study could look at several risk factors (alcohol and cocaine use).

Two typical disadvantages of case-control studies do not apply to this study. Exposure (alcohol or cocaine use) clearly preceded the outcome (suicide by handgun), so temporality of events is unquestioned. Cases and controls were easily identified by the Medical Examiner's office, with a low probability of missing cases.

Some disadvantages are:

- Errors may have occurred in blood measurements of cocaine and alcohol because of different amounts of time elapsing between death and examination. The presence of witnesses may have led to a shorter time lag before blood samples were taken. The presence of witnesses was also associated with Russian roulette suicides.
- Cases and controls might be misclassified if Russian roulette occurred in the absence of witnesses. The authors do not describe how they distinguished a Russian roulette case from other handgun suicides if witnesses were absent. Perhaps the appropriate control group should have been handgun suicides that took place in the presence of witnesses. A high proportion of cocaine and alcohol users might have been found in this group also.
- Incidence rates of suicide by Russian roulette, handgun, or other method among cocaine and noncocaine, alcohol and nonalcohol users cannot be calculated. Although complete numerator data may be available from death certificates, denominator data are not available. The data give no information about the overall risk of suicide by alcohol or drug use.

4. (a) We can collect information about exposure among cases and controls immediately, when the subject arises, and come up with an answer in a short period of time (six months to a year), to inform public decision-making.

   (b) Women with breast cancer diagnosed in a reasonable period of time (i.e., the last two years).

   (c) Women without the disease—women who have recently had exams (for example, mammograms) showing they are free of the disease— or a group of women willing to be screened for the study to show that they are free of the disease. However, for most diseases that are rare, this is not necessary.

(d) The controls should be restricted to women only, about a certain age (to allow comparable times for the disease to have occurred, and to be the same age as women who would have already had breast implants).

(e) It might be useful to match on socioeconomic status because women who get breast implants (and pay for them privately) are probably wealthier than a representative sample of women. Socioeconomic status might also be associated with other risk factors for the disease.

(f) When many variables are used in matching, it becomes difficult to find controls; one cannot examine the relationship between the matching variables and the disease; one may overmatch, match on a variable that is causally related to the disease, so that the groups or pairs are too similar.

(g) One could ask the women to describe their own histories or ask them to give permission to look at their medical records.

(h) Some women will be more accurate and more informative about their medical histories. Some women will not be willing to share information or give permission for the researchers to obtain medical information. Some women have moved often, or changed caregivers frequently, and this will make it difficult to obtain medical records. Older patients may have received care from physicians who are now retired or dead—again making it difficult to find out about silicone implants. All these variations can affect the classification of women as exposed or not exposed, and can be differnt in the cases and controls. This can affect the measure of effect—the odds ratio—reducing or increasing it depending on the particular circumstances.

Chapter 12

1. One must identify potential confounders in the literature and collect data on all potential confounders. One may restrict study subjects to a particular subgroup or match study subjects to controls.

2. One may use stratified analysis, multiple regression, or a combination of both techniques.

3. Biological significance refers to findings that affect many people, explain the cause of a disease, suggest new approaches to treatment or prevention, or suggest new research directions. Statistical significance means that the observed differences are greater than would be expected by chance alone.

4. The following concepts are used in assessing causality:
   - Strength of association
   - Consistency of the observed association
   - Specificity of the association
   - Temporal sequence of events
   - Dose-response relationship
   - Biological plausibility of the observed association
   - Experimental evidence

Chapter 13

1. Decision analysis can be applied to a specific clinical problem in a given patient, or it can be applied in a general way to a problem and can result in a recommendation for a group of patients.
2. Some of the limitations of decision analysis are that (a) information about probabilities of outcomes is not always available; (b) the decision tree can become very complicated, even for what appear to be simple choices; (c) it is hard to assign quantitative values to some outcomes.
3. The paper should describe (a) the study problem, (b) the study design, (c) selection of the study sample, (d) data analysis, and (e) inference and results.
4. All studies are susceptible to biases. Authors should address the ways in which their study may have been affected by bias, and how they dealt with potential biases in the design and analysis.
5. A physician can participate in epidemiologic research by participating in a collaborative study or by initiating an investigation in response to an observation of an outbreak, a new syndrome, or an out-of-the-ordinary occurrence.

AUTHOR INDEX

SUBJECT INDEX